THE MORALITY OF EMBRYO USE

Is it permissible to use a human embryo in stem cell research, or in general as a means for benefit of others? Acknowledging each embryo as an object of moral concern, Louis M. Guenin argues that it is morally permissible to decline intrauterine transfer of an embryo formed outside the body, and that from this permission and the duty of beneficence, there follows a consensus justification for using donated embryos in service of humanitarian ends. He then proceeds to show how this justification commands assent even within moral and religious views commonly thought to oppose embryo use. Beneath his moral reasoning lies a carefully constructed metaphysical foundation incorporating accounts of the ontology of development, embryos, and species. He also incisively discusses nonreprocloning, repro-cloning, ectogenesis, and related scientific frontiers. This compelling philosophical study will interest all concerned to understand virtue and obligation in the relief of suffering.

LOUIS M. GUENIN is Lecturer on Ethics in Science, Department of Microbiology and Molecular Genetics, Harvard Medical School.

D0824006

THE MORALITY OF
EMBRYO USE

LOUIS M. GUENIN

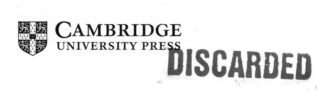

CAMBRIDGE
UNIVERSITY PRESS

CAMBRIDGE UNIVERSITY PRESS
Cambridge, New York, Melbourne, Madrid, Cape Town, Singapore, São Paulo, Delhi

Cambridge University Press
The Edinburgh Building, Cambridge CB2 8RU, UK

Published in the United States of America by Cambridge University Press, New York

www.cambridge.org
Information on this title: www.cambridge.org/9780521694278

© Louis M. Guenin 2008

09-10 BT 31.15

First published 2008

Printed in the United Kingdom at the University Press, Cambridge

A catalogue record for this publication is available from the British Library

Library of Congress Cataloguing in Publication Data

Guenin, Louis M., 1950–

09-10   The morality of embryo use / Louis M. Guenin.
273   p. ; cm.
Includes bibliographical references and index.
ISBN 978-0-521-87269-0 (hardback) – ISBN 978-0-521-69427-8 (pbk.)
1. Life and death, Power over.   2. Human embryo – Research – Moral and ethical aspects.
3. Human embryo – Therapeutic use – Moral and ethical aspects.   I. Title.
[DNLM: 1. Embryo Research – ethics.   2. Embryo Disposition – ethics.   3. Embryonic Stem Cells.
4. Embryo Transfer – ethics.   5. Personhood.   6. Cloning, Organism – ethics.   QS 620 G926m 2008]

BJ1469.G84 2008
174.2′8 – dc22   2008013429

ISBN 978-0-521-87269-0 hardback
ISBN 978-0-521-69427-8 paperback

Contents

Preface

I am concerned in this study with a moral controversy precipitated by recent scientific advances. Human ingenuity has envisioned procedures in which scientists and physicians would use human embryos in the course of attempts to overcome human disease and disability. Embryo use is the general practice of which embryonic stem cell research is a special case. As we think about the propriety of this practice, it soon appears that we must adapt our moral machinery to deal with fundamental questions about what constitutes one of us. I began this project when I glimpsed what seemed to me the grounds of a stable moral consensus. I therefore set to work on the assumption that it is feasible to construct an account that compels assent across the gamut of pertinent moral views, and in particular within views usually thought to oppose all embryo use. Mindful of those many who suffer from maladies that might yield to treatments consequent on embryo use, the motivation for this inquiry could not be more compelling.

I have been aided by the work of many philosophers to whom my debts will be apparent from the text. For their generosity in discussions over the course of the research, I am grateful to Stephen L. Darwall, E. J. Lowe, and Allen W. Wood. For illuminating conversations, comments on portions of the manuscript, and correspondence, I also thank Dagfinn Føllesdal, Jorge J. E. Gracia, David L. Hull, Joshua Hoffman, Christine M. Korsgaard, Brian F. Loar, Trenton Merricks, Alvin Plantinga, Melinda A. Roberts, Michael Ruse, Israel Scheffler, Barry Smith, and James Van Cleve. My understanding of pertinent scientific and medical matters has been aided by the guidance of Jonathan R. Beckwith, Merle J. Berger, Jonathan H. Blum, George Q. Daley, Ralph E. Dittman, John D. Gearhart, Stanley R. Glasser, Ann A. Kiessling, M. William Lensch, Paul H. Lerou, Stephanie Mel de Fontenay, R. Douglas Powers, Catherine Racowksy, Jayaraj Rajagopal, Eric J. Rubin, Gerald P. Schatten, Evan Y. Snyder, Ayalew Tefferi, and Thomas Zwaka. In envisioning probability density functions as representative of the extent of developmental potential of embryos in various situations,

I have learned much from Kevin A. Rader and Michal R. Zochowski, as well as from George DeMuth, Steven R. Finch, Oliver Knill, A. David Wunsch, and Jens C. Zorn. I thank the audiences before whom I have given talks at Schepens Eye Research Institute (whose invitation from Kenneth J. Trevett stimulated my interest), Harvard University, The Mayo Clinic, International Society for Cellular Therapy, International Society for Stem Cell Research, The George Washington University, The Burnham Institute, The Salk Institute, Brandeis University, Los Angeles Biomedical Research Institute, Genetics Policy Institute, Baylor College of Medicine, Stanford University, Children's Hospital Boston, and the University of Miami. I have benefited as well from discussions with my seminar students at Harvard Medical School. I am grateful to two anonymous reviewers for Cambridge University Press for their insightful comments. For both her thoughts and encouragement, I thank Erin V. Lehman.

I mention the following about the plan of the book, this especially for general readers interested in the controversy over embryonic stem cell research. The argument in chief, the argument from nonenablement, is set forth in Chapter 2. The analyses in Chapter 3 of individuality of the twinnable, and in Chapter 4 of respect for life forms sorted by taxa, enter into topics in metaphysics and the philosophy of science wherein arise some of the most philosophically interesting issues that I discuss. The general reader who prefers to take their moral controversy without metaphysics may pass lightly over Chapters 3 and 4 at no detriment to comprehension of what follows. Chapter 5 describes how the argument from nonenablement takes hold within influential views assumed or declared to be opponents of embryo use. Chapters 6–8 delve further into the scope of embryo use and related practices, this in respect of avenues of research and therapy, putative alternatives to embryo use, and the construction of norms.

With permission of The Royal Institute of Philosophy, Chapter 3 draws on 'The Nonindividuation Argument Against Zygotic Personhood,' *Philosophy* 81: 463–503 (2006).

By means of this work, I hope to contribute to the formation of a moral consensus that will foster efficacious means for the relief of suffering.

CHAPTER I

Preliminaries

Is it ever morally permissible to use a human embryo solely as a means for benefit of others? One should think that this question would long ago have been posed if not decisively answered. Instead it was not until the late twentieth century that anyone created a human embryo outside a human body. Or so we assume. It was then that physicians devised a procedure by which to create embryos *in vitro*. That feat has since allowed many couples experiencing infertility to bring forth children. Following this procreative innovation, scientists began to ask whether embryos created outside the body could be used in research.

In the first instance, scientists imagined experiments that might augment our knowledge of human embryology. We collectively still know relatively little about early human development. For long it was believed that conception occurs by the mixing of semen and maternal blood. Aristotle and others so concluded upon observing that when pregnancy begins, menses ceases. Then entered the theory of preformation. In its most famous version, preformation portrayed a sperm head as containing a homunculus, a 'tiny human' that needs only to enlarge to develop. Not until 1827 was it observed that there exist oocytes released from human ovaries. An explanation for the penury of our ancestors' knowledge is not hard to find. Observational barriers constrained what they could discover.

Now that there exist embryos observable *in vitro*, scientists think of observing early development. They think of what they might learn that could amplify our understanding of fundamental biological processes, that could avail in facilitating reproduction, or that could lead to preventing or treating developmental abnormalities. They also think of derivatives of embryos. Here lies an avenue that has roused great hopes for curing dreadful maladies. Scientific ingenuity has devised ways in which experiments performed on derivatives of embryos might yield fundamental knowledge. Methods have also been envisioned in which embryonic derivatives would serve as vehicles by which physicians deliver therapies. The prospects for

such advances surged when, late in the twentieth century, biologists succeeded for the first time in deriving and culturing human embryonic stem
cells. While these investigators did not wish to foster false hopes, they began
to imagine a new era of regenerative medicine. They began to envision
interventions that could constitute some of the most effective therapeutic
advances in modern history.

<h2 style="text-align:center">1.1 EMBRYO USE</h2>

I shall employ 'embryo use' to denote the use of an embryo solely as a
means. My use of 'embryo' will refer, except where otherwise indicated, to
the human. On the permissibility of embryo use in research and therapy,
the counsels of common sense are divided. Some people would condemn
every instance of embryo use, regardless of expected benefit. In their view,
hopes that medicine may succeed in a mission of mercy attach to means
that we must abjure. Other people approve the use of donated embryos
primarily by reason of the expected benefits. Still others approve use of all
and only embryos left over from fertility care in the belief that otherwise
those embryos would perish as waste.

Observers who have chronicled skirmishes over embryo use have often
spoken of irreconcilable moral positions argued to a draw. The controversy
about embryo use, they say, merely rehearses the controversy over abortion. Scratch an opponent of embryo use, they remark, and one will find
an opponent of abortion. Serious thinkers have debated the use of various categories of embryo, among them the surplus embryo, the clone, the
embryo formed in research, the parthenote. Thus far this discussion has
been fragmented. As some commentators portray things, it probably does
not lie within our ability to cobble together a consistent collective stance on
embryo use and related practices such as abortion, assisted reproduction,
and genetic intervention in reproduction. We would be well advised to forge
some compromise. If thereby we collectively saddle ourselves with inconsistency, that should not unduly disappoint us, because on these matters,
many of us are inconsistent separately.

I suggest that the foregoing gloss may stem from failure to recognize
that in a philosophical controversy, narratives of battles do not substitute
for the rigorous analysis of argument while sympathetically considering
others' views. Narratives will tell us which and how many people espouse
one view or another, or how people interact in groups and communities.
The philosopher's contribution issues from hard thought trained on assem-
bling a cohesive account sustained by compelling arguments responsive to

fundamental questions. Sometimes this work may remove seeming obstacles to agreement. 'One of the aims of moral philosophy,' as John Rawls taught us, 'is to look for possible bases of agreement where none seem to exist.'[1]

The present controversy presents compelling reasons to strive for a consensus. If the practice of embryo use were imposed as public policy by brute political machinery, that could leave a principled minority chafing under what it regards as immorality. If instead public policy thwarts the relief of suffering that a society has the ability to ameliorate, that will bring deep regret by and for all affected. Settling for either result without making a serious intellectual effort toward consensus would forsake the power of ideas.

The morality of embryo use is a question within normative ethics. Its analysis also raises questions about what we are. One prominent argument that we shall encounter beckons an understanding of what constitutes a human individual. Another line of reasoning evokes the question whether we should rest moral judgments on a particular teleology about body parts. Still another train of thought leads into the question of what ontological status a species holds, this insofar as the association of properties with species membership may be invoked as a ground for partiality. We shall also encounter the inchoate notion of developmental potential and the effect of discretion upon its extent. Within normative ethics, we shall have occasion to consider moral demands said to be placed upon us by such possible persons as it may make sense to posit in particular situations. We shall have to decide whether the duty to rescue, or any other duty, obliges a woman to undergo a transfer into her, or to allow a transfer into another, of an embryo formed outside her, this inquiry implicating the distinction between the duty to rescue and the duty of beneficence. Inasmuch as controversy over embryo use lies at the intersection of law, morals, and public policy, we shall also find reason to pause over what constraints should apply to the invocation of particular religious and moral views in the public arena. We shall as well find motivation to consider the sweep of moral views as if there were no such constraints.

I shall define a set of embryos that, so I shall argue, we may virtuously use in service of humanitarian ends. This set will consist of donated embryos that, by virtue of progenitor decisions, have permissibly been barred from entry into any natural or artificial uterus. These embryos have begun development, but they will not begin gestation. I shall argue that the use of these embryos for humanitarian ends is not only permissible and virtuous, but

---

[1] Rawls 1971a, p. 582.

that such use lies within the mandate of a collective duty. A distinguishing feature of my account will be the claim that its argument in chief commands assent even within the most prominent comprehensive views presumed to oppose embryo use. After probing to their roots the teachings of the leading presumptive opponent, we shall discover that a compelling case for donated embryo use resides there. We shall also learn that the principal argument for a contrary interpretation collapses after colliding with one of that view's bedrock beliefs.

From such lines of reasoning and their tributaries, a picture will emerge of a consensus awaiting recognition. In the work of laying the foundation for that consensus, we shall clear many conceptual brambles. Because a good case is not made better by overstatement, I shall disavow some arguments offered in support of embryo use that, according to my analysis, are unsound. Among these will be arguments asserting that twinnability precludes individuality, that imminent death is alone justificatory of embryo use, that embryo use is the utility-maximizing alternative, and that public appeals to comprehensive religious or philosophical doctrines are always out of bounds.

At various places within my discussion, embryonic stem cell research will serve as a point of entry. This field of research has brought embryo use to public prominence. But there seems no reason to assume that any one avenue of inquiry will exhaust the collective good achievable in research and therapy through use of donated embryos. In anticipation that multiple lines of fruitful inquiry may develop over time, I offer my account as a justification for the general case of embryo use in service of humanitarian ends.

I.2 THE BIOLOGICAL CONTEXT

'The student of Nature,' said the biologist T. H. Huxley, 'wonders the more and is astonished the less, the more conversant he becomes with her operations; but of all the perennial miracles she offers to his inspection, perhaps the most worthy of admiration is the development of a plant or of an animal from its embryo.'[2] The following sets forth the biological context for the discussion of embryo use that lies ahead.

Within a human ovary, the process of *oogenesis* culminates in the production of a *secondary oocyte*, one of which is released from an ovary at each ovulation. The exterior surface of each secondary oocyte is a protective

---

[2] Huxley 1894, p. 29.

shell, the *zona pellucida*. As and when a secondary oocyte is induced to begin dividing, *activation* is said to occur. In natural conception, activation occurs by fertilization, a process in which two *gametes*, a secondary oocyte and a single spermatozoon, fuse. Occurring in a fallopian tube connecting the ovary to the uterus, the process of fertilization lasts about a day. Entry of the sperm changes the oocyte into a single-cell *zygote*, which takes its name from the Greek ζυγωτοσ for 'yoke.' This name alludes to the two separated pronuclei in which at first the chromosomes from the oocyte and sperm respectively reside. Toward the end of fertilization, the pronuclei migrate together, touch, and exchange chromosomes. The ensuing merger of the paternal and maternal genomes is known as *syngamy*. The cell divides into two successor cells. After another day, the successor cells divide. Then the successors of the successors divide, and so on. This process of successive cell division is known as *cleavage* because as the number of cells increases geometrically, the average cell volume declines proportionately so that all the cells fit within the fixed volume enclosed by the zona pellucida. Each cell is a *blastomere*.

At about day 3, the whole structure compacts into a *morula*, a form that resembles a mulberry. By around day 5, the developing being has become a *blastocyst* (after βλαστο- for a bud or young growth and -κυστ for a bladder or pouch). The blastocyst consists of a spherical surface, the *trophoblast*, which will develop into the placenta, and a cluster of cells lying inside the surface, the *inner cell mass*, also known as the *embryoblast*. As cleavage continues, the blastocyst travels through the fallopian tube toward the uterus. The blastocyst hatches from the zona pellucida. The blastocyst will implant in the uterine wall, if ever, by day 7. Then follows development to the late blastocyst stage. At about day 14, there begins *gastrulation*, a process in which cells migrate and orient according to their future roles.

The foregoing postactivation events are the first steps in the human of *organismic development*. I understand organismic development as a process in which the genome, epigenetic systems, and external environment of a product of oocyte activation, or of a product of a plant propagule, interact so as to produce and transform an organism, or so as to transform a product originated as an organism, by means of phase changes occurring in a morphological sequence usual for organisms of its kind over the course of a life. A *phase change* in an individual of a given kind of substance is a change that things of that kind survive in accordance with the laws of nature.[3] When a flower blooms, a bear gains weight, or a child becomes an adolescent,

---

[3] Here I follow Lowe 1998, p. 186.

a phase change occurs. In the prenatal morphological sequence of human organismic development, the phase changes include the processes of cleavage, compaction, implantation, gastrulation, neurulation, mitotic cell division, regulated cell differentiation, and organogenesis.

To the Greeks after Homer, the fruit of the womb was known as an εμβρυον (*embruon*). The Latin term was *foetus*. Only in modern times have the extensions of these terms diverged. As I define the term, an *embryo* is a product of oocyte activation that is undergoing organismic development and that has not reached the ninth week of development. (The strict medical definition of 'embryo' demands attainment of the third week, but neither scientific usage nor common parlance imposes that condition.) A *fetus* is a prenatal product of oocyte activation that has attained the ninth week of organismic development. Moral concern would attach to an embryo insofar as it is undergoing organismic development even were it not yet an organism.

Assisted reproduction consists in a suite of procedures for initiating pregnancy by medical intervention. The techniques include *in vitro fertilization* ('IVF'), a procedure in which gametes are mixed outside the body. An IVF patient first receives daily subcutaneous injections of follicle-stimulating hormone, this to induce development of more than the usual one oocyte per month. She undergoes frequent blood tests and is otherwise followed closely by her physician. After weeks of such ovarian stimulation, the physician administers anesthesia, inserts a needle into an ovary, and extracts about a dozen follicles each containing a secondary oocyte. A laboratory technician then attempts fertilization of the oocytes by mixing them with sperm. After embryos form, the clinical embryologist examines the embryos under a microscope and, in consultation with the patient, selects several for intrauterine transfer. The physician performs the intrauterine embryo transfer within a few days after the embryos form. Then the patient waits to see whether she has become pregnant. There will commonly remain *surplus embryos*, embryos as to which intrauterine transfer has been declined. The clinic will freeze and store these embryos if the patient wishes. Patients regularly revisit the question whether to continue storing surplus embryos.[4] In the aggregate, assisted reproduction produces substantially more embryos than patients want babies.

In one technique of embryo creation that is useful in research, investigators induce asexual oocyte activation by organismic cloning. To clone is to

---

[4] In the UK, absent special pleading, an embryo must be discarded after five years (Human Fertilisation and Embryology Act 1990, c. 37, §14[1][c]). See also Brinsden 1999, pp. 215–216.

copy. 'Clone' derives from the Greek κλω'ν (*klon*) for 'twig.' A plant may be cloned by cutting and planting a shoot. In *somatic cell nuclear transfer*, an investigator activates an enucleated secondary oocyte as the investigator transfers into the oocyte a somatic cell's nucleus. The DNA of that nucleus is the *source DNA*. The result is a *clone embryo*. 'Clone embryo' is of the same form as 'mouse embryo' or 'clone adult.' (The journalistic label 'clone*d* embryo,' which reads 'copied embryo,' is a misnomer.) Somatic cell nuclear transfer is a method of organismic cloning inasmuch as it produces a product whose nuclear genome is a copy of the source's. That a somatic (nongerm) cell is the DNA source distinguishes the process from fertilization, which transfers the nucleus of a germ cell. The clone does not receive the DNA of the somatic cell's *mitochondria*, structures lying in the cytoplasm. The clone's mitochondrial genome will be that of the oocyte. *Reprocloning*, as I shall call it, consists in cloning by nuclear transfer followed by intrauterine transfer of the clone embryo. *Nonreprocloning* consists in cloning by nuclear transfer not followed by intrauterine transfer of the clone embryo. Reprocloning and nonreprocloning are mutually exclusive and jointly exhaustive of cloning by nuclear transfer. By reference to nonreprocloning and reprocloning, we may perspicuously describe research, distinguish practices for moral purposes, and express legal constraints. Stem cell research employs nonreprocloning but not reprocloning.

A product of sexual or asexual oocyte activation that is undergoing organismic development is a *conceptus*. I exclude from the extension of this term the extraembryonic supporting structures such as the placenta. (In strict medical parlance, 'conceptus' denotes a product of fertilization inclusive of supporting structures.) Some biologists have suggested that in moral debate, it avails to emphasize a distinction that I have just drawn, that between nonreprocloning and reprocloning, by ceasing altogether the use of 'cloning' for nonreprocloning, and using only the name 'nuclear transfer.' This suggestion travels in tandem with the proposal that we cease to use 'clone' and 'embryo' for a product of nonreprocloning.[5] 'Nuclear transfer' is informative so far as it goes. But it does not go far enough. According to the usage previously nourished in the scientific literature, cloning is a genetic event. That event concludes upon an oocyte's assimilation of source DNA, regardless whether there later occurs an intrauterine transfer of the clone. A clone does differ from a zygote: a clone begins with one nucleus, not two pronuclei, and a clone suffers from abnormalities in expression of imprinted genes and other defects. Even so, scientists routinely

---

[5] A fuller discussion of the response that follows is given in Guenin 2003a.

say that mature nonhuman clones (e.g., Dolly the sheep) have developed
from embryos. Withholding 'clone' and 'embryo' from life forms heretofore called by those terms risks the appearance of legerdemain, of trying to
smuggle in the creation of an embryo by not mentioning it, of switching
labels in lieu of argument. If we did not already have 'embryo' to name a
universe of moral concern, we would coin a term with like extension. It falls
to the scientist and philosopher to root out misconceptions that ordinary
language sometimes harbors, but in this case, it seems to me that ordinary
language has got things right. In a convergence of scientific expository convenience and common parlance, 'embryo' is our generic term for a prefetal
conceptus.

Parthenogenesis consists in organismic development begun upon activation of an oocyte without insertion of foreign DNA. Reptiles reproduce
in such manner. Parthenogenesis does not naturally occur in mammals.
Human parthenogenesis may be artificially initiated by electrochemical or
mechanical stimulation of an oocyte. A human parthenote will not develop
a functional placenta.

We may now sketch the role of embryos in stem cell biology. A *totipotent
stem cell* is a cell capable of developing into an entire organism with placenta.
Nontotipotent stem cells may be defined by two attributes, (a) self-renewal,
the ability of populations thereof to perpetuate by cell division throughout
the life of an organism, and (b) differentiability, the ability to issue in at
least one type of highly differentiated descendant.[6] (This is a functional
definition; in the laboratory, an investigator will apply an operational definition predicated on observables such as cell surface markers.) Stem cells
are *unipotent* if they can issue in only one type of descendant (e.g., sper-
matogenic stem cells), *multipotent* if they can issue in a few cell types (e.g.,
hematopoietic stem cells), and *pluripotent* if they can issue in cells of all
three *germ layers*, namely, the mesoderm, ectoderm, and endoderm, which
is to say cells of all types except placental. Stem cells do not transform
directly into specialized cells. Stem cells begin a differentiation sequence,
a sequence in which each successive cell type is ever more differentiated.
The sequence ends in specialized cells.

It is believed that most of the blastomeres produced during very early
cleavage are totipotent stem cells, and that after about the eight-cell stage,
totipotency has ceased. (To test for totipotency, an investigator would ascertain whether the subject can successfully implant in a uterus and develop.
But we should be hard pressed to justify experimental intrauterine transfer

---

[6] Watt and Hogan 2000. A cluster of totipotent stem cells is not self-renewing.

of what an investigator believes may be a totipotent cell, i.e., a developing embryo.) At the blastocyst stage, the blastomeres of the inner cell mass are pluripotent. They cannot generate a trophoblast.

We may think of the early blastocyst stage, the period around day 5, as a brief pluripotency interlude that succeeds totipotency and precedes differentiation. One method of extracting blastomeres from an embryo during this interlude is *immunosurgery*. Originally perfected in mice,[7] this procedure strips away the trophoblast and separates the embryoblast from the trophoblast. The procedure unavoidably destroys the embryo. It was from blastomeres extracted during this interlude that investigators first grew populations of human *embryonic stem cells*, understood as indefinitely proliferating populations of pluripotent stem cells derived from embryos.[8] The investigators accomplished this feat by hitting upon growth media and conditions that, while nurturing cells so that they continue to divide, include ingredients that avert differentiation. Because blastomeres of the inner cell mass do not self-renew *in vivo*,[9] blastomeres are not themselves stem cells (unless, contrary to our definition, we demand for stem cells only differentiability). Thus 'embryonic stem cells' does not denote blastomeres but rather the cell culture derivatives of blastomeres. 'Embryonic' here denotes 'embryo-derived.'

While embryonic stem cells are derived from living embryos, pluripotent cells of another type, *embryonic germ cells*, are derived from abortuses at a late embryonic stage.[10] A consensus justification for use of abortal tissue arises in the case of a woman who undergoes an abortion without inducement by anyone and for reasons unrelated to research, and who thereafter donates the remains.[11] A donee scientist's use of such remains may be likened to a transplant patient's acceptance of the organ of someone recently deceased, or to the use of a donated cadaver in medical education, in each case on the condition that the donee is not complicit in the death of the source. The justification of such practices in virtue of such noncomplicity has gained recognition within the fount from which emanates the notion of complicity, the teachings of the Roman Catholic Church. These acknowledge the permissibility of 'experimentation carried out on embryos which are dead,' provided that 'there be no complicity in deliberate abortion and that the risk of scandal be avoided.'[12]

---

[7] Solter and Knowles 1975.　　[8] Thomson *et al.* 1998.
[9] van der Kooy and Weiss 2000.　　[10] Shamblott *et al.* 1998.
[11] It is feasible, as in 42 U.S.C. §§289g-1(b)(2)(A),(c), and 289g-2(b) (2000), to prohibit inducement.
[12] Sacred Congregation for the Doctrine of the Faith, *Donum Vitae* § I(4).

Many diseases and disabilities result from a deficiency in specialized cells of a single type. I refer here to maladies such as diabetes, Parkinson's, heart disease, muscular dystrophy, autoimmune diseases, multiple sclerosis, Lou Gehrig's disease, other degenerative diseases, and spinal cord injury. Type 1 diabetes results from insufficiency of insulin-producing pancreatic β cells, Parkinson's from insufficiency of dopaminergic neurons, and so on.

The discovery of how to grow human embryonic stem cells in culture immediately suggested the prospect of inducing such cells to issue in transplantable cells – whether fully specialized cells, precursors, or multipotent cells – with which to augment a patient's pool of cells of a given type. Even neurons might thus be generated. The birth of Dolly by cloning then suggested a strategy for obtaining immunocompatible cells for transplant: use a skin cell of a patient to produce a clone of the patient, derive an embryonic stem cell line, then induce differentiation into specialized cells. Another strategy consists in obtaining disease-specific pluripotent stem cells, observing how the diseases begin, designing drugs to combat the diseases, and testing the drugs on the exemplifying cells. Cloning compels attention because it puts on display cellular *reprogramming* (or *dedifferentiation*), an epigenetic process in which the transferred nucleus reverts to an undifferentiated state. Reprogramming involves cytoplasmic transcription factors observed in embryonic stem cells and clones. Through embryonic stem cell research in which these factors have been observed in action, investigators have devised ways to introduce or trigger the factors in somatic cells, thereby generating *induced pluripotent stem cells*. The embryonic stem cell is the gold standard of pluripotency to which all other cell types are experimentally compared, as well as the subject of studies through which investigators probe the most fundamental questions of stem cell biology. Studies of embryos and cells derived from them could also yield insights into cellular processes in general, including cancer. Other ingenious lines of inquiry may emerge in various fields of biomedical research as the fruit of further research. A vision has developed of research and therapy enabled by observing and reprising development at its earliest stages. Thus do we find our attention drawn to embryos that will never begin gestation.

1.3 AFFECTED BEINGS AND UTILITARIANISM

The word 'person' derives from the Latin *persona*, denoting a mask worn on stage. *Persona* correlates with the verb *personare*, to resound. An actor could speak more loudly by speaking through the cavity in his mask. The phrase '*dramatis personae*' eventually came to denote not masks, but roles.

Now we use 'person' for a being recognized in a role on the stage of life. In its normative sense, 'person' designates a member of a set of objects of direct concern for some moral or legal purpose. For the plural 'persons,' it is sometimes convenient to say 'people.' There is also an ontological sense of 'person,' that which is in point when philosophers speak of personal identity, or when they assert that a person is an organism, an embodied mind, or an ensouled being. On occasion, moral questions implicating a normative sense of 'person' may motivate trying to resolve an ontological sense. For some, the ontological extension dictates the normative. But in concept, the two senses are distinct.

The point of ascribing or withholding 'person' in a normative sense usually is to declare whose actions are subjects of moral evaluation or who should receive some treatment. In this sense, 'Biggles is a person for purposes of the duty of promisekeeping' may state a conclusion reached through some line of moral reasoning. A normative sense of 'person' is always relative to a purpose. A corporation may be a person for purposes of the laws of taxation but not a person for purposes of the privilege against self-incrimination. That the extension of 'person' varies from one context to the next was partly why Bernard Williams once called this predicate 'a poor foundation for ethical thought.'[13] In any case, in the sort of normative sense that is in point here, 'person' often serves, for purposes of a treatment t, as a name for 'member of the set of beings to whom t should be accorded.' That is not to say that we use 'person' to designate every thing that would benefit from performance of a duty. We do not say that a tree is a person for purposes of our duty to protect the environment. We may have non-person-affecting duties. We also may have imperfect duties, duties that do not precisely specify either a treatment or set of recipients.

Embryo use presents us with the question, who is a person in the normative sense for purposes of the duty not to kill a person? A duty not to kill is common to a variety of moral views. Moralists variously contend that a maxim against killing is a maxim that a rational will could without contradiction will as a universal law of nature when legislating in a kingdom of ends, that a maxim against killing is a rule that in comparison to alternatives would maximize aggregate utility, that rational representative parties would choose such a rule when reasoning impartially under a veil of ignorance, or that a duty not to kill is a divine commandment. There also come to bear the duties, such as we have, not to harm a person and not to use a person solely as a means. I begin consideration of embryo use in

---

[13] Williams 1995, p. 114.

the general case with Hare's universal prescriptivism, or 'Kantian utilitarian point of view.' I turn to this in the first instance because it will be helpful in the next chapter to borrow a version of Hare's notion of possible person so as to frame opposition to embryo use in its strongest form. I also take this opportunity to consider a utilitarian analysis of embryo use.

For scientists who prefer measurements to value judgments, utilitarianism possesses immediate appeal. It strikes them as a kind of empirical anchor in judgment space. An *order homomorphism* is a function such that the values that it assigns alternatives are ordered conformably to a given binary relation on a set of alternatives. By a *positioning*, I understand a transitive, connected binary relation.[14] Within preference-based utilitarianism, individual i's utility function u_i is a real-valued order homomorphism representing or implying a positioning imposed by i on a set of alternatives. This represented or implied positioning is known as i's *preference relation*. Preference-based utilitarianism commands us to maximize *aggregate utility* defined as $\Sigma_{i \in I} u_i$, where $I = \{1, 2, \ldots, n\}$ is the *index set* of affected beings, and $(u_1, u_2, \ldots, u_i, \ldots, u_n)$ is a vector of their respective utility functions. Maximizing aggregate utility consists in maximizing aggregate preference satisfaction. In the following, if the context is the mathematics of utilitarianism, I refer to aggregate utility. If the context involves the question of whose preferences should count, I refer to aggregate preference satisfaction.

Hare takes up the objection that maximizing total rather than average utility requires overpopulating the earth. The most vigorous form of this objection has been posed by Derek Parfit as the Repugnant Conclusion: maximizing utility, or maximizing anything else deemed to make life worth living, will increase population to the point at which life is barely worth living.[15] Hare does not think it likely that adhering to utilitarianism will produce this calamity, and in the course of defending the maximization of total utility, he advances a proposition on which he will come to predicate a comprehensive view of reproduction. For moral purposes, the relevant universe of persons includes not only all 'grown persons,' but all 'possible persons.' In the argument by which he reaches this proposition, Hare adduces the universalizability requirement for moral prescriptions. A moral prescription that applies to a described person in a given situation must apply to all others similarly situated. In particular,

---

[14] An antisymmetric positioning is a linear ordering. When an agent is indifferent between some alternatives, the agent's positioning on the set of alternatives is a nonsymmetric relation. I clarify these and other transitive relations in Guenin 2001c.
[15] Parfit 1984, pp. 384–390.

The principles we adopt will have to cover the procreation of anybody. Can we restrict this by saying that they have to cover only the procreation of people who are actually procreated (that is of actual people)? I think not. . . . Actuality is a property which cannot be defined without bringing in references to individuals, and therefore no such restriction can occur in a properly universal prescription.[16]

We might quarrel with the claim that a definition of actuality requires references to individuals. Could we not define the set {all actual people at t_0}? Hare gives a better argument for his claim elsewhere,[17] but we need not pause for it.

Hare proceeds to posit a possible person *corresponding to* a conceptus. Possible persons then appear in Hare's fundamental utilitarian principle: treating everyone's preferences equally, we ought to maximize aggregate preference satisfaction for the index set of all 'people who would thereby be affected (including people who would come into existence) in the world as it is.' Coupling utilitarianism with the premise that universal prescriptions cannot be confined to actual persons, Hare reasons that we should 'give equal weight to the equal preferences of all possible people.'[18] Among alternatives, we should choose that which 'produces that set of people, of all the possible sets, which will have in sum the best life.'

Against the concept of possible person, there arises the objection that possible people do not have preferences. Hare responds that it makes sense to say 'There is a corresponding possible person' tenselessly, as when we say 'there is' in 'there is an x such that Fx.' This adverts to possibilism, a view that allows one to say that there is a possible being, a being that is not actual but could be, or, as Aristotle said, 'that which exists potentially.'[19] Against this comes W. V. Quine's warning that a 'slum of possibles' is 'a breeding ground for disorderly elements.'[20] Quine was concerned with ontologies admitting unactualized possibles so as to account for the subjects of sentences such as 'Pegasus does not exist.' Hare then suggests a way to obviate reliance on possibilism.

Hare introduces the device that I may take a sentence about a possible person corresponding to a conceptus as a sentence about an actual person, namely, me. Given a particular situation ψ affecting a conceptus x to which a possible person is said to correspond, I imagine ψ occurring for the conceptus that became me. I ask, 'What do I think about ψ on the supposition that the conceptus from which I developed was in x's

---

[16] Hare 1993, p. 72. [17] Hare 1981, p. 114.
[18] Hare 1993, p. 70; Hare 1981, p. 154. [19] *De Interpretatione* 19b3. [20] Quine 1961, p. 4.

circumstances?'[21] Epistemically, preferences of possible people lie beyond our grasp, but Hare surmises that the desire and preference to live is well nigh universal. That I now exist also confirms that it was possible that I should now exist when there formed the zygote that developed into me. So Hare concludes that when the zygote that developed into me formed, it was *my* preference to exist, even though I did not then exist. Whereupon he assigns moral significance to whatever harm occurs to whatever being comes to exist. 'Remoteness in time,' remarks Parfit, 'has, in itself, no more significance than remoteness in space.'[22] Or again, as it has elsewhere been remarked, harms 'over temporal distances' are not 'any more problematic than the more familiar cases of wrongful actions that result in harm across spatial distances.'[23] We may also lie under duties not owed to anyone in particular. Reflection on Parfit's Non-Identity Problem provides reason to think that we can have non-person-affecting duties.[24] If we can make sense of all this, we can make sense of harm to possible persons.

By 'interests,' Hare understands the best considered preferences of a fully informed diachronic person.[25] It is interests that Hare bids us honor. We must consider the interests of actual people, of possible people into which embryos and fetuses are capable of developing, and in some circumstances, even of a possible person into which some pair of a couple's uncombined gametes could develop.[26] With his sights trained on corresponding possible people, Hare concludes that 'we need not waste any more ink' on 'the wild goose chase' of deciding when a conceptus becomes a human being or a person.[27] We should instead ask, 'How ought we to treat this conceptus?' By Hare's lights, the following should be our guide: '*whenever* my life . . . began, anything that would have interfered with my developing into the grown person that I now am would have been against my interest, and therefore

---

[21] Hare 1993, pp. 86–88, 173–174. The intricacies of this are studied in Gensler 1986 and Wilson, B. 1988.

[22] Parfit 1984, p. 357.   [23] Buchanan *et al.* 2000, p. 228.

[24] Parfit 1984, pp. 351–390, and Kavka 1982. In unusual cases, wrong may occur without constituting harm to the affected being. In a case given in Parfit 1976, p. 374, it could be wrong for prospective parents to conceive during a time interval in which, so they are informed, it is highly probable that any offspring that they conceive will suffer from a genetic abnormality that brings about a severe disability. If they conceive during that interval anyway, and bring forth a child that experiences a life worth living despite a severe disability, they cannot have harmed the child, this because if they had prevented the disability, they would have prevented the child from existing. They could be said to have violated a non-person-affecting duty not to engage in reproduction by a means or at a time such that one has reason to believe it likely that the offspring will be burdened by a genetic defect that will result in a life so miserable as not to be worth living, or in a severe deformity.

[25] Hare 1993, pp. 56–57, and Hare 1981, pp. 105–106, but cf. Hare 1997, p. 77.

[26] Hare 1993, pp. 89–90, 116, 157.   [27] *Ibid.*, pp. 93–94, 130, 169ff.

pro tanto wrong.'[28] Since excising cells from an embryo or performing an abortion will effect harm to a possible person, those practices are *pro tanto* wrong. Contraception also serves to 'prevent the existence of a grown person who has an interest in existing,' and therefore is *pro tanto* wrong. But since contraception operates only on gametes, and gametes are not objects of affection, contraception is less wrong than abortion.[29]

Then comes the question whether an act or practice that is wrong *pro tanto* is wrong all things considered. Hare sets himself apart from others in urging that we honor not only the inferable preferences of the possible person corresponding to a given embryo, but also the preferences of many other possible persons. 'Contraception, abstinence, the destruction of embryos, abortion, and even infanticide ought to be controlled . . . by the interests of possible future developed people who there might otherwise be.' 'The number of these,' he continues, 'ought to be decided by finding the right population and family planning policy,' a policy that 'produces that set of people, of all the possible sets, which will have in sum the best life.'[30] The interests of actual and possible persons 'have to be balanced against one another within the limits of what we can do.'[31]

What does this all entail? Within a utilitarian account, is destruction of embryos and fetuses permissible or not? The wrong of killing inheres in violating a universalizable prescription at which utilitarianism arrives upon heeding the prevailing preference to live. Each of us can compare existence to nonexistence, and we, most of us at least, prefer existence. The utilitarian appeals to a calculation revealing that a universal prescription against killing will, in comparison with alternative prescriptions, produce the greatest aggregate preference satisfaction. To Hare it seems evident that among persons affected by a policy on embryo use will be corresponding possible people who prefer life over death. 'What makes the moral difference is what the consequences of different treatments of embryos will be for the people into whom they might turn.' So Hare concludes that 'the preservation of embryos . . . is important just because if they are preserved they will turn into grown people who will benefit from existing. . . .' In respect of conceptuses in general, 'the interest of the possible future grown person into whom they might turn . . . imposes on us, in normal cases, a duty to preserve them.'[32]

This leads Hare to a 'presumptive policy' declaring that 'abortions in general ought to be avoided.'[33] Or, without reference to possible people,

---

[28] *Ibid.*, pp. 93, 130. [29] *Ibid.*, pp. 91, 159–160. [30] *Ibid.*, pp. 89–90, 95, 163–164.
[31] *Ibid.*, pp. 90, 181. [32] *Ibid.*, pp. 87, 93. [33] *Ibid.*, p. 159.

he holds that 'if we are glad that nobody terminated the pregnancy that resulted in our birth,' then, *ceteris paribus*, we cannot declare abortion wrong for us without declaring abortion wrong for others were it to thwart the sort of experiences that have made us glad.[34] Abortion therefore would be wrong as to the 'vast majority' of pregnancies, though right as to some. But, he asks, 'Is there any reason for giving precedence to some of these [possible] people over others?'[35] Hare finds no reason for preferring a conceptus in development to other possible future children. Despite his general presumption against abortion, he concludes that it is sometimes appropriate for couples to imagine a choice between 'having this child now and having another child later.' A couple might permissibly procure an abortion if the expected quality of life by dint of a chromosomal defect of the possible person corresponding to a fetus in gestation is substantially less than the expected quality of life of a healthy child that the parents, having decided on a bound to the size of their family, would conceive if and only if the present fetus is not born. For such reasoning, parents perforce rely on probability estimates about fetal and neonatal health. Hare concedes that given present knowledge, such reasoning is guesswork. But it is not dispositive that a fetus in gestation already exists. There is always some other possible child that could come into being 'in the demography.'[36] On this view, whether abortion is right in a given case depends on the interests of all affected – including the mother, the father, the possible person corresponding, and other possible persons who may have an interest.

But when Hare considers the morality of eating animals, the practice gives him pause, enough so that he revises his fundamental utilitarian precept to demand an even larger index set: we must maximize the aggregate preference satisfaction of 'beings capable of forming preferences.' The implication is that some nonhuman animals form preferences. If we sometimes find it difficult to infer the preferences of our fellow citizens, we shall surely hesitate if asked to discern preferences of nonhuman self-conscious animals. We shall encounter more difficulty if we try to *weight* the preferences of fellow humans *vis-à-vis* those of nonhuman animals. Hare quickly retreats from his new precept and embraces a population policy encompassing the universe of concern that Bentham recognized. He settles upon maximizing the number of quality-adjusted life years of sentient beings.[37]

Embryos are not sentient. An embryo or presentient fetus, Hare writes, 'does not *currently* possess any properties that could be morally relevant to its

[34] *Ibid.*, pp. 153–154.   [35] *Ibid.*, pp. 91, 181–183.   [36] *Ibid.*, pp. 157, 182–183.
[37] *Ibid.*, pp. 226–228, cf. pp. 82, 68–69; Hare 1981, pp. 90–91.

treatment and which are not possessed equally by oysters and earthworms.'[38] His point here is that such invertebrates are not sentient. Nor do embryos have the intellectual ability to form preferences that any action by us could frustrate. '*They,*' writes Hare, 'do not want not to be killed.' Thus Hare declares that 'embryos do not as such have interests.'[39] A man and woman could act so as to maximize the number of quality-adjusted life years of sentient beings by sacrificing an extant embryo and later nurturing another to maturity. When an embryo is sacrificed,

> No harm is . . . done to the subject as such by destroying it, but only to the person that it might turn into; and this may be compensated for by the bringing into being of some other person.[40]

In respect of harm 'to the person that it might turn into,' suppose that Mary and John wish to donate a surplus embryo to research and that they decline to bring forth any other offspring. As we have seen, for purposes of computing aggregate utility, Hare includes possible persons corresponding to embryos in the index set and imputes to them a preference for life over death. In the case of Mary and John, the enormous disutility to the corresponding possible person of sacrificing the embryo will not be compensated by birth of any other offspring. But Mary and John may reasonably expect that indefinitely propagating lines of stem cells, or other benefits derived from embryos, will contribute to medical advances that avail many people. If recognizing their discretion to donate embryos is that alternative among those available for which aggregate expected utility is the greatest, utilitarianism commands that recognition.

1.4 A COMPUTATIONAL WATERLOO

Mention of compensation for harm, or of replacing an extant conceptus with one later conceived, reminds opponents why they reject utilitarianism. Utilitarianism is a sum-ranking version of consequentialism. Some opposing views do not conceive of morality as the maximization of any maximand. They no more expect preference-based accounts of welfare to yield the correct principles of right conduct than they would expect a poll of committee members to yield an analysis as compelling as what one reflective scholar could produce alone. The utilitarian rejoins that some of the hypothetical situations posed against utilitarianism are fantastic examples

---

[38] Hare 1993, p. 172.   [39] *Ibid.*, pp. 90, 128, 168, 171, 181.

[40] *Ibid.*, p. 95. Hare imagines in the first instance only destruction of nonsentients, and secondarily, he adverts to procedures on sentients in which anesthesia fully precludes pain (pp. 95, 128, 168).

contrived so as to paint the utilitarian as a moral monster, whereas in many ordinary situations, utilitarianism yields the same verdicts as those reached by other theories. For example, a utilitarian may predicate use of developed humans as research subjects on informed consent, this on the ground that each of us, and parents for their children, are the best judge of what satisfies our preferences. Should it be thought strategic to travel under the banner of a right against bodily intrusion, utilitarianism can fly that flag too. But talk of compensating for harms cannot be explained away, and the case of Mary and John is not far-fetched. The utilitarian must stand on the comparison of aggregate utilities.

The computational situation is the following. When the issue is population policy or the distribution of economic benefits, utilitarianism takes the form of a theory of distributive justice. It defines a social welfare function consisting of an unweighted sum of individual utility functions (in utilitarianism's Benthamite form) or a weighted sum of individual utility functions (in its general form), each individual utility function defined on a domain of social states. In the case of utilitarianism as a theory of right conduct, utilitarians often find it convenient to restrict the aggregate utility function to a subdomain containing only the few alternative moral prescriptions that seem applicable to a given situation, everything else being held constant. Since there exist infinitely many multidimensional social states, one might think that as between the aggregate utility function invoked by utilitarianism as a theory of right conduct and the utilitarian social welfare function, the latter is the greater computational beast. But even for the theory of right conduct, and even if the domain is only a handful of alternatives, implementation of a prescription about reproduction will involve and affect multitudinous people of reproductive age, not to mention possible people corresponding to conceptuses. It will affect people who hold strong views on reproductive issues despite no direct encounter with such issues in their own lives. It will affect those many people who hold preferences about embryo use. The universe of persons that might benefit from embryo research is huge. For a domain of alternative prescriptions about reproduction, utilitarianism seems compelled to include in the index set just about everybody. Inasmuch as the outcome of applying any prescription is uncertain, the utilitarian must calculate and sum expected utilities. The expected utility of a prescription is the sum of expected utilities of the possible outcomes. Each outcome's expected utility is the product of the outcome's utility and the outcome's probability.

The scale of this computation renders its execution doubtful. Such is the case even before an old chestnut enters to place the computation beyond redemption by the usual excuses. Given an individual's utility function representing their positioning on a set of alternatives, there exist infinitely many other utility functions that represent that positioning. A utilitarian may meaningfully sum utility functions of two or more individuals only if their respective utility functions constitute interpersonally comparable measures. In the absence of such measures, the utilitarian would have no basis for comparing the zero points or units of one individual's utility function with those of another's. In such case, to use an analogy drawn by Stephen Strasnick, 'trying to compare the utility numbers of different individuals would be just as meaningless as trying to construct an unknown object from a set of blueprints of its components that had no points of reference or units of scale.'[41] Utilitarianism is brought up short by the interpersonal incommensurability of utilities.

Hare ventures that his account escapes this fatal flaw, but his argument serves only to clarify the defect. Hare points out that for purposes of maximizing aggregate utility, one need only compare *differences* in utilities.[42] That is true. But utility differences are comparable only if the individual utility functions are at least unit comparable interval scale measures, which is to say that each function u_i is unique up to transformations of the form $t(u_i) = \alpha(u_i) + \beta$ for $\alpha > 0$. For a given domain of alternative moral prescriptions, no one will have constructed individual utility functions, much less unit comparable measures. In the absence of unit comparable measures, the maxima of the aggregate utility function $\Sigma_{i \in I}\, u_i$ will perversely differ between equivalent utility vectors.[43] Whereupon the utilitarian cannot meaningfully compute the aggregate utilities of alternatives. The utilitarian, Paul Samuelson once remarked, is 'drunk on poorly understood post-Newtonian mathematical moonshine.' In order to take the wind out of the utilitarian's sails, an opponent need only ask for the values of the aggregate utility function.

Utilitarianism's beleaguered exponents are accustomed to deflecting attention from this defect in hopes that for many in their audience, the flaw is too technical to give pause. A peculiar mercy for the utilitarian occurs when smoke from the broadsides of the purportedly fantastic

---

[41] Strasnick 1981, p. 77.

[42] Hare 1981, pp. 124, 128. He also says that 'it is not so important' that quality-adjusted life years are difficult to measure because 'after all, before weighing machines with numerical scales were invented, people could all the same pick up two sacks of corn and tell which was the heavier' (Hare 1993, pp. 186, 227). So too we always know from a represented preference relation how a given individual regards two alternatives in relation to each other, even if their utility values are arbitrary. But this says nothing about interpersonal comparability of utilities.

[43] A succinct demonstration of this is given in Roemer 1996, pp. 19–21.

counterexamples launched by opponents sometimes obscures the Achilles' heel. Occasionally even listeners aware of incommensurability will indulge the utilitarian. At Amity City Hall, a utilitarian advocates a new hospital before an audience of citizens whose houses occupy the proposed site. Amity has proposed to take their homes by eminent domain upon payment of fair market value and moving expenses. The utilitarian argues that a new hospital's utility for vastly many patients over its useful life will greatly exceed the disutility for homeowners of moving. The audience may take this argument seriously insofar as it appears that, for some plausible conversion ratio of units of measure, a comparison of utilities between the project and the status quo would be lopsided.

In the present discussion, the listeners whom a utilitarian proponent of embryo use needs to convince are unlikely to concede that a balance of utilities lopsidedly favors embryo sacrifice. Those listeners will challenge any claim that the utility gains of research beneficiaries will exceed the utility losses of possible people corresponding to embryos – not to mention the utility losses of citizens who oppose embryo sacrifice and would be saddened by it. Sceptical listeners have no reason to give credence to a computational argument that lacks the computation. Here utilitarianism has met its Waterloo. In this crippled state, it cannot ground a consensus for or against embryo use. In the next chapter, I look elsewhere for a foundation.

CHAPTER 2

Epidosembryos

In this chapter, I speak of donated embryos barred from the womb, and argue for their use in service of humanitarian ends. So as to take account of diverse moral concerns about embryo use, I begin by defining concepts that will allow us to pose opposition to embryo use in its strongest form, this by reference to possible persons as well as actual persons (§2.1). I then define the set of embryos whose use I shall defend (§2.2). I next present my argument for the use of such embryos (§2.3). Thereafter I distinguish this argument from other defenses of embryo use, describe the scope of what the argument justifies, and defend the argument against anticipated objections (§§2.4–2.7).

2.1 THE UNIVERSE OF CONCERN

I define a *uterine closure* as a structure consisting of a uterus and connected fallopian tubes. I shall say that an embryo becomes *enabled* if and only if the embryo originates in or enters a uterine closure. We may partition the set of embryos into

$T = \{e \mid e$ is an embryo that at some time exists inside a uterine closure$\}$,
$U = \{e \mid e$ is an embryo that never exists inside a uterine closure$\}$.

An embryo existing outside the human body is *extracorporeal*. I shall refer to members of U as *unenabled*.

An embryo formed *in vivo* must implant in the uterus by about day 7 if it is to mature. An extracorporeal embryo maintained beyond day 7 in a cell culture dish will not begin gestation. Gestation is by definition a uterine process. A dish's growth medium, however enriched, is not an adequate substitute for the uterine endometrium. In default of implantation, development in the dish will arrest after about ten days, if not earlier. The embryo will disintegrate, becoming, as it were, a mass of embryonic tissue.[1]

---

[1] I thank John Gearhart for elucidating the importance of implantation.

It is logically possible that a rocket travels faster than the speed of light. It is logically possible, as Ovid imagined in the *Metamorphoses*, that the statue carved by Pygmalion becomes a woman, or that Daphne the nymph becomes a laurel tree. In logic, 'possible' is the alethic mode equivalent to 'not necessarily not.' In scientific discourse, there commonly appears a more restricted sense of 'possible.' Where ϕ is an event or condition, we say that ϕ is *nomologically possible* in a situation ψ if and only if ϕ's occurring or obtaining in ψ is consistent with the laws of nature of the actual world. Kant referred to nomological possibility as 'real possibility.'[2] Nomological possibility relative to a situation is also known as 'physical possibility.' This is the notion that a scientist plausibly invokes when declaring an event or condition 'physically impossible.'

We often use 'can' or 'cannot' *tout court* in respect of a situation about which there obtains a shared understanding about what is nomologically possible. Thus we say that orchids cannot grow in the Arctic. In this instance biology alone is decisive. In other cases, human decisions may shape the situation in respect of which we predicate nomological possibility or impossibility of some event or condition. A case in point is that it is nomologically impossible for an unenabled embryo to develop into an infant.[3] Nomological possibility lies in the background of much of our moral reasoning. While it is logically and metaphysically possible for humans to fly unaided, we believe such feat nomologically impossible, and hence would condemn any act of shoving someone out an airplane door.

I earlier defined a phase change in an individual of a given kind of substance as a change that things of that kind survive in accordance with the laws of nature. A *substance* may be understood as a concrete object that subsists without depending for its identity on anything else. More will be said of substance in §3.6(b). A *substantial change* in respect of an individual x of a given kind of substance is a change in which either (1) x ceases to exist or x comes to be, or (2) while persisting, x changes into an individual of a different kind of substance. A case of (1) occurs when, as a result of combustion, a pile of wood ceases to exist and ashes are left in its place. Since a change in a persisting substance in accordance with the laws of nature will be a phase change, the effect of including (2) in the foregoing definition is to countenance as a metaphysical possibility that a protean substance survives a metamorphosis that defies the laws of nature.[4] But,

---

[2] *Critique of Pure Reason* A218–219/B265–267, A244/B302, A596n/B624n.

[3] On the other hand, some ostensibly modal sentences are best understood as descriptions of probabilities (e.g., 'There is a possibility that the dean will arrive in time for the lecture').

[4] Such a change is countenanced in Lowe 1998, pp. 55, 174, 184, 186–187.

pace Ovid, we need not presently concern ourselves with changes that defy the laws of nature. Assuming that the laws of nature prevail, a substantial change will consist in cessation or origination of a substance. A substantial change will change what substances exist.[5]

Substantial and phase changes correlate with the applicability to substances of *sortals*. A sortal is a count noun such as 'dog' or 'table.' One can form the plural of count nouns and count their referents. Thus we are apt to mention 'two tables.' Not so with bulk terms such as 'snow' or 'gold.' We would not say 'two golds.' 'Sortal' sounds like a neologism of contemporary philosophy, but the term originated with Locke, who formed it from 'sort,' likening the coinage to that of 'general' from 'genus.'[6] The concept harkens to Aristotle's observation that a species or genus 'does not signify simply a certain qualification, as *white* does. *White* signifies nothing but a qualification, whereas species and genus mark off the kind of substance – they signify what sort of substance.'[7] A substance is often denoted by a *substance sortal*. Embedded in our grasp of the concept associated with a substance sortal are conditions of applicability and persistence, the latter governing 'what can and cannot befall any *x* in its extension' and 'what changes *x* tolerates without there ceasing to exist such a thing as *x*.'[8] A substance sortal will cease to be applicable to a referent only if the referent ceases to exist (or if the substance, while slipping the bonds of natural law, metamorphosizes into a substance of another kind). A *phase sortal* is a sortal such that an individual of a given kind of substance may cease to fall under the sortal while persisting as an individual of that kind. 'Embryo,' 'morula,' and 'blastocyst' are phase sortals restricting the substance sortal 'human.' Since natural changes to persisting entities are phase changes, they go hand in hand with changes in applicability of phase sortals.

Not all biological development is organismic. We may understand *development* in general as a process consisting of sequential phase changes, consequent on interaction of genome, epigenetic systems, and environment, that transform a living thing into successive stages of a living thing of its kind.

Suppose that, within a given view, we have a definition of 'person' in the ontological sense or in the normative sense for a given purpose. We may then say the following.

---

[5] So put in Lowe 2003c, p. 141.   [6] *Essay Concerning Human Understanding*, III, iii, 15.
[7] *Categories* 3b17–21, as rendered in Wiggins 2001, p. 21.
[8] Wiggins 2001, p. 70, D(iv).

Nomologically Possible Person. For a situation ψ and a substance x, a nomologically possible person corresponds to x if and only if, in ψ, it is nomologically possible that, without there occurring any substantial change in respect of x, a person or an organism constituting the body of a person will develop from x.

The expression 'or an organism constituting the body of a person' leaves room for views holding that a person is an embodied mind, Cartesian union of mind and body, or ensouled being. To denote a nomologically possible person, for brevity's sake I shall use 'possible person.'

Talk of possible persons again invites the question of how there are things that are not actual. In order to take account of moral considerations sometimes couched in terms of possible persons, let us assume for the sake of argument a possibilist account responsive to that question. Recognizing possible persons does not require ascribing preferences or volitions. Calculations predicated upon ascriptions thereof are peculiar to preference-based accounts of welfare.

To embryos in various situations, possible persons may be said to correspond. These include not only the situations of embryos *in vivo* but also situations of embryos *in vitro* about which no decision against intrauterine transfer has been taken. On the other hand, no possible persons correspond to oocytes, gamete pairs, somatic cells, or embryonic stem cells. It is not nomologically possible for any such body parts to develop into an organism, or, in respect of personhood, to acquire any morally significant property not already possessed, unless there occurs a substantial change in which the body parts cease. We might mistakenly infer otherwise from the biological expression 'oocyte activation.' This phrase may seem to suggest that, upon activation, an oocyte undergoes a mere phase change through which it persists. To be sure, it may be said that as fertilization begins, an oocyte persists for a matter of hours. The oocyte's messenger RNA continues to run the show as the oocyte undergoes alterations initiated by entry of sperm. But as the pronuclei exchange chromosomes, the cytoplasm changes, and the cell divides, the oocyte and sperm cease to exist. There comes into existence a product of the fusion of oocyte and sperm. That product I shall refer to as an 'individual of humankind,' a characterization that I shall defend fully in Chapter 3. The nascent individual of humankind possesses a different genome than the genome of either gamete. As a result of biochemical activity, the nascent individual's cytoplasm also differs from that of the oocyte. Fertilization has thus effected a substantial change. At the outset there existed two human body parts, and in the end there exists one human individual. Cloning also begins with two body parts, nucleus and enucleated oocyte. As these parts fuse they cease, and there comes to be one human individual.

Oocyte activation may also occur spontaneously. But the only products of spontaneous oocyte activation that manifest *in vivo* are degenerate growths, namely, dermoid cysts and ovarian teratomas. Formation of such a degenerate might be characterized as a substantial change, stimulated by the oocyte's environment, in which the oocyte ceases. Or it might be viewed as a phase change of the oocyte into a degenerate. In either case, the degenerate will not undergo organismic development. It is not nomologically possible for a product of spontaneous or induced oocyte activation into which no foreign DNA enters to develop beyond the first stage at which the product requires placenta-mediated nourishment. The degenerate cannot develop a functional placenta. This limitation appears to result from lack of any paternal genetic contribution. A product of spontaneous oocyte activation, in its bounded growth, will not acquire any morally significant property not possessed at inception. It follows that spontaneous oocyte activation cannot result either in a person or in an organism constituting the body of a person unless the product of activation is a person at inception, in which case it would be pointless to assert the correspondence of a possible person. In the alternative, an investigator could in theory perform extensive genetic engineering, concomitantly with artificially inducing parthenogenesis, so as to replace multitudinous alleles in hopes of averting abnormalities in a resultant parthenote. (An allele is one of two or more alternative forms of a gene.) But if foreign DNA were thus fused with an oocyte, there would occur a substantial change. The oocyte and foreign DNA would cease to exist. A product of their fusion would come into being.

Thus a person or an organism constituting the body of a person cannot come into existence from an oocyte, a pair of gametes, or cell nucleus without there occurring a substantial change in which such body part or parts cease and a product of oocyte activation comes into being. 'Human gamete,' 'human somatic cell nucleus,' and 'human' are substance sortals. On my rendering of the condition under which a possible person corresponds to something, we recognize a possible person only if a conceptus comes into existence.

Other accounts may hypothesize a larger universe of possible persons. Hare recognizes a possible person corresponding to a future pair of gametes that could fuse were a couple who elects an abortion later to initiate another pregnancy. In considering population policy or stewardship of the environment, we may consider possible people living in later decades, this without reference to the details of their origination. For anyone who wishes to frame a case against the use of extant embryos, or against the use of embryos to be created in research, it suffices to place into consideration the possible persons corresponding to those embryos. There is no need to associate possible persons with cells that may possibly fuse.

In case it be thought arbitrary that we call a change from morula to blastocyst a phase change of a human, but call a change from human body part to human individual a substantial change, we may observe as to the former change that it is not plausible that a conceptus ceases to exist when it changes from morula to blastocyst. In respect of the latter change, it is not plausible that a human oocyte is the same thing as a fusion product half of whose genome the oocyte lacked,[9] and which product's cytoplasm also differs from the oocyte's. A sperm also ceases after contributing to the zygote's genome and leaving no other trace. The process of gamete development involves a meiotic cell cycle. Only in a product of activation does there begin a mitotic process of organismic development.

Two lines of opposition to embryo use present themselves. In the first, possible persons are said to place moral demands upon us as follows.

> *Duty of Noninterference.* In respect of any being to which corresponds a possible person, there obtains a duty *pro tanto* not to interfere with any current process of development that in circumstances such as the circumstances of such being usually results in a person or in an organism constituting the body of a person.

This duty may be asserted from within any view that pays heed to developmental potential, of which more shortly.

Let a *developmental successor* of x be any entity, whether in a prenatal or postnatal stage, into which x has developed through a process of development. Referring to an entity's developmental successors allows one to avoid begging the question of transtemporal identity. It leaves room for both a Heraclitean view in which every change brings into existence a successor that is a new entity, as well as for the view that a product of oocyte activation is identical to one or more developmental successors.

The second line of opposition to embryo use asserts the following.

> *Zygotic Personhood.* An embryo and any developmental successor thereof is a person for purposes of the duty not to harm and duty not to kill.

According to this deontic precept, an embryo is not merely a correspondent of a person *in posse*. An embryo is a person *in esse*. The name 'zygotic' emphasizes how soon in development personhood is said to begin.

---

[9] I am grateful to E. J. Lowe for insights concerning this.

'Zygotic' in one respect is unduly restrictive, as the term leaves out a clone and parthenote. But Zygotic Personhood is asserted as to a clone and parthenote insofar as each begins as a product of oocyte activation undergoing organismic development, hence as an embryo (as defined in §1.2).

The strategic significance of asserting the Duty of Noninterference arises because of opposition to Zygotic Personhood. For many philosophers who have studied 'person' as an ontological category, the set of embryos and the set of persons are disjoint. Locke held that a person is 'a thinking intelligent being, that has reason and reflection, and can consider itself as itself, the same thinking thing, in different times and places.'[10] When thinking of personhood, philosophers have variously demanded the following mental attributes: self-consciousness (including ability to envision having a past and a future), reason (or, in Boethius's phrase, 'individual substance of rational nature'), autonomy, preferences (including especially a preference to live), and second-order volitions. Arguments in defense of Zygotic Personhood will receive our attention in due course. But insofar as any view constrains the extension of 'person' so as to parry Zygotic Personhood, we must consider the putative Duty of Noninterference if we are to take account of opposition to embryo use in its strongest form.

2.2 THE SET OF ELIGIBLE SUBJECTS

After the Greek *epidosis*, for an Athenian's beneficence to the common weal, I define the following.

> *Epidosembryo.* An epidosembryo is a human embryo as to which the following obtain:
> (a) the embryo was created outside the human body, and
> (b) the progenitors who contributed the gametes or other cells from which to form the embryo have donated the embryo, as of or after its creation, on the condition, set forth in written instructions accepted by the recipient, that (i) the recipient shall use the embryo solely in medical research or therapy, and (ii) never may the embryo or any totipotent cell taken from the embryo be transferred into a woman or into an artificial uterus.

An artificial uterus may be understood as any device capable of nurturing development past what is achievable by cell culture techniques in the dish. I shall say something more about an artificial uterus in §8.4.

---

[10] *Essay*, II, xxvii, 9.

What a recipient of an epidosembryo donation initially receives may be either an extant embryo or cells from which to form an embryo, governed in either case by a binding donative restriction forbidding intrauterine transfer. Let

$$E = \{e \mid e \text{ is an epidosembryo}\}.$$

We observe that $E \subset U$. We may define a partition of E consisting of

$$R = \{e \in E \mid e \text{ is donated as of } e\text{'s creation}\},$$
$$S = \{e \in E \mid e \text{ is not donated as of } e\text{'s creation}\}.$$

Epidosembryos formed by scientists from contributed cells belong to R. Surplus embryos donated as epidosembryos after creation belong to S.

Presumed in the concept of a donation is that the progenitors act of their own volition whilst fully informed. (Here and elsewhere, I sometimes speak in the plural of 'progenitors' and 'donors,' this to avoid distracting us with the question of how those who contribute cells from which an extracorporeal embryo forms should share authority and responsibility concerning the embryo. That is an important question, but not one that I discuss here. When intending to refer separately to a contributor of cells, I sometimes use the expression 'coprogenitor.') An epidosembryo donor does not merely *consent* to someone else's conduct, a donor *directs* what is done with an epidosembryo. Because a decision on so sensitive a matter ought to be revocable, a donation is not deemed effective until revocation is infeasible. Revocation may become infeasible as of such time as the embryo does not lie within direct or indirect progenitor control.

To illustrate donation of a member of S, we may imagine Dr. Smith, a physician specializing in reproductive endocrinology, or what I shall call more simply a 'fertility physician.' Professor Brown, a stem cell biologist, has informed Smith of an interest in receiving embryo donations. As most fertility clinics do, Smith's clinic charges an annual fee for storage of frozen embryos in liquid nitrogen tanks. The clinic periodically queries patients whether they wish to continue storing embryos. Whenever a patient instructs Smith to destroy a surplus embryo, Smith directs a technician to heat the embryo in an autoclave. If a patient expresses an interest in donating embryos to medicine, Smith provides the patient with a copy of Brown's written description of the Brown laboratory's research. If thereafter the patient executes an instrument donating epidosembryos, Smith sends the embryos to Brown, or to any other recipient designated by the patient, transmitting with them a certificate setting forth the patient's instructions, this without disclosing the patient's identity. The recipient executes a written acceptance of the donation on such terms. Upon receipt of a donated embryo, the Brown laboratory seeks to derive from it a line of embryonic stem cells. The laboratory then conducts studies of such cells. By virtue of the usual practices in Smith's clinic, a donated embryo would likely have perished sooner had it not been donated.

On another occasion, a woman enters Smith's care seeking to contribute oocytes to scientists performing nonreprocloning. Smith's assistants interview her so as to ascertain that no financial or other inducements incline her to take on burdens and risks adversely to her well-being. If the clinicians are satisfied with the results of this interview, she then undergoes, as would a fertility patient, a program of ovarian stimulation by means of follicle-stimulating hormone, then an oocyte retrieval procedure. Smith transmits recovered oocytes to the investigator designated by the patient, sending a certificate and obtaining an acceptance as in the first case.

2.3 THE ARGUMENT FROM NONENABLEMENT

I now offer a justification for the choice to donate an epidosembryo, as of or after its formation, and for the recipient's use of the epidosembryo in accordance with the donative instructions.

(a) Developmental potential and discretionary action

Recognizing a possible person corresponding to an embryo recognizes the developmental potential to attain a stage with which a given moral view associates personhood. Ever since Aristotle spoke of a block of wood as a potential statue of Hermes,[11] potential has been thought of as constitutive of or bound up with possibility. *Developmental potential* of a living thing in a situation ψ may be understood as the capacity to undergo in ψ a nomologically possible process of development. It is not anomalous that developmental potential should be a function of situation. We define gravitational potential energy and electrical potential energy as properties of a body relative to a situation (viz., the field created by another body and distance between the bodies). In the biological case, since we are not contemplating a conservative force, we need a different concept of potential. An embryo's situation may be understood as specifiable by the device – such as tissue culture dish, artificial uterus, and natural

---

[11] *Metaphysics* 1048b1–3.

uterine closure – in which the embryo is located. Such devices may differ in structure and ambient conditions maintained. The extent of embryonic developmental potential in a given device may be represented by a probability density function of a continuous random variable defined on a set of outcomes each of which is a latest developmental stage attained in the device. The integral of this probability density function over an interval of its domain will equal the probability that an embryo's development will end at some developmental stage within that interval. A stage s represents an upper bound on the developmental potential of embryos in a given device if, as shown by the density function, the probability is zero that development of an embryo in that device will reach any interval whose opening endpoint lies beyond s. The least element of a set of upper bounds is the least upper bound. Given the probability density function for each member of a set of devices, we may compare the least upper bounds on embryonic developmental potential in the respective devices.

Among situation-conditioning events that can affect developmental potential are discretionary acts. By a discretionary act, I understand an act chosen in an autonomous choice to which the agent is not obliged. Unless there occurs the discretionary action of intrauterine transfer, it is not nomologically possible for an extracorporeal embryo to develop into an infant. The least upper bound on developmental potential of an unenabled embryo nurtured by cell culture techniques in a device such as a dish falls in the neighborhood of day 10 – well short of sentience or even the formation of limbs or organs. The developmental potential of such an embryo lies a discretionary step behind that of an embryo formed by natural conception.

The probability distribution for a natural uterine closure, which may be modeled as a mixture of Weibull and normal distributions, is such that the density function is twin-peaked: a substantial proportion of conceptuses expire within two weeks of fertilization, only a small proportion are lost to miscarriage after the first trimester, and another substantial proportion, in the neighborhood of one-quarter, develop to term. The least upper bound on developmental potential within a mother's body is fetal maturity.

In opposition to views that assign significance to potential, it has been contended that 'everything that can be said about the potential of the embryo can also be said about the potential of the egg and sperm.'[12] The suggestion is that moral recognition of a possible person corresponding to an embryo in virtue of its potential commits one to the absurd result of having to recognize a possible person for every pair of unjoined gametes,

---

[12] E.g., Singer 2002, pp. 185, 201–202, 204.

and, it may be added, for every oocyte and somatic cell – since a significant probability obtains of producing a zygote if gametes are mixed, and of producing a clone or parthenote upon activating an oocyte. In reply, I observe these different potentials: for immature oocytes, potential to mature to the point of being ovulated; for cells undergoing spermatogenesis, potential to mature into sperm; for many cells, potential to perform specialized functions or to issue in cells. In §2.1, we drew a metaphysical distinction – based on what is nomologically possible in the absence of substantial change – between conceptuses, to which possible persons are said to correspond, and body parts. Gametes and somatic cells will not contribute to a process of development by which it is nomologically possible to produce an organism, or to exemplify any property of a person that such parts do not already possess, unless discretionary action such as gamete mixing or artificial oocyte activation effects substantial change in respect of such parts. Hence no possible persons correspond to gametes or somatic cells, and the Duty of Noninterference does not apply to them.

Another admonition concerning talk of potential would remind us that in deciding how we should treat things, we are not obliged to regard the possible as the actual. An acorn is not an oak. Or as Jonathan Glover has remarked, if a customer orders chicken in a restaurant and the waiter brings an omelette of fertilized eggs, the customer has grounds for complaint. The Duty of Noninterference is not a mere injunction to treat the potential as the actual. If one were to take an axe to all positions grounded on potential, as some philosophers would do, one would fell what some discussants, especially some religious believers, regard as deontic barriers against abortion and infanticide. That move would demolish any prospect of drawing those discussants into a consensus on embryo use. I shall continue to take account of potential. I shall do so by recognizing possible persons corresponding to enabled conceptuses, as well as possible persons corresponding to extracorporeal embryos whose progenitors have not permissibly and irrevocably decided against intrauterine transfer.

(b) Permissibility of declining intrauterine transfer

The woman from whose oocyte an extracorporeal embryo originates is the only person in the world, save for the coprogenitor by veto, who is privileged to decide whether the embryo will be transferred into her. Suppose an embryo that has been created, either in fertility care or in research, from one of Alice's oocytes. A discussant poses for consideration that Alice lies under a duty to undergo intrauterine transfer of any embryo created from one of her oocytes. This duty strikes Alice as onerous. She replies by posing the maxim, 'When an embryo has been created from one of my oocytes, I may decide as I wish, in light of my situation, whether to have it transferred into me.'[13] We first ask, as will any moral theory, whether this maxim is universalizable. Without contradiction in conception, or in the will, we can will the generalization of this maxim as a law applicable to all of us. We can will that were any of us the progenitor of an extracorporeal embryo, we would have the discretion to decline an invasive medical procedure, to decline initiating a pregnancy. Universalizability free of contradiction will not, without more, establish that the maxim is binding, but our moral intuitions strongly suggest that it is on target. No leading moral view holds that a woman lies under a duty to undergo a transfer into her of an embryo lying outside her. Even in the vanguard of opposition to abortion, it is not held that there obtains a duty to initiate a pregnancy. Because the Roman Catholic Church disapproves all nonconjugal methods of procreation, it does not even consider intrauterine transfer of an extracorporeal embryo permissible.[14] Whether to undergo an invasive medical procedure, whether to initiate a pregnancy – these are decisions that lie within an autonomous agent's discretion.

But, our discussant asks, supposing that in the exercise of discretion, Alice declines intrauterine transfer of an embryo into herself, might there obtain a duty to allow someone else to adopt the embryo? Suppose that one or more women eager to become mothers offer to bear the embryo. It is urged upon Alice and her coprogenitor Bob that the duty to rescue compels assistance to a person encountered in peril when one can provide assistance without incurring an unreasonable risk or burden. If Alice and Bob were to allow adoption of the embryo, they would incur no financial cost. Someone else would take on the burden of raising a child. Even though Alice and Bob would prefer that the embryo not be borne by another woman, why is it right to indulge that preference?[15] By implementing their preference, they deny the embryo an opportunity to develop into someone who enjoys a long and fulfilling life.

According to one account of causation, if an agent's inaction is an indispensable member of a set of conditions jointly sufficient to effect a harm that rescue could have averted, the agent has caused that harm.[16] A contrary view characterizes an agent who fails to rescue a person in peril of severe harm as allowing rather than causing the harm. The latter view, joined with

[13] I am indebted to Stephen Darwall for discussion of this.
[14] Sacred Congregation for the Doctrine of the Faith, *Donum Vitae*.
[15] I am grateful to an anonymous reviewer for Cambridge University Press for comments related to this question.
[16] As discussed in McIntyre 1994.

another that characterizes declining to rescue as a declination to confer a morally optional benefit, underlies the refusal of most common law jurisdictions to recognize a legal duty to rescue a stranger. Against this refusal, and in support of both a moral and legal duty to rescue, Joel Feinberg has presented a concept of obligatory benefit. The obligatory benefit consists in the prevention of harm. Feinberg points out that in a case of life-threatening peril, 'to escape with one's life is not to become better off than one was before one's life was imperiled.'[17] A bystander who fails to rescue a drowning swimmer fails to restore the victim to the victim's baseline state, to wit, survival. If the rescue would have been easy, then the bystander has not merely omitted to confer a benefit of the morally optional sort, the bystander has wrongfully harmed the victim. A bystander's knowing omission to do what it is reasonable to expect an agent to do may sometimes be cited for moral purposes as a contributing cause in harm's occurrence. When a threatened harm is extreme and the effort needed to avert it minimal, it would be quibbling to contend that the bystander has allowed rather than caused harm. 'The duty to attempt an easy rescue, to call the police or summon an ambulance, seems every bit as stringent . . . as the corresponding duty not to cause the harm directly by one's own action.'[18]

Let us assume the following.

> *Duty to Rescue.* If an agent encounters a person in peril of severe harm, the agent must attempt to avert the harm if and to the extent that the agent can do so without incurring an unreasonable risk or burden.

Even opponents of this duty for the general case usually concede the duty when there obtains a special relationship between the agent and the imperiled, of which the relationship between parent and child is an example. Suppose that by appeal to the Duty to Rescue, the following is proposed.

> *Duty of Intrauterine Transfer.* Any woman and coprogenitor who contribute cells from which an extracorporeal embryo is formed must arrange or allow transfer of the embryo into her or into another woman.

To ascertain whether it is permissible to decline intrauterine transfer of an embryo, I shall consider whether the Duty of Intrauterine Transfer follows from the Duty to Rescue, or from the Duty of Noninterference, Zygotic Personhood, or other source.

We may first observe that the Duty of Intrauterine Transfer draws no support whence one might expect it. In vigilance concerning early human life,

---

[17] Feinberg 1984, pp. 54, 126, 138, 143, 159–163.   [18] *Ibid.*, p. 168.

the Roman Catholic Church stands foremost, but in its view, intrauterine transfer of an extracorporeal embryo is illicit. That verdict does not change for the case of extracorporeal embryos that have already been created. Allied views opposed to abortion approve assisted reproduction while also rejecting the Duty of Intrauterine Transfer, this because assisted reproduction inevitably creates more embryos than patients want transferred into them.

The Duty to Rescue commands that we respond to peril of severe harm. But according to the following argument, an embryo cannot be harmed by death. Harm consists in a wrongful setback to an interest. Interests originate in wants, in desires.[19] Only a conscious being possesses the capacity to want or desire. A nonconscious embryo has no capacity to desire continuing to live, hence no interest therein. An embryo has no interests that could be set back. A second argument asserts that only conscious beings fare better or worse, hence that only to them does the concept of welfare apply.[20] A nonconscious being has no condition that can be worsened so as to be harmed. A third argument asserts that only a self-conscious being is aware of a self.[21] A being that is not self-conscious, whether at maturity (e.g., an oyster), or at an early stage (e.g., the embryonic), cannot be harmed by loss of a future, as it is not aware of itself having a future. For proponents of the foregoing arguments, no duty to avert harm lends support to the Duty of Intrauterine Transfer.

So as to consider the strongest case for the Duty of Intrauterine Transfer, let us heed a view according to which an embryo *can* be harmed. Conceding that nonconscious beings lack wants or desires, and do not conceive of a self, this view challenges the second argument of the preceding paragraph. This view holds that something can be good for a nonsentient being while other things are bad, that a nonconscious being can fare better or worse, that its condition can be improved or worsened, that it has welfare, more or less. What is good for a being may be understood as what it is rational for someone who cares for that being to want for the being for its sake.[22] For a tree, light is good and improves its condition, insect infestation is bad

---

[19] *Ibid.*, pp. 34–45, 52–55, 84; p. 96 ('death to a fetus before it has any actual interests . . . is no harm to it'); Hare 1993, p. 95 (referring to lack of preferences).

[20] Arneson 1999, pp. 104–105.

[21] This view, after Locke, may be found in Tooley 1972, Parfit 1984, p. 202, and Singer 2002, pp. 118, 136–137.

[22] Darwall 2002, adverting to what is good for beings other than moral agents. Darwall holds that welfare is not the same as interests, that some interests of conscious beings may not conduce to, or not even affect, their welfare (pp. 40, 53).

and worsens its condition.[23] It may be said that an embryo's development to maturity is good for it. But it has been objected by Jeff McMahan that if a person is essentially an embodied mind, maturation could not be good for an embryo. If a person is essentially an embodied mind, the developed organism into which an embryo grows is not a person but only the bodily component of a person. McMahan infers from the putative nonidentity between developed organism and person that growth to maturity cannot be said to be good for an embryo.[24] On the contrary, it may be replied, it is rational to want for an embryo, for its sake, that the embryo develop to the stage of being conjoined with a mind, this because a mind will enhance its life. An embryo's development may also be good for a corresponding possible person.

Acknowledging harm to beings of a given kind is one thing, fashioning duties regarding them another. One may recognize the welfare of trees but exclude nonsentients from the set of persons for purposes of the Duty to Rescue. But suppose it is the eve of an embryo's scheduled transfer into a fertility patient. A disgruntled laboratory technician maliciously inserts a damaging chemical into the medium nurturing the embryo. The embryo survives and develops into a child, but by effect of the chemical, the child is mentally impaired. Someone who rationally cares for the embryo could judge not only that the technician harmed a corresponding possible person, and harmed the child eventually born, but that the technician worsened the embryo's condition, that the technician harmed the embryo. If a coworker had at the time observed the technician on the verge of injecting the chemical and the coworker was able to intervene at not unreasonable risk or burden, then, so it may be argued, the coworker was obliged by the Duty to Rescue to attempt a rescue. The extracorporeal embryo was then a person for purposes of the Duty to Rescue. A successful rescue would have consisted in averting contamination of the medium. That feat would have maintained the embryo at its baseline, at life as an embryo in a dish.

The question for Alice and Bob is whether there obtains a duty of transfer from the dish into a woman. In support of the view that the aid obliged by the Duty to Rescue consists of that mandated by the Duty of Intrauterine Transfer, it might be urged that to create an embryo outside the body is to place the embryo in peril *ab initio*, and that a duty to avert serious harm

---

[23] Korsgaard describes something as good for a plant if it enables the plant to function well in maintaining itself (2005, p. 102).

[24] McMahan 2002, pp. 68, 88, 305. A like argument, met with a reply like that which follows in the text, could be given for the theory of a person qua ensouled being or qua embodied psychological substance when ensoulment or the psychological conditions of personhood eventuate after conception.

demands more of an originator than of a bystander. Anyone encountering a person in peril must also take account of that person's condition. The embryo is changing such that soon it will require a uterine environment if its condition is not to fall below its baseline of survival. The action obliged by the Duty to Rescue includes preventing a person from falling below the baseline of survival. When the threatened harm is death, such prevention is not gratuitous. Such prevention is an obligatory benefit such that failure to attempt it effects harm.[25] Obligatory prevention, it may further be urged, sometimes includes effecting a change in environment. If while walking in the woods during a winter storm, we come upon a boy who, having lost his way the previous night, is huddled beneath a tree and shivering, the aid enjoined by the Duty to Rescue includes getting him indoors.

To this I would reply that an embryo in a dish is not a being whose life is suddenly placed in peril because of some change in circumstances, as when Hugh falls into a river and cannot swim. If rescued from the river, Hugh will continue to live as before; Hugh will not by virtue of the rescue become different from what he was. Every living thing lives for only a finite time, and the expected lifetime of an embryo in the dish is short. Transferring the embryo to a uterus would not be a rescue from peril, but an enablement of a developmental transformation. The transformation would advance the embryo's welfare above its locus-dependent baseline. That baseline is only such existence as is nomologically possible in the dish. Enabled development to a more advanced stage, even though by means of phase rather than substantial change, would result in a longer life than what in the natural course would occur at the embryo's baseline. Rescue consists in action needed quickly in response to a peril quickly avoidable. Parenthood extends over decades. A progenitor who declines enablement only declines conferral of a gratuitous benefit. An alternative means is available for averting the threatened harm of death. One could freeze the embryo indefinitely. For these reasons, I conclude that placing an extracorporeal embryo into a woman's body is beyond the scope of aid mandated by the Duty to Rescue.

I now turn from the scope of mandatory aid to the burden that would be imposed by enjoining intrauterine transfer. The Duty of Intrauterine Transfer would command gestation of all embryos created in fertility care. (If instead the duty were applied only to embryos contemplated for use

---

[25] Feinberg's sense of obligatory 'benefit$_1$,' failure to confer which is 'harm$_2$' (1984, pp. 138–139, 143), could support a claim of harm redefined as an effect upon a condition of a nonconscious being rather than upon an interest of a conscious being.

in research, that would yield the perverse result that people may sacrifice embryos in vain but not for good.) Alice must choose between bearing the embryo that she does not wish to bear and becoming its remote mother. Pregnancy and parenthood constitute a great and unusual burden not heretofore imagined as reasonable to expect in a rescue. The burden of pregnancy and raising a child is obvious. Compelled remote parenthood would impose on remote parents the burden of anxiety and remorse in not knowing how their child is being raised, not knowing the child's welfare over time, not wanting to confuse the child by inserting themselves into the child's life, and perhaps not wanting the child to confront them as parents. The child might feel abandoned, desirous of knowing its parents or biological siblings, and confused. Such burdens are often assumed when, after discretionary conduct risking and producing a pregnancy, parents give up a child for adoption. But in authorizing creation of an extracorporeal embryo, Alice and Bob did not take a discretionary step risking pregnancy. The direct burden of imposing the Duty of Intrauterine Transfer on them seems unreasonable in the sense thereof that we would understand in reading the Duty to Rescue.

Now comes the rejoinder that the disvalue of compelled parenthood is less than the disvalue for an embryo of death. But such a quantitative comparison wants for a foundation. On what scales are such values defined, and are they commensurable? If one presses the comparison, one encounters the following. In an account offered by McMahan, the disvalue of an embryo's death 'is proportional to' the 'strength' of 'what there is most reason to care about *for its own sake now*,' its 'time-relative interest' in continuing to live.[26] The embryo's time-relative interest in continuing to live equals the sum of the discounted values of the events of the life that would be lived. That an embryo cannot desire anything does not matter; in any future event that someone else has reason to want for an embryo for its sake, the embryo is taken to have an interest as of the time of the event. An event's discounted value is the product of (a) the value of the event at the time of occurrence and (b) a number $r \in [0, 1]$ representing the 'strength' of the 'prudential unity relations' that would connect the embryo to itself in the future, were the embryo to live. Here 'prudential' signifies 'self-interested.' The relations to which McMahan refers are psychological connectedness and psychological continuity as defined by Parfit.[27] Unlike the capacity to want, these relations may obtain to varying degrees. For an

---

[26] McMahan 2002, pp. 79–80, 98, 105–106, 170–171, 184, 268, 275, 297, 307–308, 317, 321–322.
[27] Parfit 1984, p. 206.

adult, it may be that $r = 1$. An adult who dies is 'strongly related, in the ways that matter, to the person who would have been the subject of the good' if life had continued. The adult's future could have fulfilled interests, made meaningful past goal-directed efforts, accorded just deserts for past actions, and completed the 'narrative unity' of a life. Only by reckoning r for an embryo may we ascertain 'the extent to which it matters, for his sake now or from his present point of view, that he should continue to live.' The embryo 'is unaware of itself, unaware that it has a future; it therefore has no future-directed mental states; no desires or intentions for its future.' An embryo that dies is 'only weakly related, in the ways that matter, to the subject of the good that is lost.' The value of r is very low. By reason of 'the virtual absence of potential psychological connections to the life that is lost,' McMahan says of an embryo that 'it is almost as if the future it loses might just as well have belonged to someone else.'

The quantitative variables imagined in the foregoing account cannot be reckoned in any precise way. So it remains in doubt whether parental burden and the future life of an offspring are commensurable. Among people not daunted by incommensurability, some may confidently say that the parental burden is the lesser in absolute value. Others may contend that the parental burden is the greater. But the following intuition seems inescapable. The loss of a future life cannot be damaging *for* an embryo in the way that cessation of experience is damaging for someone who has had experiences and looks forward to more. Since an embryo has not had experiences, an agent who cares about the embryo has little data from which to conjecture what would be the future of the embryo, hence scant reason by which to want a future that is more than an idealization. We must also bear in mind that although it is rational to want for an embryo's sake that it develop into a mature human that enjoys a long and full life, this condition establishes only the recognition of such development as a good for the embryo, not an obligation to enable such development. It is also rational to be content for an extracorporeal embryo's sake that over the remainder of its life, the embryo will not experience discomfort, frustration, or any sense of a lost future, this by virtue of the progenitors' decision that they will not assume a burden that it would be unreasonable to demand, and that the embryo will not enter an environment in which it could attain sentience or birth, but instead that the embryo will be used for benefit of others, others for whom it is rational to want medical relief for their sakes.

What it is reasonable to expect people to do – that is the standard set forth in the Duty to Rescue's condition concerning burden. When we judge a case of killing in self-defense, we do not countenance a claim that one person's life holds more value than another's. Instead we consider what, in the circumstances, it was reasonable for the threatened person to do. Taking account of the beings affected, including corresponding possible persons, the analysis in which we are presently engaged must answer the question what progenitors may reasonably do. Rational care extends to all the people around us. Loved ones care deeply about spouses, children, and friends who are sick. Embryo progenitors may be keenly aware that we have overpopulated the Earth. They may embrace Parfit's view that we are obliged to make people happy, not to make happy people.[28] It is progenitors who would bear an appreciable loss in the death of an embryo. *Ex hypothesi*, epidosembryo donors will accept such loss. It is rational to want for progenitors for their sakes that remote parenthood not be imposed, and as well that they fulfill their desire to help others by epidosembryo donation. No cogent rationale so far appears for mandating that instead progenitors must effect or allow transfer of every embryo to a womb.

In considering the burden of imposing the Duty of Intrauterine Transfer, it might be thought that a fertility patient could minimize the effect on her if she instructed her physician to create only so many embryos as she would want transferred into her. The Duty of Intrauterine Transfer imposes an incentive to attempt just that, and thereby to risk deleterious consequences. Fertility physicians aim to transfer at one time that number of embryos n that will maximize the chances of one but only one healthy birth. They take account of the probabilities that their attempt to fertilize will fail as to some portion of secondary oocytes recovered, and that some embryos formed will die or be found defective. They therefore recommend recovering and attempting to fertilize, per cycle of ovarian stimulation, some number of oocytes $m > n$. At this writing, it seems generally thought that $n \approx 3$, $m \geq 12$. If transfer of n embryos does not result in a pregnancy, the patient must undergo another cycle. Each cycle involves daily injections of ovarian stimulation drugs, this for a period of weeks, then oocyte retrieval, then later intrauterine transfer. The drug regimen is burdensome and discomforting. The regimen poses a nontrivial risk of ovarian hyperstimulation syndrome whose effects may range from mild illness to life-threatening complications. The fewer the cycles, the better. Assume now the Duty of Intrauterine Transfer. A patient reflects on the number of oocytes for which she will authorize an attempt to fertilize. She encounters a dilemma enclosing another dilemma. (a) She can authorize the

---

[28] Parfit 1976, p. 371.

recommended *m* attempted fertilizations, in which case she runs the risk
that more than *n* embryos will survive, whereupon she must choose between
(i) transfer of more than *n* embryos into her, incurring a greater risk of
multiple births or necessitating multiple pregnancies, and (ii) remote parenthood. (b) She can authorize fewer than *m* attempted fertilizations, in
which case she decreases her chances of pregnancy and increases her probable number of cycles. By imposing this dilemma, imposing the Duty of
Intrauterine Transfer would distort fertility care. It would deny a woman
the reasonable expectation that she may undergo fertility treatment in the
belief that she may decide all matters concerning her care by following
her physician's best advice for the welfare of herself and such number of
offspring as she wishes to bear, and that no one else will bear her offspring.

I now want to draw out another consequence of imposing the Duty
of Intrauterine Transfer. According to clinical standards, many surplus
embryos are not even of sufficient quality for intrauterine transfer.[29] They
possess morphological defects that manifest to the fertility clinician when
examined under the microscope. They may also possess chromosomal
abnormalities or alleles implicated in disease that will manifest in the life
of the offspring and might presently be detectable by genetic testing. Some
embryos will be cleaving but such that the best medical advice is not to
transfer them. If, as the Duty of Intrauterine Transfer commands, the progenitors arrange for transfer of all embryos, they will impose the risks of
untoward consequences. That may put them in violation of moral and legal
duties. A moral duty for which there obtains a compelling case is a duty not
to select and transfer an embryo burdened by a genetic defect making likely
either a life not worth living or a life diminished by a severe deformity.[30]
Should any offspring born to the progenitors or to an adoptive mother
suffer any deformity, there may also lie against the progenitors a cause of
action for wrongful life. It is unreasonable to demand that progenitors violate the aforementioned moral duty, or commit a tort, by arranging for
gestation against their wishes. The proponent of the Duty of Intrauterine
Transfer might propose to carve an exception thereto as to embryos that
are defective, this on the theory that an attempt to rescue is not obligatory
if the effort clearly would be futile, but there may occur many cases as to
which the applicability of 'defective' is debatable. Any leeway granted in
construing 'defective' would undermine the claim that the Duty to Rescue implies the Duty of Intrauterine Transfer, since the former is a perfect

---

[29] I thank Joshua Rothschild for drawing my attention to this.
[30] As asserted in Buchanan *et al.* 2000, pp. 226–256, principles M and N.

duty. When the Duty to Rescue applies, it commands rescue of the very victim encountered. It does not allow leeway to rescue someone else later. Conceding an exception as to less healthy embryos would also undermine any claim that the embryo bears a right to life by virtue of intrinsic worth. Intrinsic worth would not seem diminished by poor health.

Compelled parenthood would constitute an unreasonable burden upon progenitors of embryos created in research just as it would upon progenitors of surplus embryos. It would be yet more unreasonable for the former if the embryos were produced asexually. Clones are so abnormal that intrauterine transfer would impose unwarranted risks for mother and offspring. This obtains *a fortiori* as to parthenotes.[31] Imposing the Duty of Intrauterine Transfer would effectively impose a duty not to create embryos in research, since rational agents wishing to donate cells toward embryo creation and use in research would not choose to do so if they would be compelled to allow intrauterine transfer of any resultant embryos. For this reason, someone might observe that imposing the Duty of Intrauterine Transfer would not impose compelled parenthood on any prospective donor to research. This observation would not lend support to a duty not to create embryos in research unless it were shown that, all other things considered, the Duty of Intrauterine Transfer has been tenably imposed.

Thus not only does it appear that initiating gestation and the ensuing decades-long relationship of parenthood is beyond the aid mandated by the Duty to Rescue, but it may further be held that for three reasons, the Duty of Intrauterine Transfer does not follow from the Duty to Rescue, and that the Duty of Intrauterine Transfer is objectionable. First, the Duty of Intrauterine Transfer requires progenitors of extracorporeal embryos to choose between raising a child themselves and remote parenthood. I agree with Feinberg that the Duty to Rescue does not compel a burden 'of uncertain or controversial reasonableness.'[32] Compelled parenthood is not a transitory and reasonable burden of rescue, but an open-ended burden whose imposition would be more than controversial. Second, imposing the Duty of Intrauterine Transfer would erect incentives to distort an important field of medical care. Such duty, by its threat of compelled remote parenthood, would encourage many fertility patients either to increase the odds of becoming mothers of more children than they wish, or to increase the probable number of cycles. Regardless whether one approves of assisted reproduction, it must be acknowledged that such distortions would be

---

[31] I explain in §7.4 why I take a parthenote to fall within the definition of 'embryo' introduced in §1.2.
[32] Feinberg 1984, p. 157.

detrimental to women and to some of their offspring. Third, the Duty of Intrauterine Transfer would impose on progenitors the jeopardy of bringing about the births of severely impaired offspring as the progenitors act contrarily to medical advice and moral and legal duty. The duty admits of no apparent exception that does not undermine the duty's supposed ground and render its implementation arbitrary. The first and third of the foregoing are reasons that the burden of intrauterine transfer does not meet the standard of reasonableness of the agent's burden on which rests the Duty to Rescue. The second is a reason why the threat of that burden makes imposition of the Duty of Intrauterine Transfer unreasonable. Even for a discussant prepared to overlook the second reason,[33] the first and third reasons suffice to render it implausible that the Duty to Rescue sustains the Duty of Intrauterine Transfer. The third reason strongly suggests that no other ground could warrant imposition of the Duty of Intrauterine Transfer.

Turning to consideration of possible people, might the Duty of Intrauterine Transfer be sustained by the Duty of Noninterference? Even for a discussant sceptical that a nonconscious being can suffer harm, it cannot escape notice that it is nomologically possible that a person or the body of a person will develop from any embryo for which (as we assume at this stage of the argument) enablement has not decisively been precluded. What 'usually results,' in the language of the Duty of Noninterference, may be understood as what most often occurs in the ordinary course absent external intervention by volitional action. The Duty of Noninterference would render abortion wrong *pro tanto*. That duty also accounts in part for the wrongfulness of the conduct of the disgruntled laboratory technician. The patient-physician plan to transfer the embryo into the patient effectively coupled cleavage in the dish and contemplated gestation, compelling recognition of a process that usually results in a person. But in a case in which no such plan has been adopted, we must distinguish cleavage in the dish from gestation. It cannot be claimed that cleavage and gestation are obligatorily coupled, as that would beg the question whether intrauterine transfer is obligatory. Cleavage in the dish is not a process that usually results in a person. It is not plausible that if an embryo is not already a person, it becomes one by any process in the dish. As we shall see in Chapter 3, it is mistaken to think that individuation does not coincide with fertilization.

---

[33] The experiment of making intrauterine transfer into self a legal duty has been conducted, to great consternation, in a small minority of jurisdictions (e.g., Italian Law 40/2004, Article 14[2], allowing creation of no more than three embryos at a time and mandating transfer of all created).

In all events, declining to initiate gestation is not interference with anything. Nonenablement is not interference. The Duty of Noninterference does not sustain the Duty of Intrauterine Transfer.

Perhaps, it might be ventured, the Duty of Noninterference is too weak. Should we bring to bear Hare's duty to preserve conceptuses 'in normal cases'? If a conceptus in the womb is a normal case, a conceptus in the dish is not. Nor is there a duty to actualize the potential of all living things. Such a duty would compel fertilization of every oocyte. Nor should there obtain a duty not to harm a gamete. No possible person corresponds thereto. The Duty of Noninterference is already a strong and nuanced duty in respect of possible persons. The duty provides as strong a protection for conceptuses as would be sought by one who rationally cares for others for their sake. It is pertinent to rational care for extracorporeal embryos that loss of a future cannot be damaging for them in the way that cessation of experience is damaging for beings like us who have had experiences and look forward to more. Rational care also extends to progenitors.

Nor will Zygotic Personhood establish the Duty of Intrauterine Transfer. Nonenablement is neither killing nor an act of harming. Zygotic Personhood will not compel intrauterine transfer unless it implies an obligation to prevent threatened harm, which is to say an obligation to rescue. As to that one would have to ask what is reasonable in view of the burden, and this is what we have just analyzed.

A choice to create an embryo in the dish is not a choice to initiate a process that usually results in a birth. As we take account of burden on those affected, including the embryo, there is insufficient reason to hold that the first choice obliges the second. All things considered, the putative Duty of Intrauterine Transfer does not obtain. There is no duty to initiate gestation, no duty to enable. Intrauterine transfer, into self or other, lies within the discretion of progenitors.

(c) Collective redistribution indefensible

Someone might interject that as we have vested in the state the authority to take custody of abused and neglected children – to place them in foster care and arrange for their adoption – so we should empower the state to provide unwanted embryos the only environment in which they can survive. The state should take protective custody of any embryo as to which intrauterine transfer is declined, and, to the extent possible, arrange for gestation in an adoptive mother. Pending adoption, the state should store the embryo.

If we were thus to empower the state to take custody of unwanted embryos and to arrange for their adoption, this against their progenitors' wishes, we would venture into deep water from which we would best extricate ourselves quickly. Such action by the state would alarmingly intrude into procreative liberty and privacy. Consider Mill's *harm principle*, declaring that 'the only purpose for which power can be rightfully exercised over any member of a civilized community, against his will, is to prevent harm to others.'[34] Assuming that embryos or corresponding possible persons can be harmed, a progenitor who decides against intrauterine embryo transfer does not perpetrate a wrongful harm.[35] It is morally permissible, so I have just argued, for a progenitor to decline intrauterine transfer. State seizure of embryos would not be action preventing a wrongful harm. It would be an illegitimate exercise of state power. That exercise would be illegitimate even when judged by the precept described by Feinberg as *legal moralism*, the precept that it can be morally legitimate for the state to prohibit harmless action constituting immorality.

There are many sorts of state action that we can justify on grounds other than the prevention of harm or immorality. Mill himself endorses taxation for the purpose of financing public goods and redistributing income and wealth. But the reasons for which the Duty of Intrauterine Transfer does not obtain as a moral duty stand also against state seizure and allocation of embryos. State redistribution would impose the burdens that the moral duty would impose, and wreak more havoc. Shall the state effect the adoption of every embryo over which it has jurisdiction? If not, on what grounds and by means of what investigation, morphological or genetic or other, shall the state choose which embryos are adopted? On what grounds shall the state decide which embryos shall go to whom? Will the state answer in damages for wrongful life when asserted by offspring burdened with abnormalities?

Mill plausibly applies the harm principle not only to state action but to 'the moral coercion of public opinion.' The reasons just given against state custody, joined with the need to preserve public order, also tell against allowing citizens or associations to seize embryos of which they are not the progenitors.

(d) No possible person corresponds to an epidosembryo

In their instructions, epidosembryo donors forbid intrauterine transfer and direct that each epidosembryo shall be used in a program of research

---

[34] *On Liberty*, p. 14.
[35] Here I follow the formulation of the harm principle in Feinberg 1984, pp. 26, 105–106.

and nothing else. An attending physician could refuse, on grounds of conscience, to implement such instructions, but we may presume that in such case, the progenitors will ask another physician to carry out their wishes. Whereupon a donee investigator may act in the belief that a progenitor decision against enablement is a *fait accompli*. There being no one privileged to countermand that decision, the decision is irrefragable. Only by impermissible donee conduct could an epidosembryo become enabled. Assuming compliance with the donor instructions, the epidosembryo is unenabled. It is nomologically impossible for the epidosembryo to develop to any significant further extent. The epidosembryo cannot develop so as to approach sentience, self-consciousness, or an expectation of a future. *Ex utero*, an embryo cannot acquire any morally significant property that it does not already have. If the epidosembryo is not already a person, nothing can happen to make it one. Hence no possible person corresponds to an epidosembryo. This obtains in consequence of a permissible exercise of discretion.

(e) Epidosembryo personhood untenable

Suppose now that a proponent of Zygotic Personhood contends that even if intrauterine transfer is discretionary, a progenitor who refuses intrauterine transfer is not privileged to kill the epidosembryo. The proponent contends that the embryo will be harmed by being killed, or in the alternative, that killing the embryo would be a wrong to self in the Kantian sense, a demeaning of oneself in destroying a potentially rational being. Or the proponent might restate Zygotic Personhood as a non-person-affecting principle.

The situation is as follows. Given the epidosembryo donor's permissible decision against intrauterine transfer, the rest of us cannot offer the embryo gestation. That is barred by the donative instructions. We cannot spare it discomfort, frustration of preferences, or failure to achieve ends, since it could not experience any of these. In fact nothing can be accomplished for an epidosembryo – or for any other being in the universe – by declining to use the epidosembryo for benefit of others. It would not avail an epidosembryo, or anyone else, to arrange that it perish as waste in an autoclave rather than in aid of others, or that it be frozen. Freezing would risk damage upon thawing, and thereafter the alternatives would remain the same, viz., benefit to others and perishing in vain (unless the embryo were frozen forever, which would as effectively preclude any life experience as would consumption in experiment). Were we to abjure use of a surplus embryo for others' benefit, we could only assure that the embryo dies in vain. In comparison with the fruitless alternatives of being destroyed in an autoclave or disintegrating in a dish, medical use of the embryo in research or therapy is Pareto superior. Here I am not mistaking Pareto superiority for a principle of right conduct. Rather the Pareto relation furnishes a basis for saying whether, assuming that rational care for embryos and other beings defines for each being a positioning on the set of pertinent alternatives, a gain will result by choosing one alternative over another.[36] It is no worse for a surplus embryo, and it is better for beneficiaries of medical research and therapy, that the embryo be consumed in an endeavor that presents the prospect of helping others, than that the embryo perish as waste. For an epidosembryo created in research, we compare its existence with nonexistence. We are acquainted with such comparisons from tragic cases in which severe genetic defects leave an infant in such misery that it is said that life is not worth living, that not having been born would have been better. Many adults suffering from terminal illnesses also know what it is like to compare existence and nonexistence and to prefer the latter. We more happily observe cases in which a child who suffers from substantial infirmities is unquestionably happy such that life is clearly better than not having been born. Because an epidosembryo, as a nonsentient being, will never experience any discomfort, frustration, or sense of a lost future, its creation and use in research will not be worse for the embryo than the embryo's not having been created. The epidosembryo's creation and use will be better for those who may benefit from its use. Hence for the set of all affected beings inclusive of the epidosembryo, the creation and use of an epidosembryo in research is Pareto superior to not creating it. It is also superior to creating but not using it, this by the reasoning above for a surplus embryo.

Thus one cannot accomplish anything, for anyone, by asserting that an embryo as to which progenitors refuse intrauterine transfer, and that they wish to give to medicine, is a person for purposes of the duty not to harm or duty not to kill. Once progenitors have barred an embryo from the womb, its developmental potential is bounded such that the foregoing situation will not change. The embryo will not acquire any morally significant attribute that it does not already possess. I therefore hold, against

---

[36] x is Pareto superior to y if and only if x is no worse than y for all affected beings and x is better than y for at least one affected being. Economists who define efficiency as absence of a Pareto superior alternative take 'better than' to be a preference relation. But the binary Pareto relation just stated is defined when 'better than' is any positioning, regardless of the criteria by which constructed.

Zygotic Personhood, that an epidosembryo is not a person for purposes of the duty not to harm or duty not to kill.

Some people will instinctively resist this conclusion in the belief that it does not square with respect for human life. They may surmise that the fact that the embryo is human somehow should change the analysis. They may surmise that an epidosembryo's membership in the human species establishes that Zygotic Personhood does hold as to an epidosembryo, or even that such membership installs the Duty of Intrauterine Transfer. I reply that throughout the foregoing discussion, it has been understood that the embryos in question are human. An embryo's membership in the human species does not alter the analysis just given. I elaborate upon this in Chapter 4.

(f) Fulfilling the collective duty of beneficence

I shall use 'epidosembryo use' for the use of an epidosembryo in accordance with donor instructions. I now argue that epidosembryo use is not only virtuous but collectively obligatory. For this purpose I invoke the following duty held in common across the range of leading moral views.

> *Duty of Beneficence.* We have a duty, insofar as we can do so without imposing an unreasonable burden upon ourselves or others, to contribute to the provision of assistance to those in need.

Philosophers have given other formulations of what I have rendered as the command 'to contribute to the provision of assistance to those in need' and the condition of 'unreasonable burden.' In respect of epidosembryos, I shall confine myself in what follows to an argument applicable across the various formulations. Kant argues for beneficence as one of our principal duties to others, of which more anon. Rawls adverts to the comfort of knowing that others will honor a duty to assist us. Hume adduces a rationale of reciprocity. Hare likens his route to this duty, via embracing others' preferences as one's own, to Kant's reasoning from the premise that we must make others' ends our own. (To this it must be said that preferences and ends are not the same, but this point need not concern us here.) Religious traditions know the Duty of Beneficence as the duty of charity. Beneficence may also be asserted, as by Parfit, as a non-person-affecting duty.

Because the Duty of Beneficence obliges us to contribute to the provision of assistance, it applies to needs of people whom we do not directly encounter and that are of such magnitude that each of us alone could alleviate only a small part of the need. As a wide or imperfect duty, its burden is reasonable because of the leeway allowed. The leeway permits self-apportionment to one's means.

Because the Duty of Beneficence was conceived long before anyone imagined a welfare state, it is usually presented as an individual duty. It is sometimes not even mentioned as a collective duty. For example, in Rawls's justice as fairness, beneficence is posterior to and dissociated from the principles of justice for the basic structure. Of the individual duty, it is common to say that because the duty is wide and owed to everyone in general but not owed to anyone in particular, failure to fulfill it will not wrong anyone, will not violate anyone's rights. So at least some would say, although Feinberg argues that failure to attempt to help any of those in need wrongs each of them.[37] I understand the Duty of Beneficence as both an individual and collective duty. If justice is an attribute of society and institutions, so may beneficence be.

We have just seen that we cannot achieve anything, for any actual being, by treating epidosembryos as persons for purposes of the duty not to harm or duty not to kill, and that no possible persons correspond to epidosembryos. The consumption of epidosembryos will not bring about any detriment to actual or possible persons. Because no possible persons correspond to epidosembryos, the Duty of Noninterference is inapplicable to them. Were we to forego epidosembryo use, we would forsake a means by which to aid others who suffer, and yet not one more baby would likely be born. Embryos that might have been used in a work of beneficence would be disposed of as waste or would not be created, and thus would society suffer a significant opportunity cost. We have good reason to believe that if we use epidosembryos in regenerative medicine, we may contribute significantly to the relief of our neighbors who suffer from disease and disability. We may even do so on a large scale. It is virtuous to eliminate suffering when we may do so at no cost in thwarting development of beings to which possible persons correspond, or in lives of beings for which we could achieve anything by ascribing personhood for purposes of the duty not to harm. Epidosembryo use manifests the virtue of benevolence. Hence epidosembryo use is not only permissible, but praiseworthy.

The wide individual Duty of Beneficence does not dictate which embryos should be donated. Latitude allowed by this duty permits agents to choose the occasions and means of contributing to assistance of others. The collective duty does not tell us in general how much of the polity's collective resources we should devote to each pressing need. Given scarcity of resources, we have hard choices to make. But the collective duty does not

---

37 Feinberg 1984, p. 147.

allow much leeway when citizens of the polity lie in dire physical need and (i) a resource has been donated to the common weal, (ii) the resource possesses a high probability of contributing to the relief of those citizens, (iii) the resource may be devoted to such relief at virtually no financial cost, and (iv) the use of the resource will impose no cost in lives of actual persons or in thwarting development of beings to which possible persons correspond. We may establish (i) by the fact of epidosembryo donation, while (ii) follows from our reasonable beliefs about the relevant biology. I have just argued for (iv) in subsections (d) and (e) and the previous paragraph. It happens that (iii) obtains within industrialized democracies devoting vast financial resources to medical research in general. The number of investigators who work in embryo research is relatively small. Embryo research could be supported with funds already in the coffers and committed to medical research. If need be, some funds allocated to other fields could be shifted to embryo research. If some of the expectations for embryo research are fulfilled, the polity will even realize savings in aggregate health care costs. The distributive concern that arises in deciding about this practice is not so much competition for resources as it is waste. Failure to fund embryo research would waste a precious resource given to the common weal. I conclude that under these circumstances, the Duty of Beneficence commands use of that resource in medical research and therapy.

For many individuals, the taxes that they pay greatly exceed what they can afford to give to charity. In their stance on public welfare policies, they express their will on the extent to which the large portion of their income devoted to taxes will assist others in need. It can be wrong not to support policies providing for the poor. Or the sick.

Against this the objection might be posed that it is inconsistent to say that we must contribute to assistance to others who suffer but that a mother has no duty to rescue an embryo by bearing it or allowing its adoption. I reply that no inconsistency obtains. The Duty to Rescue is that special case[38] of the Duty of Beneficence applicable when an agent directly encounters a person in peril and the agent is the only agent, or one of a few, who can prevent the imminent harm. As noted, the Duty to Rescue is a perfect duty such that it is owed to a particular person now and does not allow latitude to rescue someone else later. We saw that while the Duty to Rescue applies to the colleague of the disgruntled laboratory technician, it does not imply the Duty of Intrauterine Transfer. No different conclusion follows from the Duty of Beneficence directly. As a wide or imperfect duty, the Duty of

---

[38] Kant's account makes this architecture conspicuous. The wide duty of beneficence is explicitly developed, but one arrives at a duty to rescue only by 'transition' thereto in a particular situation (*The Metaphysics of Morals* 6:468–469; Wood 1999, p. 328).

Beneficence would not in any event oblige aid to a particular being at a particular time.

Epidosembryo donors act virtuously and deserve praise for their benevolence and generosity. So do recipients of their gifts who work in fulfillment of our collective duty.

2.4 OTHER DEFENSES OF EMBRYO USE DISTINGUISHED

In the remainder of this chapter, I bring the argument from nonenablement into relief by noting differences from other defenses of embryo use, by replying to objections, and by remarking on the scope of what the argument justifies.

We sometimes hear expressed the intuition that use of surplus embryos in research and therapy is justified in part because their progenitors initially intended to bring forth a child. My view is that whether initial procreative intent obtained neither avails nor constrains in reckoning whether a surplus or other embryo may be used as means. In my account, the universe of eligible research subjects E is not confined to embryos formed with procreative intent.

Suppose one Publius who praises the practice of assisted reproduction as an appropriate method for overcoming infertility. Publius describes surplus embryo use as a means of turning to a good end the unintended consequences of worthy intentions to beget children. He goes on to say that not only does initial procreative intent furnish a reason for concluding that surplus embryo use is permissible, but that initial procreative intent is a necessary condition of any permissible embryo creation or use. He condemns the creation of embryos 'for research purposes.'

Let us consider Publius's view. Fertility patients do not usually intend that they will nurture to birth every embryo created. They intend to create multiple candidates for intrauterine transfer. They understand that their clinicians will reject some candidates after a look under the microscope, that the number of ostensibly healthy candidates may exceed the number of babies that they as prospective parents want, that no embryo can mature outside a uterus, that they must pay periodic fees for storage of embryos, and that embryos no longer stored are usually destroyed. Such procreative intent of the progenitors as may plausibly be associated in a one-to-one correspondence with candidates is noncommittal. It is also ephemeral. In respect of those many embryos rejected within a day or two after fertilization, we may better say that procreative intent never attaches. Publius would like to think that a fertility patient's conative stance is an admixture of procreative intent distributed in a diffuse way across the set of candidates. Publius would add that the fertility patient's stance differs markedly from the conative stance of a scientist who, in creating embryos, harbors no thought of procreation. But when we compare the conative stance of a fertility patient who donates surplus embryos with that of a progenitor who donates cells for the purpose of embryo creation in research, we find that they do not differ as to whether embryo destruction is intended or approved. They differ only as to the method of destruction and the proportion of embryos to be destroyed. In approving use of surplus embryos and those alone, Publius either does not insist on initial procreative intent as a condition of permissible embryo creation or use, or insists on it inconsistently.

Why does Publius think that the fact of initial procreative intent would avail in the defense of surplus embryo use? His thinking seems to resemble, though it does not precisely follow, the principle of double effect. This precept asserts that when one or more of an act's unintended but foreseeable effects would otherwise render the act impermissible, the act may be rendered permissible by virtue of its intended effects. A physician may be justified in prescribing medication with the intention of relieving a patient's pain even as the physician foresees but does not intend that the medication will hasten the patient's death. This precept is not embraced within all moral views, and its formulation differs from one exponent to another. Another consideration influencing Publius may be the embryo's purportedly imminent death. When surplus embryo use has recently been defended in the public arena, it has often been asserted that the surplus embryos exist already and would die anyway. Because an unenabled embryo is doomed, its sacrifice in experiment will not meet the 'but for' standard of causation that applies in the law of negligence as to whether an agent is liable for another's death. The experiment might even nurture the embryo in culture for longer than the embryo would otherwise live. Yet our concern is not tort theory. Our concern is the more demanding standard of morality. On a sultry afternoon in yesteryear, a tired McCoy arrives on horseback at a railroad siding. Dismounting, McCoy sits down, then proceeds to fall asleep. As a train approaches at high speed, the switch is open to the siding, and the snoozing McCoy lies between the tracks. Onto the scene rides Hatfield, McCoy's archenemy. Hatfield gallops toward McCoy and, just a moment before the train arrives, yanks McCoy from the tracks. Then Hatfield, eager for the satisfaction of dispatching his enemy by his own hand, pulls out his rifle and kills McCoy. Hatfield, we should say, is guilty of wrongful killing – even though the train would have killed McCoy moments earlier. Imminence of death by one means does not alone justify the killing of a person by another means.

In reply to this, Publius might say that part of what is going on in our condemnation of Hatfield's conduct consists in our disapproval of his villainous motive – we do not approve of a killing motivated by hate or revenge – but that some killings are justified. We condone killing in some circumstances in self-defense, and some of us condone euthanasia from the motives of mercy and trying to do what the patient would wish in the face of imminent death. But embryos pose no threat, nor experience any suffering that mercy might relieve. If Publius has in mind a defense of embryo use predicated on a putatively worthy motive in circumstances of the subject's imminent death, he must travel a long distance from the special cases of self-defense and euthanasia. We need only imagine the effect of allowing that for some end, say, the end of aiding individuals in acute need, or of aiding humanity through research, an agent may kill beings whose death seems imminent. Through the door thereby opened, much mischief could enter. We should have to fear that people would often kill others when the imminence of their victims' deaths was implausibly imagined if not contrived. In ostensibly obvious circumstances of imminent death, death does not always soon occur, or occur at all. An earthquake could derail the train shortly before it reaches McCoy. Taking the long view of matters at hand, everyone's death is always imminent. Such are the vagaries of accepting imminent death as alone a justification for killing.

If imminent death alone is thus not a sufficient condition for permissible embryo use, neither is it a necessary condition. Relative to the time horizon applicable to an embryo in the dish, the death of a frozen epidosembryo is not imminent, yet by virtue of the argument from nonenablement, its use is permissible. I do not say that imminent death in no way bears upon the morality of embryo use. Earlier, in anticipating the claim that we might gain something for an epidosembryo if we refrained from using it, I remarked that forbearance could only assure that the epidosembryo dies in vain. What I maintain is that imminent death is not alone justificatory. The justification for epidosembryo use starts with a discretionary decision against intrauterine transfer. As a result of that decision, it is nomologically impossible for the embryo to develop to a later stage. It is not that death is imminent, it is that developmental potential is bounded.

I return to the claim that initial procreative intent is a necessary condition of permissible embryo creation or use. If it is permissible to create embryos while intending to procreate and thereby overcome infertility, why would it not be permissible to create embryos while intending not to procreate but to overcome some other disease that is life-threatening? In both cases, embryos will be destroyed. It seems untenable to hold that infertile couples enjoy a moral privilege to form and destroy embryos but that people who wish to help others through research do not. Why, we might ask, would Publius believe that initial procreative intent is a necessary condition of permissible embryo creation or use? A likely explanation is the supposition that the singular purpose of human oocytes is reproduction. God made gametes for the purpose of making babies, and for nothing else. Therefore it is wrong to appropriate oocytes for any use other than reproduction. We shall meet this view, which I call 'the teleological objection,' in Chapter 6. I summarize its refutation here. The teleological objection appeals to a teleology that, since Darwin, has lost its grip on our thought. The objection's premise of a single purpose is belied by a continuous stream of discoveries, discoveries that reveal the remarkable adaptability of cells and tissues to perform multiple functions. The objection also involves an implausible assumption about divine will. It seems unlikely that an all-merciful supreme being would endow humans with reason, and endow every human female with vastly more (of the order 10^5) oocytes than she could ever ovulate, and yet would prefer that we not use our reason, and that no use be made of a surfeit of oocytes, in helping our neighbors.

2.5 TWO SUBSETS, ONE JUSTIFICATION

In the argument from nonenablement, as in the definitions of E and its subsets S and R, procreative intent plays no role. According to my account, the morality of embryo use does not depend on whether a donor previously intended pregnancy. Permissibility of epidosembryo use follows from the embryo's presently bounded developmental potential and the end to be served by using the embryo. Boundedness of developmental potential imposed by a permissible prohibition of intrauterine transfer obtains for surplus epidosembryos, clone epidosembryos, and other epidosembryos created in research. The embryo formed from Alice's oocyte, the embryo whose treatment is at stake in the argument from nonenablement, enters the argument as having been created either in fertility care or in research. While probable consequences for fertility patients were given as a reason for rejecting the putative Duty of Intrauterine Transfer, that argument also developed the point that the burden of intrauterine transfer would be unreasonable if that duty were imposed as to embryos formed in research. The argument therefore rejected imposition of the Duty of Intrauterine Transfer as to embryos formed in research. If instead we were to impose the Duty of Intrauterine Transfer only for embryos formed in research, we would effectively permit sacrifice of surplus embryos in vain while forbidding sacrifice of embryos in hopes of accomplishing good. No one who rationally cares for an embryo has reason to want that. Anyone who cares for an embryo belonging to *R* cannot rationally regret that there will be lost a future life that the embryo would experience if the Duty of Intrauterine Transfer compelled the embryo's gestation; if the Duty of Intrauterine Transfer obtained as to members of *R*, no members of *R* would exist. People would not donate cells for creation of embryos in research if intrauterine transfer were obligatory. If a possible person corresponded to an embryo of *R*, for that possible person the alternative that such embryo perishes in experiment while nonsentient would be no worse than the alternative that the embryo never exists.

Once we have rejected the putative Duty of Intrauterine Transfer, once we have recognized the discretion of a progenitor to decline intrauterine transfer, the justification of epidosembryo use follows from the remainder of the argument from nonenablement. By virtue of this argument, epidosembryo use is permissible and virtuous in fulfillment of a progenitor postconception desire to help others, and so too is the use of an epidosembryo created from cells donated by progenitors who intend from the beginning only to help others. The argument from nonenablement thereby innovates within a debate in which it is common to hear a defense for use of members of *S* separately from a defense for use of members of *R*. Some discussants have thought that initial procreative intent renders the use of surplus embryos the only, or the easier, practice to defend. Others have thought that the abnormalities of clones and parthenotes make their use the only, or easier, practice to defend. My account justifies all epidosembryo use by the same argument. Neither the use of members of *S* nor the use of members of *R* rests on higher moral ground than the other. They both rest on the ground of permissible nonenablement that bounds developmental potential.

2.6 REPLIES TO OBJECTIONS RELATING TO POTENTIAL

It might be objected that the argument from nonenablement turns on an embryo's locus and that an embryo's locus is a morally arbitrary attribute. My response is that locus is not always morally arbitrary and that in this case, a permissibly determined locus constitutes the spacetime coordinates of a situation that affects the extent of developmental potential. The objector might reply that developmental potential relative to a situation is a relational property, not an intrinsic property of the embryo, and that an embryo possesses an intrinsic potential to develop into an infant. I answer firstly that to hold that developmental potential is entirely intrinsic and independent of situation would amount to genetic determinism, and secondly that extrinsic properties often cogently ground moral conclusions. 'Married' is a relational extrinsic property. In rationing food during a famine, an adult's greater weight may warrant a greater ration than that allotted a child, yet weight is a function of the earth's gravitational field and locus within it. That we govern our conduct by reference to the extracorporeal locus of an embryo does not entail that we regard that embryo as of any less intrinsic value than an embryo in the womb.[39] We merely recognize occasions on which, in consequence of a permissible decision, an embryo's developmental potential is bounded.

Another objection might begin with an acknowledgment that an unenabled embryo's developmental potential in the dish is bounded by the laws of nature, then continue with the complaint that epidosembryo donors have brought it about that unenabled embryos exist in that situation. The donors have procured fertility treatment incurring the risk that embryos created will be left over, or they have donated cells to scientists for use in creating research subjects. How can progenitors claim a situation of their making as justification for sacrificing an embryo? Again we may take rational care for an embryo to define a positioning on the set of pertinent alternatives. In the dish, an embryo cannot experience discomfort, frustration, or sense of a lost future. Creation of an embryo that will always be nonsentient is no worse for the embryo than not having been created; for others who would benefit from the embryo's use in medical research or therapy, the embryo's creation will be better than its not having been created. Hence for the set of affected beings inclusive of the epidosembryo, the situation of the progenitors' making is a Pareto improvement over the *status quo ante*. The progenitor decision that confines the embryo to the dish is shown by the argument from nonenablement to be a permissible exercise of discretion.[40]

It is sometimes argued that because vastly many embryos die in the fallopian tubes or uterus during the first week, a process that Aristotle

---

[39] I am indebted to Stephen Darwall for this point.
[40] A defense of embryo use vulnerable to the line of objection just posed is the claim that an embryo that never becomes conscious lacks moral status (Harman 2007). Apart from the need to show that no preconscious attributes suffice for moral status, this defense stands in need of an argument that an agent may permissibly arrange that an extracorporeal embryo will never be conscious.

called 'effluxion,'[41] and because we do not mourn them, we ought not regret sacrifice of extracorporeal embryos at or prior to the blastocyst stage. I do not endorse this argument. The argument may be refuted by noting that we have no ability to prevent the deaths of early embryos of which we do not know, whereas progenitors of extracorporeal embryos have the opportunity to choose against death of those embryos. Another argument that I am not making asserts that embryo use, and abortion, are permissible merely because an embryo is a microscopic being that lacks organs, lacks a brain, and cannot feel sensation. That argument plays straight into the hands of an opponent of embryo use invoking developmental potential. What matters in the case of an epidosembryo is not that the embryo presently lacks properties of a developed organism, but that its potential to develop is permissibly bounded.

It has on occasion been suggested that condoning embryo use commits one to condoning experiments on fetuses in the womb, incompetent adults, sleeping or anesthetized people, or others who lack preferences or aspirations. This claim falls as first we observe that humans who have begun or completed gestation either possess in their situation the developmental potential to acquire, or at some point in their lives have acquired, capacities for self-consciousness, forming preferences, and setting ends, and we then affirm that possession of such capacities, or of the developmental potential therefor, constrains how others may treat the possessors. To approve epidosembryo use is only to approve the use of beings that, by virtue of permissibly bounded developmental potential, lack the potential ever to acquire any such capacities.

Someone accustomed to speaking of a right to life might suggest that my account does not consider that right. I have instead spoken of the obligations of agents toward beings that, within other accounts, would be described as bearers of rights. I have done so by virtue of a general aversion to the practice of facilely ascribing rights, a practice that often leaves a given ascribed right locked in unresolved conflict with another, and because I take the view that tenable ascription even of an unopposed right serves as shorthand for specifying the duties of agents other than the right bearer. Regardless of one's view on this, what I have argued may be translated, by anyone who wishes, into a demarcation of the rights borne by the embryos referenced.

Lastly, the use as means of epidosembryos lies athwart the morality of abortion, but the practices are distinct. My account does not purport to

---

[41] *Historia Animalium* 583b12.

resolve a woman's moral obligations in respect of a conceptus inside her. It does affirm her discretion as to a conceptus outside her.

2.7 IN SERVICE OF HUMANITARIAN ENDS

Someone might urge that progenitors may permissibly devote extracorporeal embryos to any ends that they choose. For my part, having described as humanitarian the use of donated embryos in assisting our neighbors in need, I wish to add that this is the only embryo use that I am here considering. 'Humanitarian' of course is vague. If we learned that use of embryonic derivatives for toxicity tests of industrial chemicals would spare conscious nonhuman animals from being used in such tests, someone might respond that restriction of embryo use to humanitarian ends is too restrictive. I have argued here only for epidosembryo use, which by definition is restricted to medical research and therapy. I am concerned not only to understand right conduct, but to foster a public consensus. Symbolism therefore matters greatly. Epidosembryo use constitutes the use of human life solely in aid of human life. Others may wish to explore the rationale for a wider range of uses, but I do not delve into that here. Pursuing ends that are not beneficent would require some ground other than the Duty of Beneficence.

We may hear the concern that epidosembryo use even as I have confined it may undermine respect for embryos to an extent that eventually people will exploit embryos for any purpose whatsoever. Hence we may be urged to refrain altogether from embryo use, this so as to avert a race to the ethical bottom. It is understandable that people would regard with a measure of dread any interventions affecting early human individuals. Even the most far-sighted of us may not anticipate what our descendants come to see as the ill effects of our innovations. Mendel would have been appalled to see what was wrought during the twentieth century in the name of eugenics. Even so, we possess the collective ability, and have frequently shown the resolve, to constrain biotechnology. We have the power through legal institutions to constrain embryo use in particular, as recent political history amply evidences. I shall illustrate in the final chapter how we may fashion constraints pertinent to epidosembryo use.

The argument from nonenablement has not invoked premises peculiar to any particular moral or religious view. The Duty of Beneficence, the autonomous discretion of persons to elect whether they shall undergo medical procedures – these are common to all leading moral and religious views. Yet it remains to be shown how my case for epidosembryo use compels assent within comprehensive moral views often presumed to oppose all embryo use. I shall attempt to show in Chapter 5 why Kantian morality and Catholicism, the former sometimes interpreted, and the latter usually interpreted, as opposed to embryo use, should be understood as members of a consensus supporting epidosembryo use. Before doing so, I shall explore in the next chapter an argument that would buttress, and in the succeeding chapter an argument that would undermine, the reasoning thus far given.

CHAPTER 3

Individuation

There arises an argument whose arrival has been thought by many scientists and others to clinch the case for the humanitarian use of donated embryos. From the point of view of exponents of this new argument, the argument from nonenablement's response to Zygotic Personhood does not go far enough. The argument from nonenablement relies on the contingent circumstance that an epidosembryo donor has forbidden intrauterine transfer into self or other, an exercise of discretion that I have argued to be permissible. It has permissibly come about that nothing can be accomplished by asserting Zygotic Personhood as to an epidosembryo. From this it is concluded that an epidosembryo is not a person for purposes of the duty not to harm or duty not to kill. The newly arriving argument is more fundamental. On the understanding that only a human individual can be a person, the new argument avers that an embryo in the earliest developmental stages is not a human individual. In this chapter, I study this argument, its shortcomings, the prospects for its rehabilitation, and where things stand in its aftermath.

3.1 THE ONTOLOGICAL CHALLENGE

During early embryogenesis, it sometimes happens that an embryo splits into monozygotic twins. It also sometimes happens that monozygotic or fraternal twins fuse. Monozygotic twinning will occur, and twins will fuse, if at all, prior to formation of *the primitive streak*. This is a longitudinal axis of organization that forms in the embryo at about day 14, as gastrulation begins.

I shall call any embryo in which the primitive streak has not formed an *early embryo*. I define a *human individual* as an individual of humankind, a natural kind identical to or corresponding to our species. Human individuals exist at various developmental stages.

The argument with which I am concerned is the following.

Nonindividuation Argument Against Zygotic Personhood ('NA').
(1) A necessary condition for a being to be a person is that the being is a human individual.
(2) An early human embryo is not a human individual.
(3) Therefore an early embryo is not a person.
In support of (2), there have been offered three subarguments that I sketch here and state more fully hereafter.

[a] An individual is not divisible into surviving individuals of the same kind as itself. It can happen that an early human embryo divides into twins. Therefore an early embryo is not a human individual.

[b] If an early human embryo is a human individual, what occurs in monozygotic twinning may be given one of three characterizations: the embryo that splits survives as one twin but not as the other, the embryo survives as both twins, and the embryo dies without leaving a corpse. None of these characterizations is tenable. Hence in virtue of its capability of splitting into twins, an early embryo is not a human individual.

[c] For such time as an early human embryo is constituted of totipotent blastomeres, each blastomere has the potential to become a human individual. Not until there vanishes the opportunity for totipotent blastomeres to separate may it be said how many human individuals exist in the early embryo.

In the foregoing statement of *NA* and in fuller statements below of the arguments for (2), I have combined, for maximal persuasive effect, contentions adduced by various proponents. Seldom does one hear any one proponent advance all these contentions together. From scientists offering *NA*, one will usually hear a lucid explanation of twinning, then the assertion that divisibility is inconsistent with individuality, and there the matter will be left.

I mention in passing two claims that so quickly fail that we would distort *NA* by associating them with it. The first asserts that, because conjoint twins or an engulfed twin can form even *after* the primitive streak forms, a human individual could not exist prior to the time at which ends the possibility of those eventualities. This claim is farfetched inasmuch as, for every implanted embryo, the claim would deny individuality by reason of the chance (which happens to be very small) of a usually fatal event. The claim reduces to denying individuality because of the chance of death. The second is the notion that what we call 'an early embryo' is sometimes, unbeknowst to us, more than one embryo. This notion does not hold water. The embryo possesses a boundary and structure such that under the microscope it is easily distinguished from others of its kind and from its nutritive environment.

Attractive to scientists and nonscientists alike, *NA*'s biological sophistication has fostered the belief that on scientific grounds alone, *NA* deals a decisive blow to Zygotic Personhood and thus clinches the case for embryo use. One hears *NA*'s conclusion reiterated, and some of its implications drawn out, by remarks such as the following:

> Whatever else has varied in our confused moral tradition, it has been consistent in affirming that, without discrete individuality, there can be no moral or legal personality. . . . In the period of cellular cleavage, before the embryo is formed, individuality is not yet.[1]

Day 14 is 'the onset of human individual development.' 'The "embryo" as a continuous entity could be traced back from birth only as far as the primitive streak stage. . . .'[2] It makes no more sense to say that there exists a person if one cannot say how many than to say that there exists an individual if one cannot say how many. A supposed embryonic person that has not reached day 14 is not yet one; it might be two, or none.

Even some Catholic theologians have concluded that personhood or ensoulment does not obtain until the possibility of nonconjoint twinning ceases.[3] After *NA*'s embrace by the Warnock Committee,[4] Parliament enacted the rule that no embryo may be kept or used beyond the earlier of the appearance of the primitive streak and day 14 of development.[5] Bernard Williams endorsed this rule on the ground that although it 'is not . . . uniquely reasonable, it is nevertheless reasonable to draw a line there. . . .'[6]

I have myself invoked *NA*.[7] I no longer believe the argument sound. Despite their scientific patina, premises (1) and (2) are not scientific but metaphysical. I shall not be challenging, but rather assuming, (1). Premise (2), that an early human embryo is not a human individual, is ripe for dispute. I shall review the three arguments offered for (2), and then another argument for (3) that does not invoke (2). I shall argue that each of these

[1] Dunstan 1988, p. 55. This remark presupposes that 'embryo' does not apply until the third week.
[2] McLaren 1986, p. 14. For the case in point, G. E. M. Anscombe answers the question posed by the title of her paper 'Were You a Zygote?', with 'No, I was an identical twin,' though she allows that identical twins 'jointly were once a zygote' (Anscombe 1985). *NA* is also offered in van Inwagen 1990, p. 154.
[3] Ford 1988 and other works cited in Guenin 2006, p. 466, n. 6.
[4] Warnock 1985, pp. 65–66, stating that formation of the primitive streak 'marks the beginning of individual development of the embryo.'
[5] Human Fertilisation and Embryology Act 1990, c. 37, §3(3)(a).
[6] Williams 1986, p. 190.   [7] Guenin 2001a.

arguments fails. To inquire whether other plausible support obtains for (2), I shall then canvass various ontological accounts and explore individuality of living things in search of any requisite of individuality that an embryo lacks. Finding no compelling reason to deny that an early embryo is a human individual, I shall clarify where that leaves matters.

I begin with the metaphysical concepts as to which our inquiry will require clarity.

3.2 IDENTITY

The *identity relation* on a set A is the set $I = \{\langle x, x \rangle \mid x \in A\}$. A thing is identical to itself and to nothing else. This led Wittgenstein to remark that statements of identity are either trivial or false.[8] But the significance of an identity relation inheres in the circumstance that more than one name sometimes pertains to 'only one thing' (to use Kant's phrase for expressing *numerica identitas*).[9] Or, as we sometimes say, more than one name designates 'one and the same' object. ('Identity' is a contraction of *idem et idem*). 'The utility of language,' explains Quine, 'lies partly in its very failure to copy reality in any one-thing-one-name fashion. The notion of identity is then needed to take up the slack.'[10]

When philosophers designate a relation I by the term 'numerical identity,' at first 'numerical' seems peculiar. We do not ordinarily think of any number by reference to which identity obtains – unless, that is, in using 'one and the same,' we prosaically lay stress on 'one.' Therein lies precisely why 'numerical' is apt. Numerical identity bears upon counting. As we count a given universe, if we encounter 'x' and 'y' and discover that the object named by 'x' is identical to the object named by 'y,' we increment by one, not two. When we count expressions in $\{4^3, 8^2, \pi\}$, the total is three; when we count real numbers, the total is two. 'Numerical identity' signifies identity properly so called, and hence I shall mention it simply as 'identity.' We use 'distinct' for 'not identical.' No two objects are identical. What authors have sometimes called 'qualitative identity' consists in exact similarity, as if by virtue of copying. That, Quine remarks, is 'better called resemblance.'[11]

For some sets A, there obtains an *identity criterion*, an explicit membership criterion for I. For example, the axiom of extensionality – two sets are identical if and only they have the same members – constitutes an

---

[8] *Tractatus Logico Philosophicus* 5.5303.
[9] *Critique of Pure Reason* A263/B319. The Latin expression was introduced by Leibniz.
[10] Quine 1959, p. 209.   [11] Quine 1960, p. 53. An instance in biology is homology.

identity criterion for sets. On the other hand, many an identity relation is well-defined although no identity criterion is apparent.

3.3 UNDERSTANDING INDIVIDUATION

Some ontological theories conceive a *particular* as an instance – of a universal, kind, type, property, general term, or in general, of an instantiable. Other theories conceive a particular as something other than an instance – as a trope, existent having attributes that are tropes, existent explained by thisness, impredicable subject of predication, mereological sum, or simply a particular. By all accounts, a necessary condition of being a particular is noninstantiability.[12]

As *NA*'s name makes plain, its target is individuation. But 'individuation' has been used in multiple senses. I review these with a view to identifying which is at stake in *NA*.

(*i*) *Relation of Universals to Particulars.* For those who countenance universals, individuation may be understood as the origination of particulars from universals or as the origination of what appear as particulars. Individuation is 'what it takes for a universal to become' particular.[13] Mechanisms of origination and those positing them include partaking in transcendent Forms (Plato), bundling of universals (Russell), and instantiation as a directly apprehended primitive (Armstrong).

(*ii*) *Achievement of Particularity.* Individuation has also been understood to consist in particularization in the general sense of the satisfaction of necessary and sufficient conditions for being a particular.[14] One proffered condition is 'having a locus in spacetime.' Another is 'thisness.' The

---

[12] An exception to this requirement of noninstantiability is a peculiar classification devolving within Nelson Goodman's mereological constructive nominalism (Goodman 1977, pp. 159, 162, 177–179, 206). Goodman is concerned to treat every existent as an individual. He so defines terms that the predicate 'universal' applies to what he calls an 'individual' (what I call a 'particular') just in case the individual contains no complex that is unrepeatable. (An individual, understood as a mereological sum of one or more atomic qualia, is a complex if and only if every two discrete parts of it are together, as 'together' is rigorously defined. A complex is repeatable if and only if it or some other complex of its category, or kind, has instances.) What he thus calls a 'universal particular' is an individual with instances. By contrast, other nominalists dispose of universals by denying their existence or by reducing them to similarities among paradigm individuals – without saying that any particular (or individual) *is* an instantiable. As we shall later see, this classification by Goodman does not suggest that an early embryo is not a human individual.

[13] Gracia 1988, pp. 18, 84.

[14] Gracia refers to individuation not only as the satisfaction of conditions of individuality but as the process of becoming an individual (1988, pp. 4, 18, 84, 141). (In his lexicon, 'individuality' and 'particularity' are synonymous [p. 53].) But in Gracia's comprehensive taxonomy of views about what individuates (pp. 143–178), as well as in that of Lowe 2003, pp. 75–93, all candidate individuators are attributes or conditions.

conditions depend upon how particularity is understood. Noninstantiability consistently appears among them. It is no part of the brief of an *NA*
proponent to deny that particularization obtains in the case of an extant
embryo. But neither the concept of particular nor accounts of the realiza-
tion of particularity (whether in terms of instances or other) specify in a
given case *how many* particulars of a given kind exist, or their distinctness.
What it is to be *one* of something is a precondition for counting. In theory,
E. J. Lowe points out, there could exist a homogeneous material γ that is
infinitely divisible in the sense that any bit of γ is divisible into two or more
bits of γ (this contrary to physical theory supposing that divisibility ends
at fundamental particles). Without more, particularization of the kind 'bit
of γ' achieved in some lump of γ will not settle how many particulars of
the kind 'bit of γ' that lump comprises. This obtains because, although
distinctness of any two bits may be well-defined, there is no smallest bit
of γ. Lowe uses the expressions 'dividual' and 'quasi-individual' for a bit
of an infinitely divisible homogeneous material such as γ. A dividual, he
imagines, is 'matter without form.'[15] Whether there exist dividuals need
not detain us, but the concept does bring into relief the contrast between
particularization and the next sense of individuation.

    (*iii*)   *Discrete Particularization.* I define discrete particularization as the
condition of, or the effectuation of the condition of, being one particular –
being a discrete *unit* particular – of a given kind. Here particularization is
understood as just above described. 'Discrete' signifies distinctness by virtue
of an identity relation. An identity relation will report when we are using
two names for the same object. A human synchronic identity relation contains ordered pairs of names and definite descriptions (e.g., ⟨Ethelred the
Unready, the penultimate Anglo-Saxon king⟩), of legal names and nick-
names (e.g., ⟨Charles, Charlie⟩), of maiden names and married names,
and so on. A human diachronic identity relation (containing such ordered
pairs as ⟨Napoleon at Elba, Napoleon at Waterloo⟩) is a relation for which
theories of transtemporal personal identity state a generating criterion:
they describe in what transtemporal personal identity consists.[16] In general, according to accounts treating particulars as instances, an identity
relation's domain is a set of instances. According to accounts that do not

[15] Lowe 1998, pp. 72–74, 77, 161, 201; Lowe 2003b.
[16] In the absence of a nontrivial and noncircular generating criterion, one could take the existence of a
diachronic personal identity relation to be unanalyzable and primitive (as in Lowe 1996, pp. 41–42;
Lowe 1989, p. 137; Lowe 1998, pp. 44, 60, 77, 154, 169–173). Wiggins has pointed out that in practice,
the considerations that underlie synchronic and diachronic identity relations for a given kind are
the same (Wiggins 2001, pp. 9n., 71).

render particulars as instances, a particular may still belong to a kind for which an identity relation obtains. A particular may instantiate more than one instantiable, or fall within more than one kind. A robin in flight is both a bird and a flying object.

A distinguishing characteristic of discrete units is that one may count them. We often think that of a given kind of physical object, we have observed units whose discreteness is apparent from separation in Euclidean space (e.g., units of 'orange' in the grocery store). In other cases, it may be more difficult to discern how many units of a given kind exist.

Discrete particularization is the sense of individuation at stake in *NA*. Suppose one Nindy who is a proponent of *NA*. About unclarity on number of units, Nindy takes an early embryo to be a case in point. As Nindy would have it, an early embryo is, in respect of humankind, a blob. The embryo is not infinitely divisible, hence not a dividual. It may be a particular, even a discrete particular, of the kind 'blob,' but not a discrete particular of humankind. As to humankind, it is unindividuated.

Discrete particularization is the sense of individuation that Quine supposes in saying, 'We have an acceptable notion of class, or physical object, or attribute, or any other sort of object, only insofar as we have an acceptable principle of individuation for that sort of object. There is no entity without identity.'[17] For x to be an entity of kind K, there must be a fact of the matter whether x is the same entity of K as y. For as Quine elsewhere observes, 'The statements of identity . . . consist of unlike singular terms that refer to the same thing.'[18] That *singular* terms are the relata of the identity relation reveals that for individuation, Quine demands not only an identity relation but discrete particularization. Without discrete particularization, we do not have an acceptable notion of 'horse' or 'star.'

When individuation is discrete particularization, as I shall take it to be, we say that an *individual* of a kind is a discrete unit particular of the kind. Individuality is unit particularity. Or again, an individual is a member of the set of all and only those existents that are individuated. A human individual is a discrete unit particular of humankind.

Some philosophers take 'individual' and 'particular' to be synonymous, but as I have defined terms, the set of individuals is a proper subset of the

---

[17] Quine 1981, p. 102. Quine refers to an identity criterion as a 'principle of individuation,' noting that attributes lack one (p. 100). See also Quine 1969, p. 23, and Quine 1995, p. 75. For reasons that will become clear in the discussion that follows, I was mistaken on a prior occasion (Guenin 2001a, p. 1660) to think that 'no entity without identity' lends support to *NA*.

[18] Quine 1960, p. 117.

set of particulars.[19] *NA* does not challenge particularization but lays siege to human individuation, this by alleging failure of discrete particularization. I conclude this section by noting three other senses of individuation from which discrete particularization must be distinguished.

(*iv*) *Achievement of Unit Status Sans Distinctness.* Individuation might be rendered as a particular's being or becoming a unit of a given kind for which no identity relation obtains. Lowe has posed an unusual case that evokes this sense of individuation. Lowe supposes that in a superposed state of quantum entanglement, the electrons of a helium atom are countable even though there is no fact of the matter whether each of two singular terms used for the electrons names a distinct thing. He holds that countability and identity are independent so that in this case countability obtains even though distinctness is indeterminate.[20] Does this, contrarily to 'no entity without identity,' imply individuation without distinctness? Whether the truth value of any '*x* is identical to *y*' could be indeterminate is a subject of dispute. In any case, if we are given a list and it is indeterminate whether one or more of the list's entries denote the same thing, we cannot count the entries. If we are able to count the number of electrons in a helium atom as two, it would seem that we have relied on an identity relation. We may have inferred distinctness and number in the same observation (e.g., by ionizing).

Lowe elsewhere says that an individual is 'a countably distinct instance of its kind.' Reading 'countably distinct' to impose the requirement of countability in the mathematical sense would untenably exclude from recognition as individuals the real numbers or anything else the cardinality of whose kind exceeds that of the natural numbers. But if 'countably distinct' is understood as 'discrete,' then this concept of an individual is, within ontologies in which a particular is an instance, extensionally equivalent to the concept of a discrete unit particular of a kind. Supposing individuality thus understood, if attainment of countability were to suffice for individuation but sometimes to obtain without distinctness,[21] then some things individuated would not be individuals. Lowe's account will avert

[19] Nonsynonymous use of these terms may also be found in Lowe 1998, pp. 160–161, and Goodman 1977, pp. 178–179.
[20] Lowe 1998, pp. 33, 61ff., 74–75, 78, 160–161, 200. In mathematics, a set is said to be countable if and only if the set is finite or denumerable. Denumerability obtains if and only if there exists a bijection from the set into the set of natural numbers. By contrast, when metaphysicians speak of countability, often they are not concerned with how large is the relevant set. Rather they are pondering whether it is clear what to count (e.g., dividuals?) or whether the circumstances (e.g., of electrons) will allow counting.
[21] Lowe calls the superposed electrons 'quasi-objects.' He does not say that they are individuals.

this anomaly only if, in distinguishing attainment of countability from individuation, it demands distinctness for individuation. In all events, unit status independently of distinctness would seem to have no prospect of application to life forms above the subatomic scale.

(*v*) *Differentiation.* In another sense, individuation of *x* consists in specifying what about *x* makes *x* different from others of some relevant kind. This sense travels with the view that individuality consists in being different from others.[22] This view seemingly presupposes discrete particularization of *x* – if *x* were not a unit distinct from others, how could *x* be said to differ from others? – but this view understands more by individuation. As Lowe puts it, 'What "individuates" is whatever it is that makes it the single object that it is – what it is that makes it *one* object, distinct from others, and the very object that it is as opposed to any other thing.'[23] On this understanding, individuation effects differences in attributes.

What differentiates? In scholastic philosophy, this was the question of what is the *principium individuationis* when individuation was taken to be differentiation. Metaphysicians have nominated categories of what differentiates – matter and form (two of Aristotle's four causes of change), dimensions, a bundle of features, and spacetime coordinates. Of physical objects, Quine remarks,

They all have their impeccable principle of individuation: physical objects are identical if and only if coextensive. . . . Physical objects are well individuated, whatever else they are not. We know what it takes to distinguish them, even where we cannot detect it.[24]

It has been said that physical objects self-differentiate.[25] Some of the foregoing categories are reducible to spacetime coordinates (assuming a reference frame), but what differentiates need not fall into any one category.[26] It may take all the attributes of a physical object to differentiate it from all others of its kind. That is, it may take the object itself.

[22] 'Apart from contemporary figures,' observes Gracia, 'most modern and many medieval authors either explicitly interpret individuality as difference or fail to distinguish between the two' (1988, pp. 33 and 247). See, e.g., Strawson 1959, ch. 3, §4.

[23] Lowe 2003a.

[24] Quine 1981, p. 101. Here by reference to both individuation and distinguishing of physical objects, Quine effectively says that physical objects meet both the stronger condition of being differentiated and the weaker condition of discrete particularization.

[25] Lowe's term is 'self-individuate,' but in the account in which he uses that term (Lowe 2003a), he takes individuation to be differentiation.

[26] One thread in the history of metaphysics concerns whether or how properties within the foregoing categories effect particularity (or individuality). One reason why various candidates may not is failure to account for noninstantiability.

The indiscernibility of identicals (Leibniz's law) entails that two entities differing in properties are distinct.[27] If we assume the converse, the identity of indiscernibles,[28] we would deduce from its contrapositive, the dissimilarity of the diverse, that distinct relata must differ in some property. Why not therefore understand individuation as differentiation? Endurance through change would refute the diachronic application of Leibniz's law. Views differ on what version of the identity of indiscernibles obtains. In order to be fair to *NA*, we should not assume either principle, but instead assume it possible for things to satisfy discrete particularization without satisfying differentiation. Consider that two top quarks may have the same nonrelational properties. Differentiation is a stronger condition than what *NA* must deny.[29] *NA* succeeds if it disproves discrete particularization. In urging *NA*, Nindy need not suggest a lack of differentiating features.

(*vi*)   *An Epistemic Process.* 'Individuate' has also been used to describe what we do when, as observers of reality and speakers of a language, we distinguish individuals. Quine also writes, 'When we do propound identity conditions for bodies or persons or classes, we are using the prior concept of identity in the special task of clarifying the term "body" or "person" or "class"; for an essential part of the clarification of a term is clarification of the standard by which we individuate its denotata.'[30] This sense will not figure in our discussion. *NA* purports to speak of what is.

In scrutinizing *NA*, I shall in consequence of the foregoing take individuation to be discrete particularization, and individuality to be discrete unit particularity.

3.4 ARGUMENTS AGAINST EARLY EMBRYONIC INDIVIDUALITY

(a) Demanding indivisibility

The general question posed by *NA*'s appeal to twinning is whether discrete particularity may be contingent on what may occur to a particular or by means of a particular in the future. At first blush, it seems straightforward that whether a being now constitutes a discrete unit of a given kind admits

---

[27] $\forall x \forall y (x = y \rightarrow \forall F [Fx \equiv Fy])$, here applying the contrapositive.
[28] $\forall x \forall y (\forall F [Fx \equiv Fy] \rightarrow x = y)$. *F* has been read to range over all properties (in the weak version), over nonrelational properties (in Leibniz's version), and over qualitative properties (in other versions). It is also debated whether any version is necessarily true.
[29] In their leading statement of *NA*, Helga Kuhse and Peter Singer challenge the existence of 'a particular, identifiable individual' and of 'distinct individuals' (1990, pp. 66, 68). As addressed to a Platonic realist, *NA* challenges the discreteness of an apparent individual.
[30] Quine 1972. Quine similarly describes the individuation of propositions (Quine 1970, p. 8).

of an answer regardless of the possibilities of what in the future befalls the being, how the being develops, or what the being does. But to assess in its most favorable light argument [a] for *NA*'s premise (2), I review the association of indivisibility with individuality.

In the ontology of Parmenides, reality was one rather than many. To this Parmenides added the thesis 'What is is indivisible.' After opponents ridiculed him, his student Zeno paid them back in their own coin. Zeno presented the following argument against divisibility of individual objects. Assume that individual objects of finite volume are divisible. We take an object of finite volume and split it in half. We retain one half and put the other half in a bin. According to our assumption, any part of the individual object, being itself an individual object of finite volume, is divisible, and any part of a part of this object is divisible, and so on. The object is infinitely divisible. So we take the retained half and divide it, retaining one of its halves and putting the other in the bin. We keep repeating this process of splitting, retaining, and putting a part into the bin *ad infinitum*. The size of the retained parts gets ever smaller as we go. Each of the parts in the bin must be of nonzero volume, since otherwise they would be nothing. As the process of splitting continues without end, the volume of the parts in the bin will be the sum of infinitely many nonzero volumes. Therefore the original object's volume must be infinite. This contradicts the opening premise that the object's volume is finite. Since the object in question was arbitrarily chosen, the same result follows for any other individual object of finite volume. Hence it is false, as initially assumed, that individual objects of finite volume are divisible.

As Zeno did not know, some infinite series converge. Let v be the volume of the finite object with which we began. The volume of the parts in the bin is

$$v\left(\frac{1}{2} + \frac{1}{4} + \ldots\right) = v\sum_{n=1}^{\infty}\frac{1}{2^n} = v.$$

Divisibility does not lead to any contradiction of the assumed finite volume.[31] Hence Zeno's argument fails. While it could be true that matter is not infinitely divisible – that there exist indivisible elementary particles, and that spacetime is granular – Zeno did not show infinite divisibility impossible.

'Indivisible' and 'individual' both derive from the Latin *dividere*. Some medieval philosophers, using 'divide' in a way that seems inapt to the

[31] I have benefited on this point from Sainsbury 1995, pp. 7–11.

modern ear, held that a distinctive characteristic of a universal is that it is 'divided into' individuals. A realist about universals would nowadays instead say that a universal is multiply instantiated. As medievals would say that an individual is 'indivisible,' we would nowadays say that an individual is noninstantiable. Since none of this casts doubt on a noninstantiable's divisibility in the sense of fissionability, we may leave this aside.

Other medieval philosophers harkened to a notion of individuality as indivisibility into parts. For Duns Scotus, the question was whether a candidate something is 'of its very nature numerically one, incapable of division into several individuals.' Scotus answered that an individual is 'a this, to which any sort of division is abhorrent.'[32] 'An individual is incompossible with being divided into subjective parts.' Suarez also understood individuality as a sort of indivisibility. Aquinas remarked that 'the individual in itself is undivided.'[33]

These scholastic formulations seem untenable unless one understands their use of 'indivisibility' as shorthand for some more nuanced concept. For if, contra Zeno, infinite divisibility is possible, so too must be divisibility once. Most of the garden variety things that we recognize as individuals – desks, rocks, and even, if we are reminded of Procrustes, adult humans – are divisible. They are no less distinct individuals for that susceptibility. After we have split a desk or rock, the object does not seem to have been any less an individual before division by virtue of the fact that it was later divided. Indivisibility *simpliciter* fails as a condition of individuality because at least some individuals are divisible.

To put a sympathetic interpretation on the notion that individuality demands indivisibility, we might read Scotus and Aquinas to say that indivisibility is the quality of being one – of not being two or more distinct beings – for counting purposes. Two things of the same kind stuck together and separable by pulling apart would not satisfy indivisibility as being one thing for counting purposes. But in urging *NA*, Nindy wants to say more than that being two things stuck together is inconsistent with individuality. Nindy wants to insist that divisibility in another sense is inconsistent with individuality. So Nindy advances a more nuanced claim, a claim that becomes the opening premise of the argument to which we now turn.

Argument [a] for *NA* premise (2), the premise that an early embryo is not a human individual, runs as follows.

(4) An individual is not divisible into surviving individuals of the same kind as itself.

---

[32] Quoted in Park 1988, p. 112.   [33] *Summa Theologiae* I, q. 29, art. 4, obj. 4.

(5) A human individual is not divisible into surviving individuals of the same kind as itself.

(6) An early human embryo is divisible into surviving early human embryos.

(7) Therefore an early human embryo is not a human individual.

In respect of (4), Nindy points out that if we split a table, we shall not have two things of the same kind as the original table. We shall have but two remnants of a table. If (4) is true, (5) follows as a special case. In support of (6), Nindy correctly adduces the possibility of monozygotic twinning. A human individual and an early human embryo are said by (5) and (6) to differ in a modal property. That, in conjunction with Leibniz's law, implies (7).

Mitosis is the routine process, in our bodies and in virtually all organisms whose cells have nuclei, in which two somatic cells originate by division of a somatic cell that has replicated its chromosomes. Suppose at time t_0 a cell c undergoing mitosis.[34] As of a later time t_1, c has completed the process of division, c no longer exists as such, and there now exist c's separated daughter cells, d_1 and d_2. As we look back on history from t_0 to t_1, we have no doubt that at all times prior to its division, c was an individual cell. Plainly c had the capability of dividing, and in fact, c did divide, but it is not incoherent to say, and we unhesitatingly do say, that for so long as c existed, c was an individual cell. Similar reasoning applies to amoebae and bacteria. They divide into individuals of the same kind. In fact they reproduce by division. Neither the possibility nor actuality of dividing and separating impugns their individuality. These biological counterexamples show (4) false. Just as it is the case that the possibility or actuality of c's dividing mitotically into daughters surviving as individual cells does not impugn c's cellular individuality, neither the possibility nor actuality of a human individual i's dividing into twins surviving as individual humans impugns i's human's individuality. There is no anomaly in saying that an embryo is a human individual capable of dividing. Or that an embryo that did divide was a human individual before it divided. Hence (5) is unsustained, and argument [a] does not go through.

Suppose that Nindy, in hopes of rescuing argument [a], responds by weakening (4), replacing it with

(4′) A finite individual is not divisible without change in itself into surviving beings of the same kind and quantitative extent as itself.

---

[34] The case of mitosis is posed in Oderberg 1997, p. 268, in reply to argument [a].

This premise does not fall to the counterexamples of dividing cells, amoebae, and bacteria. Each of their daughters possesses less cytoplasm than the progenitor possesses (although because the progenitor expands prior to division to approximately double its previous size, each daughter receives roughly the volume of cytoplasm of the preexpansion progenitor).[35] 'Finite' appears in (4′) to block what would otherwise be the counterexample of infinitely extended beings, including sets of infinite cardinality, which happen to be divisible into individuals of the same kind and infinite extent.[36] (For example, the set ω of natural numbers, an individual, may be partitioned into X, the set of even natural numbers, and Y, the set of odd natural numbers. In set theory there is proven the counterintuitive result that, where 'card' is the cardinality or size of a set, card ω = card X = card Y = $\aleph_0$.) Upon substituting (4′), Nindy modifies (5) and (6) *mutatis mutandis* to

(5′) A human individual is not divisible into surviving beings of the same kind and quantitative extent as itself.

(6′) An early human embryo is divisible into surviving early human embryos of the same quantitative extent as itself.

We now observe that a monozygotic twin possesses only about one-half the mass of the early embryo from which it comes. An early embryo is not divisible into surviving early embryos of the same quantitative extent as itself, i.e., (6′) is false. Substituting (4′)–(6′) has not saved the argument.

Nindy next urges (5) independently of (4), saying that (5) does not need the support of a generalization so broad as to encompass things of all kinds. In order to entail (7), (5) and (6) must state *de re* properties of a human individual and early human embryo, respectively.[37] Such premises must not be merely *de dicto* statements manifesting how we, or at least some of us, use words. Leibniz's law refers to properties of things, not to the truth value of statements that we utter. Word usage could easily mistake intrinsic properties of things. So Nindy asserts that it is not in the nature of a multicellular organism to divide. Someone then points to a plant any of whose shoots, when broken off and planted in the ground, will grow into a

[35] I am indebted to Roberto Kolter for explanation of this.

[36] A counterexample adduced in Gracia 1988, p. 31.

[37] That is, (5) would be '$\forall x(Hx \rightarrow \neg\Diamond Dxs)$,' and (6) would be '$\forall x(Ex \rightarrow \Diamond Dxs)$,' where H is 'human individual,' D is 'divides into,' s is 'surviving individuals of the same kind as itself,' and E is 'early human embryo.' Assertion of a *de re* property occurs because an unbound variable occurs within the scope of the possibility operator '$\Diamond$.' This is to say nothing of general objections that Nindy must meet to arguments advancing nonidentity conclusions using premises about purported modal properties of concrete things. Were Nindy to replace (5) and (6) with premises concerning non-modal *de re* properties (referencing, say, cellular mechanisms), the analysis that follows would still apply.

new plant. Perhaps then, Nindy rejoins, it is not in the nature of animals to divide. Whereupon a discussant mentions worms. If divided, a flatworm of the genus *planaria* will draw on a reservoir of stem cells at both termini to accomplish a regeneration process that results in two surviving flatworms. In all the cases just mentioned, divisibility into survivors of the same kind does not impugn individuality of the divisible. So as we observe an early human embryo to be divisible, Nindy's appeal to the claim that a human individual is not at any stage divisible appears to be *ad hoc*.

(b) Embryo splitting and personal identity

Argument [b], in two versions, poses a puzzle about identity. Each version purportedly shows that if one assumes that every early embryo is a human individual, one will be caught up short by the question of what happens to such an individual when monozygotic twinning occurs.

The first version begins by assuming, contrary to (2), that an early embryo is a human individual, then proceeds as follows. Suppose that an early embryo splits into monozygotic twins. We try to characterize what occurs. Consider

(8) The embryo survives as and is identical to one but not both of the twins.

This is implausible. Monozygotic twinning is symmetrical. The twins exactly resemble each other and are often called 'identical twins.' We have no apparent explanation why an embryo that splits would survive as one of the twins but not as the other. So we consider next

(9) The embryo survives as and is identical to each of the twins.

This is impossible. An identity relation is an equivalence relation, which is to say that it is transitive, symmetric, and reflexive. The twins cannot both be identical to the original embryo unless they are identical to each other. Instead the visibly separate twins are distinct. Thus we are left with

(10) The embryo does not survive.

This seems to say that the embryo has died without leaving earthly remains. Dying without leaving a corpse is a feat of which no human individual is capable. In default of a coherent life history of the putative human individual – assuming none of the alternatives in the foregoing trichotomy plausible – it is concluded that the initial premise that every early embryo is a human individual is false. No mention has been made of early embryos that do not split, but this purported *reductio* has been taken to show that, in respect of any embryo for which the possibility of twinning remains, human individuality has not been established.

In the second version of [b], Kuhse and Singer begin not merely with the assumption that an early embryo is a human individual, but with a stronger assumption, the Identity Thesis.[38] This is the claim that a product of oocyte activation and its developmental successors are identical, that they are one and the same individual. Put the other way round, the Identity Thesis entails that any developed human individual is identical to its developmental predecessors – as far back as the embryo. A *developmental predecessor* of *i* is an entity of which *i* is a developmental successor. According to the Identity Thesis, I am identical to the zygote from which I developed.

Kuhse and Singer argue as follows. Because, according to the same reasoning given in [b]'s first version, neither (8) nor (9) is true, the Identity Thesis must be false as to embryos that split, and since the remaining possibility (10) entails the absurd consequence of death without a corpse, it is false that every early embryo is a human individual. They go on to argue in the same vein that when fraternal twins (twins developed from distinct oocytes) fuse, it cannot be that one twin but not the other is identical to the emergent embryo, since the emergent embryo will contain a genomic contribution from each twin. Nor can the twins both be identical to the emergent embryo, since the twins were distinct, and hence there remains only the absurd result that one or both twins has died without leaving a corpse. So it must not have been the case that the twins were human individuals. This version too says nothing about embryos that neither split nor fuse with others, but Kuhse and Singer suggest that we could best make sense of the failure of the Identity Thesis for monozygotic and fused twins by concluding that no early embryo is a human individual.

Kuhse and Singer portray the Identity Thesis as a linchpin in the debate about embryo use, but they do not ascribe the Identity Thesis to anyone in particular. An opponent of embryo use could disavow the Identity Thesis and assert only Zygotic Personhood. But since the Identity Thesis could avail a proponent of Zygotic Personhood, we ought not regard the Identity Thesis as a straw man. The Identity Thesis enables the claim that if, as most of us think, an adult human individual is a person, then its zygotic predecessor, because it is one and the same individual, is a person. This offers a proponent of Zygotic Personhood a response to the contention that a developing human only gradually becomes a person. Absent the Identity Thesis, the proponent of Zygotic Personhood is committed to an ontology of at least two persons per adult. For if one assumes Zygotic Personhood but denies the Identity Thesis, then the zygote that became

---

[38] Kuhse and Singer 1990, pp. 65–68; see also Singer *et al.* 1990, pp. 107–108, n. 7.

me was a person, but a different person than I, whereas if the Identity Thesis holds, mine is a life story of only one person. Still it is the case that, notwithstanding this affinity between Zygotic Personhood and the Identity Thesis, the first version of [b] attacks the human individuality of an early embryo without regard to the Identity Thesis.

Taking up the first version of [b], one might think of challenging its dismissal of (8). Contrary to popular misconception, monozygotic twins are not identical in genome.[39] The degree of homology is extremely high, but sometimes a monozygote inherits a genetic disposition to a disease while its twin does not. On rare occasions, monozygotes even differ in sex. Genetic dissimilarities between cells in the embryo may contribute to the occurrence of monozygotic twinning. Nor is the process of twinning perfectly symmetrical: it may distribute matter unequally. Hence one might entertain (8). But we must recognize that there occur many cases in which *NA*'s analysis of (8) stands. These are cases in which, even though monozygotes do not exactly resemble each other, they are so similar that one could not muster a plausible case that one and only one twin is transtemporally identical to the original embryo.

Where argument [b] goes wrong is in dismissing (10). Death is not the only process by which a life form may cease to exist as such. In §2.1 we saw in the case of gametes that fusion is another. Fission is yet another. Parfit remarks of fission and death that 'to regard these as the same is to confuse two with zero.'[40] After an embryo splits into twins, there is no corpse. The embryo that split was one human individual before it split, a substantial change occurred in which that individual ceased to exist but did not die, and two human individuals have succeeded the one that ceased. In monozygotic twinning, (10) is the outcome. Thus does the conundrum dissolve. Not every plant begins as a seed; some plants begin as shoots taken from other plants. Not every human individual begins by fertilization or as an activated oocyte. Twins begin at twinning – although we can 'trace' each to an activated oocyte. Anne McLaren is correct to say, of an embryo that eventually splits, that 'the "embryo" that develops from fertilization onwards is a different entity, which includes and gives rise to the "embryo" that grows into a foetus and neonate but is in no way coextensive with it.' She is incorrect to say this of an embryo that does not split. That someone does not lament cessation upon twinning would not tell against their opposing embryo use, which is a moral choice as twinning is not.

---

[39] Machin 1996.   [40] Parfit 1984, p. 262.

The foregoing response to the first version of argument [b] also applies to Kuhse and Singer's version in respect of embryos that have split. We may explain the event that Kuhse and Singer pose in which two fraternal twins fuse as an event in which two human individuals cease without either dying. Each twin's contribution to the successor's genome makes untenable the notion that one but not the other twin is identical to the successor, while the distinctness of the twins precludes their both being identical to the successor. The successor is a new human individual.

In the general case, we can trace an adult to a zygote, whereupon the Identity Thesis could hold. In the special case of an embryo that splits, we have said that the original human individual ceases to exist upon splitting, two new human individuals succeed it, each twin's existence begins at twinning, and each twin's origin can be traced to the embryo. One might try to say that the Identity Thesis holds in this case, that each twin is identical to its predecessors, by recognizing as each twin's first predecessor the dividing embryo. But since the dividing embryo has a zygote as predecessor, that zygote is a predecessor of each twin. It is more plausible to abandon the Identity Thesis in the case of monozygotic twins. A monozygotic twin is not identical to its predecessor zygote whose successor ceased. This may sacrifice the economy of associating only one human individual with a life history, but the biological fact that monozygotic twinning occurs warrants it.

Thus twinning is consistent with human individuality of the dividing early embryo. If the case of an embryo that does split resolves in this way, no impediment arises to human individuality of an early embryo that never splits.

(c) Totipotency of blastomere components

It might seem that Nindy would be tempted to confound opponents by urging the following. Because a single totipotent blastomere is fully capable of developing into an infant, any two-cell embryo is two individuals, any four-cell embryo is four individuals, and so on. But this contention would concede unit particularity, that which Nindy seeks to deny. Worse, it would commit Nindy to a count of more than one individual, a count that, in a routine case in which an embryo never splits and there develops one infant, could not easily be explained by an advocate of [b] who has declared it absurd that a human individual could cease without leaving a corpse.

Instead argument [c] for *NA* premise (2) begins from the observation that, for so long as an embryo consists of totipotent blastomeres, the embryo is spontaneously divisible into surviving embryos. (I say 'spontaneously' to distinguish natural twinning from blastomere separation by external intervention, the latter a method of cloning in animal husbandry.) The argument then proceeds to say that so long as an embryo remains divisible by blastomere separation into surviving individuals, the embryo is not a human individual. The potential to become multiple individuals precludes the present individuality of any. Not until it is no longer possible for a separated cell to survive can one say that individuals exist, or how many. 'An early human embryo,' Kuhse and Singer conclude, 'is not one particular individual, but rather has the potential to become one or more different individuals.'

The first thing to say about this argument is that totipotency ends around day 4. So if the argument were sound, it would only disprove human individuation prior to day 4; it would not raise doubt whether a five-day-old blastocyst, from which embryonic stem cells may be derived, is a human individual. In the second place, as Oderberg writes, 'The potential of each cell in an embryo, early in its development, to become a distinct human individual is not the same as each cell's *being* a distinct human individual while it subserves the embryo of which it is a part.'[41] The potential to become multiple individuals does not preclude the individuality of the extant embryo. It makes sense to say that an embryo is a human individual; the embryo does not fail to be such because each of its blastomeres is an individual blastomere or has the potential to become a human individual. It is no more anomalous to recognize the human individuality of a divisible embryo than to recognize the individuality of a plant each of whose shoots can develop into a plant.

Another decisive consideration against argument [c] is that spontaneous separation of totipotent blastomeres constitutes the mechanism of monozygotic twinning. Argument [c] asserts that an embryo is not an individual so long as it remains divisible into surviving individuals. To say that is merely to repeat argument [a] for the special case of embryos that have not reached the blastocyst stage.

3.5 DIVISIBILITY AND PERSONHOOD

Suppose that Nindy, still determined to find a place for indivisibility in our thought, proposes that indivisibility is intrinsic to personhood even if not intrinsic to individuality.[42] So Nindy argues as follows:

---

[41] Oderberg 1997, p. 280.   [42] I am grateful to George Daley for adumbrating this claim.

(11) A being divisible into surviving beings of the same kind as itself cannot
      be a person or the body of a person.
 (6) An early embryo is divisible into surviving early embryos.
(12) Therefore an early embryo is not a person or the body of a person.

Granting (6), let us scrutinize (11) by reference to what a given view takes
a person to be. Consider first the view that a person is a body. 'A person
is something indivisible,' remarked Thomas Reid. A part of a person 'is a
manifest absurdity.'[43] To support these remarks, Reid says only that 'when
a man loses his estate, his health, his strength,' or 'if he has a leg or an arm
cut off,' in either case 'he is the same person as he was before.' The severed
limb would not 'have a right to a part of his estate.' Surely Reid is correct
that such losses would not alter the man's personhood or personal identity,
or make the limb a person. But that observation does not provide support
for (11).

We have seen from various examples that there exists a nonempty set D
of living things divisible into survivors of the same kind. Suppose that it is
proposed that a duty bears upon us to refrain from wanton destruction of
members of some subset P of D. Each member of P is defined as a person
for purposes of this duty. Whatever we may come to think of the proposed
duty, classification of living things as members of P is not incoherent by
reason of their divisibility. Yet in (11) we have the assertion that a thing that
is divisible into surviving beings of the same kind *cannot* be a person. For a
person qua body, (11) lacks evident support both as a claim of metaphysical
impossibility of personhood in the ontological sense, and as a claim about
what we may rationally decide by way of classifying beings as persons for
normative purposes. We may rationally choose to regard a divisible being
as a person for some purpose.

We consider next those views holding that a person is not identical
to a body. As various accounts would have it, a person is an embodied
mind, Cartesian union of mind and body, or, as envisioned by Hume
and Parfit, a unified succession of psychological or conscious mental states
of a biological substance. Experiences of patients who have undergone a
commissurotomy have been said to demonstrate divisibility of consciousness.[44] This procedure, performed in cases of intractable epilepsy, consists
in severing the *corpus callosum*, the thick bundle of nerves connecting the
hemispheres of the brain. The result is dual consciousness – as if there
were two brains. The left and right sides do not, as it were, know what

---

[43] *Essays on the Intellectual Powers of Man*, Essay III, ch. 4.
[44] See, e.g., Parfit 1984, pp. 245–246, 254–255.

each other is doing. Two independent streams of consciousness flow. That this manifests split consciousness, and perhaps thereby split personhood, is debatable. It has been suggested that a patient might instead possess 'a phenomenally disunified consciousness in certain special situations while retaining a unified consciousness elsewhere.'[45] By anyone who holds that a person is an embodied mind, it may also be maintained that the existence of centers of dual consciousness does not establish the existence of more than one mind.[46] Commissurotomy is not a decisive counterexample against (11). We can imagine another operation that more clearly effects split consciousness. Suppose that Tom, Dick, and Harry are triplets.[47] In an automobile accident, Tom suffers fatal internal injuries although his brain is unharmed, and Dick and Harry each die of brain injuries without suffering any other bodily harm. The physicians attending Tom perform a brain split and transplant operation. The surgeons split Tom's brain, then transfer one half to Dick's body and the other half to Harry's body. Both Dick and Harry survive. (As Peter King has observed, it is possible to survive with half a brain – though in such case one is limited to a career in politics.) After the operation, Dick and Harry experience Tom's memories. They display such psychological continuity with Tom that Dick and Harry each think that they are Tom. The question whether Dick or Harry *is* Tom has been pursued by Parfit to the conclusion that neither is Tom, although Parfit characterizes the question as empty because what matters is not personal identity, but psychological continuity and connectedness.[48] That question also does not matter for our purposes. We need only ask whether there obtains any reason to doubt that Tom was a person before the accident. There seems no reason to doubt that. Tom was a person by any account. Within the sort of view of a person that we are presently considering, Tom before the accident was a carrier of psychological continuity. That carrier was divided into surviving carriers. When a person is not essentially material, when personhood is associated with a psychological or mental existent, or succession of states, we can conceive a person being divisible into persons.

We may also show (11) false by showing that the *body of* a person could be a being divisible into surviving beings of the same kind. By all accounts, a human person has a body. The person has associated with it the body of a human individual. In praise of the diplomat Averell Harriman's preoccupation with professional matters, it was once remarked that his body

[45] Tye 2003, p. 135. See also Nagel 1975.   [46] McMahan 2002, pp. 87–88.
[47] The following is the case of My Division in Parfit 1984, pp. 254–255.
[48] Parfit 1984, pp. 259–260.

was something that he dragged around with him. Consider an occasion on which the body of a human individual *x* divides into surviving beings of the same kind as itself – either an imagined event, or an actual event of monozygotic twinning. We could plausibly offer any of the following accounts of what then transpires: the person having *x* as its body ceases as that person divides into two persons with which the surviving bodies are respectively associated; the person having *x* as its body ceases without dividing and two new persons respectively associated with the surviving bodies come into existence; no person was associated with *x* or is associated with the survivors at present, this because the division occurs at a developmental stage earlier than that at which personhood commences, but two persons will respectively come to be associated with the survivors. Thus the possibility that a person could have a divisible body.

'We find it so difficult to comprehend,' remarks Lowe, 'how a person could split or divide, since only what has parts seems capable of division.'[49] But the purport of this comment, as I understand it, is not inconsistent with the point that I have just made. Lowe supposes, after P. F. Strawson, that a person is an embodied psychological substance whose modes include not only mental states but physical states that supervene upon those of its body. Embodiment is viewed as a *sui generis* relationship different from composition. A person 'has' a body without being identical to or constituted by that body or any body part. 'Persons are not, plausibly, constituted by anything.'[50] A person is a primitive substance, a simple substance that, as Descartes thought, has no parts. Lowe's account arrives at this denial of parts not by demonstration, but as a default conclusion: there appear no plausible candidates for parts of a psychological substance; if there were parts, their identity criterion would ground an identity criterion for persons, and as there does not appear to be an identity criterion for persons, there seem to be no parts. Other accounts viewing persons as embodied psychological substances could countenance divisibility of persons without supposing that persons have predivision parts, but let us suppose that a person qua embodied simple substance is indivisible. On the understanding given in the previous paragraph, the person may have a body that is divisible into surviving beings of the same kind as itself. Divisibility of the body is compatible with indivisibility of the person.

As premise (11) is unestablished, the argument relying upon it fails. When an embryo is capable of dividing, or does divide, its divisibility

---

[49] Lowe 1989, p. 130.   [50] Lowe 1989, p. 129, and Lowe 1996, pp. 35–42.

is consistent both with its being a person and with its being the body of a person.

3.6 INDIVIDUALITY FURTHER CONSIDERED

I have argued that no notion of indivisibility states a necessary condition of individuality or personhood, that nonidentity of an early embryo with successor twins does not impugn the status of the embryo as a human individual, and that totipotency of blastomere components does not impugn that status either. But Nindy may remain unconvinced. 'Perhaps,' says Nindy, 'I have not discerned precisely the right failing, but I suspect that an early embryo fails to satisfy some important condition of being a human individual.' So let us inquire whether, apart from the premises already ventured, there circulates some metaphysical view according to which human individuality demands some attribute that an early embryo lacks. If so, and if that view happens to be an otherwise plausible metaphysical view, *NA* might be saved.

(a) Individuality within alternative ontologies

When recognized as such, individuals are said to populate sets and to admit of characterization by what have variously been described as properties, attributes, and features. For philosophers who recognize property or characterizing universals, nonsortal general terms such as 'red' apply to property instances but do not embed criteria for differentiating instances. On the other hand, a sortal is conceived as having packed within the concept thereof criteria of applicability, persistence, and identity. A realist concerning universals may also say, with Strawson, that a sortal universal supplies those criteria. The identity criterion determines when two expressions for things falling under a sortal designate the same thing. The identity criterion for objects falling under a sortal is sometimes conceived as embedded within the highest sortal in the hierarchy of sortals under which those objects fall. Someone might claim that the embedded identity criterion for the phase sortal 'early human embryo' therefore coincides with the identity criterion for the substance sortal 'human' that subsumes 'early human embryo,' and that by virtue of thereof, every early embryo is a discrete unit particular of humankind. But that claim would beg a question at issue. Nindy contends that the characteristics of an early embryo are such that 'human' does not subsume 'early human embryo.'

The history tells us that in past skirmishes, each of competing answers to the problem of universals, the conflict in which individuality is caught up, has been shown vulnerable on some flank. For each answer, there exist philosophical opponents who hold that it commits to an unparsimonious ontology, conflicts with common sense, implies some regress, or otherwise founders. But in an effort to see whether support for *NA* lies within any plausible metaphysical theory, I interrogate each of the leading ontological accounts in the following vein. Do they demand for individuality or individuation the satisfaction of some condition that an early embryo fails to satisfy? Does individuation come about through some individuator that is inoperative as to an early embryo?

Platonic realism holds that only universals exist. It denies the existence of particulars as such (which is why the view now has relatively few adherents other than proponents of the existence of mathematical objects). Plato is concerned in the main with depicting the transcendent Forms, the existents whose imitation is said to present us with the appearance of particulars. Appearing as a particular (individuation in sense [i] defined in §3.3) obtains in virtue of partaking in the Forms. That partaking, for concrete apparent particulars, must occur at spacetime loci, whereas the Forms exist outside spacetime. As the Platonist labors to flesh out the notion of instantiation by partaking, this view does not suggest any reason why an early embryo would not be a discrete apparent particular of humankind.

Immanent realism supposes that universals exist immanently – in and not apart from their particular instances and exemplifications. Versions differ as to whether there is something to an individual other than instantiated properties. The Russellian bundle theory holds that an individual *consists* of a complete complex of wholly present property universals standing in a relation of coinstantiation (or 'compresence') to each other. To the contrary is the view that a concrete object consists of an ineluctable substratum, or 'bare particular,' together with instances of properties. In D. M. Armstrong's substance-attribute account, a 'thin particular' instantiates nonrelational property universals (or ways things are) that, enfolded with the thin particular, constitute a 'thick particular.'[51] Relations (or ways things stand to each other) are instantiated by *n*-tuples of particulars. There are no kind universals. Kinds are 'true joints in nature,' but are accounted for by properties and relations. Lowe's ontology includes kinds as universals. Objects are understood as instances of kinds. Lowe's ontology also includes something else that Armstrong's does not, namely, instances of property

---

[51] Armstrong 1997.

and relation universals. These 'modes' characterize objects and *n*-tuples of objects. No substrata are supposed; objects simply have modes.[52] Property and relation universals themselves directly characterize kinds and *n*-tuples of kinds. Of the latter characterizations are built dispositional predications and natural laws.

It is implicit and sometimes emphasized in immanent realist accounts that individuals are what I have categorized as discrete particulars. The bundle and bare particular views have even been criticized for training their sights on distinctness and differentiation of individuals at the cost of neglecting to account for particularity.[53] The bundle theory may fail in explicating distinction. Because compresence is nontransitive, a complete complex of compresent universals may 'spread over more than one particular.'[54] The Russellian theory also requires some version of the identity of indiscernibles to avoid the antinomy of two objects having exactly the same properties. But early embryo individuality fares no worse under the bundle theory than does the individuality of everything else. In respect of a bare particular, Locke referred to a substratum's 'support' for properties, but a bare particular's principal effect is distinctness: Socrateity renders Socrates distinct from the rest of us. A bare particular renders an object distinct even from another with which it shares all its properties. A thin particular is a particular envisioned 'with its attributes abstracted away,' this by a mental exercise that Locke called 'partial consideration.' The thin particular is an 'individuator,' a discrete particular.[55] Lowe's account as well demands discrete particularity (described as 'determinate identity conditions' among 'countable entities') for individuality. These realist accounts are only made more clear upon distinguishing discrete particularization from differentiation. As their proponents work to justify belief in universals, explain how a universal can be wholly present in more than one place at a time,[56] or account for abstract objects, these realist accounts present no reason to doubt that early embryos are individuals of humankind.

Versions of nominalism (including conceptualism, class nominalism, resemblance nominalism, predicate nominalism, and Renford Bambrough's interpretation of Wittgenstein, which accounts for the reach of general

---

[52] Lowe 2006, esp. pp. 27–28.

[53] Gracia 1988, pp. 89–90, 93–94, 149–150. Distinctness and differentiation do not suffice for particularity; universals can be distinct and differentiated. Particularity requires noninstantiability.

[54] As argued in Armstrong 1989, pp. 70–72.   [55] Armstrong 1997, pp. 68, 96.

[56] Lowe contends that there need be no place in which universals are said to exist (2006, pp. 89, 99). Armstrong holds that spacetime consists of states of affairs of which universals are constituents (1989, pp. 98–99, 158; 1997).

terms by family resemblance) vary in how they account for that which prompts others to believe in universals. For a nominalist such as Quine, the question 'What makes something a particular?' is trivial. Because every existent is particular, the answer is existence. Since the nominalist wants to deny the existence of anything but particulars, the nominalist is not motivated to demand more for individuality than discrete particularity as demanded by my definition. One view classifiable as nominalist even conceives of particulars by reference to instantiables (i.e., universals) while maintaining that mention of universals does not imply their existence.[57] A particular is a noninstantiable instance of an instantiable. In this vein no reason is given to think that an early embryo is not a discrete instance of humankind.

Nominalist trope theory holds that properties and relations are tropes. Tropes are particulars in the sense of noninstantiables. (Except within a view that countenances universals, tropes are not instances.) D. C. Williams and Keith Campbell hold that an object consists of a bundle of compresent tropes. Against this, C. B. Martin contends that although properties are 'physically located with the object,' properties are not parts of objects, bundled or otherwise. A baseball's cover is a part of it; its sphericity is not a part of it, but a way that it is. Harkening to Locke, Martin offers an account in which objects possess tropes borne by a substratum.[58] Substratum too is not a part of an object. Rather substratum is conceived, via Lockean partial consideration, as 'that about an object that is the bearer of properties.' 'The object qua object is both the bearer of properties and the properties borne.' Without properties, 'objects are empty.' Resemblances of tropes, exact or inexact, determine trope equivalence or resemblance classes. When designated by general terms (e.g., 'sphericity'), these classes play the role in discourse of ersatz universals. Two objects having 'the same' property is not a case of universal instantiation, but of trope resemblance. Ways in which objects are, resemble others, differ from others, and relate – these are all included in Martin's economical ontology without supposing that objects consist of properties, and without supposing universals. Martin's account resembles Armstrong's in substance-attribute structure, but differs from Armstrong's insofar as Martin's has objects possessing tropes rather than instantiating universals. Since by definition, no trope is possessed by

---

[57] Gracia 1988, pp. 109, 136, 235. 'Existence,' says Gracia concerning universals, 'is a category that does not apply to them.' Gracia takes universality to be a mode, a view with antecedents in scholastic ontologies envisioning 'natures' that have 'some sort of being' short of existence (pp. 82–83, 118).

[58] Martin 1980, Martin and Heil 1999.

more than one individual, tropes may be said to differentiate individuals. So too for trope bundles. A transitive compresence relation marks off all and only tropes of one particular,[59] this without appeal to the identity of indiscernibles. It has been argued that such talk of tropes differentiating individuals is circular insofar as individuals differentiate tropes.[60] But for those many tropes that do not closely resemble each other, either direction of explanation seems plausible. Insofar as individuals differentiate tropes, substratum may be the individuator. What constitutes an individual of a kind is a discrete particular of the kind. Equipped with resources to recognize kinds, trope theory provides no reason to doubt that an early embryo is a unit of humankind.

Mereology (after μεροσ for 'part') is the study of parthood relations as they bear upon ontology. In Goodman's mereological constructive nominalism, the world is composed of individuals in a sense other than those earlier enumerated, i.e., a sense of things no two of which break down into the same atoms. An individual is a sum of its parts, and, by virtue of any property possessed by the individual, is a part of the sum of all things possessed of that property.[61] It is further said that 'an individual may be divisible into any number of parts; for individuality does not depend on indivisibility.' Divisibility is requisite for things of two ontological categories: 'an individual is "concrete" if and only if it is exhaustively divisible into concreta'; 'an individual is "particular" if and only if it is exhaustively divisible into unrepeatable complexes.'[62] Though nothing is said here of surviving things of a kind, neither is any support lent to *NA*.

When the nominalist J. H. Woodger undertakes to show that a scientific theory can be stated using only logical operators, primitives, and relations such as 'part of' and 'precedes in time,'[63] he sets forth a theory built on the concept of a cell. As the theory takes shape, it accounts for both fusion and reproduction by division.[64] Whereupon Woodger surmises that if it happens that his exemplified theory applies only to organisms and their parts, he has come close to defining biology. In a yet more detailed account of biological constructs, he supposes time slices.[65] One can step into the same river twice, but not into the same river stage twice.[66] The time slices of

---

[59] Armstrong 1989, p. 114.   [60] Lowe 2003a.

[61] Goodman 1977, ch. 2; Goodman and Quine 1947; Goodman, 'A World of Individuals,' in Goodman 1972, pp. 159–163. An atom is a thing that has no part other than itself. Another thorough account is Eberle 1970. I am indebted to Israel Scheffler for insights concerning this view.

[62] Goodman 1977, pp. 33, 150, 178–179. A concretum is any complex that is together with no individual. In the 'calculus of individuals,' an individual is 'potentially divisible' (Leonard and Goodman 1940, p. 45).

[63] Woodger 1970.   [64] *Ibid.*, pp. 512–514.   [65] Woodger 1937, pp. 58ff.   [66] Quine 1961, p. 65.

an organism or other creature, Woodger takes pains to say, include prenatal time slices. In the case of a dog, 'One state develops from preceding ones, but they are *all* dog-states.'[67] On such a view, an embryo at a given time could be a time slice of a person.

Our tranche of metaphysical theories admits of a convenient summary. Within leading ontological accounts, there does not appear any proposed requisite of individuality or individuation that, in respect of humankind, an early embryo lacks.

(b) Categories and kinds of creatures

In our everyday observations of nonliving objects, we do not find discrete particularization remarkable. Objects belong to multiple kinds, and usually we think of some kind or other of which an object that we encounter clearly seems a unit. We think that we observe discrete tables, pencils, and airplanes. We may even suppose that all particularization is discrete (though a dividual, if such exists, would give pause). The conditions that qualify something as a unit particular vary with the kind of particular. We define a unit of 'furniture' by different sorts of conditions than those by which we define a unit of 'snowstorm.'

We have seen that none of the following is a necessary condition for being a discrete unit particular of humankind: indivisibility into survivors of the same kind, identity with successor twins, and nontotipotency of components. We have not yet stated what constitutes a unit particular of humankind. We might try this enumeration of attributes: a primate with a trunk, a head, two legs, two arms, various specified organs, a 46-chromosome diploid genome with various specified sequences, all of these subject to variation within some range, including conjoint twinning. In the next chapter we shall see that the extent of variation within species is enough to confound attempts to specify such a range even before we consider prefetal stages.

For an embryonic stage, 'unit' needs some foundation. I turn to the philosophy of biology in search of insights about ontological categories and kinds insofar as they may illuminate the individuality of an embryo.

We commonly think of biological species as composed of organisms. It is very nearly the case that all living things that taxonomists classify are organisms. (Viruses are classified by species even though they are not organisms – being acellular, they lack the ability to metabolize or grow – but

---

[67] Woodger 1937, pp. 132–133.

neither, on many accounts, are viruses living.) We find reason to think further upon observing the following. Near the town of Crystal Falls in the Upper Peninsula of Michigan, there exists an enormous underground fungus – at least we may provisionally call it *a* fungus – spanning over 35 acres and thought to be approximately 1500 years old and to weigh about 100 tons. How many particulars of 'fungus' exist there? Investigators have concluded from genetic samplings that the same genome exists throughout the 'humungous fungus' expanse.[68] This has led them to characterize the expanse as one fungus. Sceptics have replied that the mass is disconnected, hence not one fungus, but many. Here we have a case in which, as we attempt to individuate in sense (vi) in respect of this expanse, we easily apprehend particularity. But we are not so sure about discrete particularity. We may also observe a colonial siphonophore such as a Portuguese man-of-war, consisting of zooids, all of the same genome, each of which zooids could be recognized as an organism if separated. Instead each zooid plays some specialized role within the whole that it subserves, a whole nearly indistinguishable from a jellyfish. Corals consist of colonies of polyps each recognizable as an organism. A lichen also seems to be one thing, but it consists of independently recognizable algae and fungi in symbiosis. Dandelions of a given patch spread across a field are distinct organisms, yet they may all possess the same genome.

One suggested way of acknowledging such life forms as these consists in taking a pluralist view of individuality. Before considering that suggestion, it bears telling what ontological categories are in point here. In scientific parlance, a substance is any material all specimens of which possess the same chemical composition and physical properties. In the argot of metaphysics, a substance is a concrete object that subsists without depending for its identity on anything else. Although metaphysicians have fashioned still other notions of substance, the foregoing has been the most enduring concept and seems the most pertinent to the concept of substantial change. An individual *s* is a substance just in case which thing *s* happens to be of *s*'s kind is not determined by which thing any other *x* happens to be of *x*'s kind.[69] A substance may depend on other things for its existence, but does not depend on anything else for its identity. Organisms are substances. Although my body could not exist without its parts, which thing of the kind 'human organism' my body is does not depend on which thing of its kind anything else is. It is metaphysically possible for my body to remain

[68] Smith, Bruhn, and Anderson 1992.
[69] A definition developed in Lowe 1998, ch. 6. See also Hoffman and Rosenkrantz 1997.

the same human organism even as one of its parts is replaced with another part of the same kind. (Interchangeability may not obtain for the parts *in toto*, as consideration of the Ship of Theseus indicates.) My body as of yesterday is the same human organism as my body as of today even though some cells of the former are gone. An object that has parts other than itself, so it is said, is a *composite*. A part of a composite substance is itself a substance if it is metaphysically possible that, following the part's removal, the part continues to exist separately without depending on anything else for its identity. The hour hand of a clock is a substance. But a thorax is not a substance, because which thing a thorax *t* happens to be of the kind 'thorax' will be determined by which thing of some kind of animal possesses *t*.

It is commonly supposed that for every substance, there exists a highest kind in the hierarchy of kinds to which the substance belongs, or a most general or ultimate substance sortal under which the substance falls, either of which embeds a criterion of identity distinguishing one substance of that sort from another. A strain of essentialism runs through the supposition that there are some properties that a substance could, and others that it could not, gain or lose while persisting. This supposition underwrites the notion that it never happens that a substance becomes a substance of a different kind while persisting. That notion must yield when we define substantial change so as to allow for metamorphosis of a persisting substance into a substance of a different kind. Thus we allow for unary substantial change in addition to binary changes such as fission and fusion. But as substance is conceived in most accounts, a persisting substance does not naturally transubstantiate. A statue does not become a woman. Metamorphosis is possible, but we encounter it only in myth and fable.

I shall say that a *constituent* of a composite is one of a sort of things upon whose loss, replacement, or joinder the composite does not persist. When a composite does not persist, some of its constituents may form a successor composite. Inasmuch as 'constituent of' is a nontransitive relation, not every part is a constituent.[70] A *colligation* is a concrete composite object composed of multiple closely resembling constituent substances tied together in some nontrivial spatiotemporal, causal agency, or sociolegal relationship. A pile of stones is a colligation of which each stone is a constituent. If I remove a stone, a different pile will come to be. If a school of porpoises loses or gains a porpoise, a successor school has come into existence. Schools, flocks, and herds of animals are scattered colligations. If the constituents of a colligation are not scatterable, the colligation is an *assemblage*.

---

[70] For thoughts on this, I am indebted to Lowe 1989, pp. 89–90, Lowe 1998, p. 119, and discussion with Lowe.

The extension of the category *organisms* may be roughly delineated as the set of living substances capable of living on their own rather than as parts of other living things. The following has been offered as an enumeration of properties that are sufficient if not necessary for being an organism.[71] An organism is a composite substance composed primarily of water and carbon-based macromolecules. It includes molecules and developmental systems capable of replicating. The organism synthesizes macromolecular parts of itself. It replaces macromolecules by using energy from external sources. Its exterior surface is a membrane through which the organism absorbs and excretes. Substances of its kind reproduce by means of replicable macromolecules. The organism's processes of synthesis, metabolism, absorption, excretion, growth, and reproduction are causally interrelated. A 'master part,' centralized or decentralized, regulates or controls the organism's life processes. An organism is not a proper part of anything else that satisfies the foregoing conditions, which is to say that an organism is not a proper part of any other organism (although an organism may occupy a niche within another organism, as does an embryo as a tenant in the amniotic cavity).[72] An organism maintains a form or organization of its parts as it persists through changes in the matter composing it. Operating as a behavioral whole, an organism exerts some control over its interaction with its environment. An organism's processes contribute to their own preservation. An organism is a homeostatic mechanism.[73] Unlike a nonliving machine whose parts must exist before the machine is assembled, a developing organism grows parts while maintaining itself.

We recognize a cell, we find the concept thereof relatively easy to define, we recognize organs and other body parts, and we recognize an organism and can give some account of what constitutes one. The humungous fungus and other unusual creatures do not seem to fit within our familiar ontological categories of living objects on an ascending scale of organization. If the humungous fungus is an organism, then its proper parts cannot be organisms. That seems puzzling: those parts would be organisms if detached. Conversely, if the proper parts are organisms, the humungous fungus cannot be an organism. That would not jibe with observations of the fungus seemingly functioning as if an organism. The same dilemma arises for coral and other colonials. Something in our conceptual scheme has to give. One option is to drop the condition that an organism cannot be a proper part of another organism. Were we to do that, and were we then to attempt

[71] As given in Hoffman and Rosenkrantz 1997, pp. 93, 105–112, 130, and Rosenkrantz 2001.
[72] Such a niche is described in Smith and Brogaard 2003, pp. 69–75.
[73] So described in Lowe 1989, pp. 101–102, and Lowe 1998, p. 187.

classifying the humungous fungus as an organism, evidently we should also have to give up the condition that an organism has a master part.[74] A more plausible move might be to abandon the supposition that every creature is an organism.

Whereupon, so it has been suggested, we might countenance multiple 'kinds of biological individuality.'[75] I demur to the notion that individuality is multivalent. 'Individuality' may be given multiple senses correlatively with senses (ii)–(v) of 'individuation,' but we need not multiply senses of that term in virtue of the diversity of living things. We do have reason to recognize some new biological kinds and categories to which individuals belong, and to refine our understanding of the conditions for qualification as such. I shall use the term 'creature' to denote an individual belonging to a species, this to avoid the implication that all such individuals are organisms. In the first move, we may subpartition our ontology more finely by recognizing the following new categories of living composite things. A *genet* is a living thing whose one or more cells possess a single genome distinct from the genomes of other things of its kind. A genet may be a scattered colligation, assemblage, or substance. A genet may have organisms as parts. A *ramet* is a constituent of a colligation of clones. A *symbiont* is a symbiotic colligation of more than one kind of closely resembling organism. We may locate the foregoing categories within an ontological hierarchy of particulars as follows. Suppose the category *concrete objects*. We take that category to be divided into *substances* and *nonsubstantial concrete objects*. A subcategory of the former is *living substances*, and a subcategory of the latter is *living nonsubstantial concrete objects*. Under *living substances* we now recognize not only *organisms* but *substantial genets*. As a substantial genet, a colonial creature is more integrated than is a highly organized assemblage. A colonial creature's integration is such that, like an organism, the creature will remain the same entity as parts are replaced. In ontological hierarchies, categories need not be mutually exclusive. So the extensions of *organisms* and *substantial genets* intersect but are not coincident. Some organisms (mosaics and chimeras) are not substantial genets; some substantial genets (colonial creatures) are not organisms. Under *living nonsubstantial concrete objects*, we introduce the categories *ramets, nonsubstantial genets, symbionts*, and *body parts*. Nonsubstantial genets and symbionts are colligations. Each's identity changes if constituents are replaced. We would likewise revise a realist hierarchy of universals by adding, for each of the foregoing new

---

[74] Hoffman and Rosenkrantz 1997, p. 147, and Rosenkrantz 2001, p. 131.
[75] Wilson, J. 1999, p. 59.

categories, a category under *substantial natural kinds* or *nonsubstantial natural kinds*.

Secondly, if a kind is a type of thing, a natural kind is a type of naturally-occurring thing. Natural kinds have been construed by some as universals and by others as sets, of which more in the next chapter. Under each of the foregoing ontological categories there fall natural kinds, including biological kinds. Insofar as kinds are denoted by sortals (e.g., 'human,' 'fungus'), the criteria for constituting an individual of a kind may include sortal applicability and persistence conditions, conditions that sortals are understood to have packed within them. It is not supposed that we can capture such conditions in formulae, nor that the conditions are immune from vagueness, but reflection on unusual creatures suggests some applicable types of conditions. A *develope* is a successor in development of an activated oocyte (or of a propagule in the case of a plant). A mosaic (a product of a single activated oocyte not all of whose cells have the same genotype) is a develope that is not a genet. A *connected entity* is an entity spatiotemporally connected save only for microscopic spatial gaps. Sortal applicability and persistence conditions will vary from one kind to another. Another classification, though perhaps neither a fundamental ontological category nor a sortal condition, is that of *interactor*, a unit of a kind that is directly selected in natural selection.

The humungous fungus, so we may now say, is an individual substantial genet of the kind 'fungus.' The individual is composed of multiple organisms and ramets. A parallel classification obtains for individuals of the kinds 'fern' and 'bamboo.' A colonial siphonophore is a substantial genet within which a zooid is the largest develope. Many asexually-reproducing plants issue in ramets that are separate organisms but together form one nonsubstantial genet. A sexually-produced dandelion and its scattered asexually-produced clones together constitute a nonsubstantial genet and, so it has been argued, an interactor. Each dandelion is an organism, ramet, and connected unit. A lichen is a symbiont.

Such variation in ontological categories into which creatures fall is not common within the set of metazoans (higher animals). A metazoan will typically constitute an organism and a substantial genet. A metazoan will be an individual of a kind that falls under the category *organisms* and an individual of another kind under the category *substantial genets*. The body of Socrates is an individual of a kind named 'human' under the former category and an individual of another kind also named 'human' under the latter category. A metazoan will also be a develope, connected entity, and interactor.

(c) The embryo as organism

What holds for human prenatal stages? We have the question whether an embryo is an organism. By consensus, there exist one-cell organisms (e.g., amoebae). In Jack Wilson's account, the human zygote is a one-cell 'functional individual,' a locution used indistinguishably from 'organism.' After oocyte activation, 'the zygote divides' into two cells, they into four, and so on. Each of the blastomeres is, like the zygote, causally integrated. Hence each blastomere qualifies as a functional unit. (Apparently Wilson assumes totipotency, in default of which there would be no capacity to reproduce. Totipotency ceases before the blastocyst stage, but this I leave aside.) Until the blastocyst stage, the cells are merely 'stuck together' such that 'removing a cell does not have a significant effect on other cells' insofar as survival is concerned. So Wilson concludes that what we call the *cleaving ovum*, the embryo during the interval from the two-cell stage to gastrulation, is a mere agglomeration of cells. Hence the cleaving ovum is not a functional individual. Wilson envisions that sometime during or after gastrulation, the hundreds of cells composing the aggregate combine into a single functional individual. He goes on to say that a human individual *is* a functional individual.[76] Together, the foregoing characterizations imply that a cleaving ovum is not a human individual. According to this picture, a life history begins with a single human individual, that entity is succeeded by multiple human individuals, and they are succeeded by a single human individual.

According to an alternative view of things, the zygote would otherwise qualify as an organism, but since it is 'predestined to undergo fission,' the zygote is not an organism. The transition from zygote to two-cell stage is taken to be a substantial change by fission. The blastocyst, for putative lack of heterogeneity and for lack of a mechanism for restoring stability in case of external disturbance, is not an organism either. An organism first appears in a substantial change, an 'almost instantaneous' process, during gastrulation.[77]

We recall from §2.1 that in a substantial change, either a substance ceases to exist or comes into existence, or a substance metamorphosizes into a substance of a different kind. I shall refer to the above mentioned changes from zygote to cleaving ovum, and from cleaving ovum to postgastrulation

---

[76] Wilson, J. 1999, pp. 62–63, 90, 96, 106, 111.

[77] Smith and Brogaard 2003, pp. 60–62, 75. Another account in which a zygote is said to divide is given in van Inwagen 1990, pp. 152–153.

organism, as 'the transitions.' The two pictures just painted suggest for consideration three alternative ways to construe the transitions.

(SC1) Each of the transitions is a substantial change in which the number of extant substances within the category *organisms* changes.

(SC2) Each of the transitions is a substantial change in which an individual of the human kind of organism within the category *living substances* is succeeded by, or succeeds, some individual of a kind of nonorganism within that category.

(PC) Each of the transitions is a phase change in an individual of the kind of substance to which the embryo belongs.

Fission of a substance effects the substance's cessation and originates successors and is therefore a substantial change. So is fusion or unification of two or more substances. But to say 'the zygote divides' is a loose way of speaking. Rather it is the case that inside a zygote's zona pellucida, its shell, the single cell (bounded by its own membrane separate from the shell) divides into two daughters, this occurring at the end of fertilization. The daughters too lie within the shell. When $n \geq 2$ and cells inside the shell of an n-cell embryo divide, we do not say that the embryo divides or fragments. The reasoning is the same for $n = 1$. Assuming that the zygote is an organism, there persists one and only one organism as the cells successively divide inside the shell. There is no multiplicity of organisms that later combine. When the blastocyst hatches from the shell at around day 5, the blastocyst keeps its shape within a well-defined boundary. Upon implanting around day 7, if it does, the blastocyst will be integrated enough to burrow into the uterine wall. The embryo is one substance from fertilization through gastrulation and beyond. (SC1) is false.

If (SC2) were to hold, then early embryogenesis would be a scenario of now an organism, now a nonorganism, now an organism again. Substantial change would occur if the one-cell human organism x were to cease and be replaced by a cleaving ovum y, or if y were to cease and be replaced by a later-stage organism z, while $x \neq y$ or $y \neq z$. But it does not seem plausible that either the one-cell x or cleaving ovum y would cease to exist. We have just seen that x will not cease in consequence of zygote fission, which does not occur. Nor is a postblastocyst transition from cleaving ovum y to later stage z plausibly cast as the cessation of y – any more than is the morphologically much more extensive transition from tadpole to frog plausibly cast as the cessation of the tadpole. Rather it would seem that y changes and persists. (The view might be adduced that a living thing can exist intermittently, as when a thing is first alive, then frozen and nonliving, then thawed and revived.[78] If it were also assumed that a living thing is essentially living, intermittent existence might be ventured so as to entail that $x \neq y$ and $y \neq z$ but $x = z$. But a cleaving ovum does not undergo anything like freezing. Its life is not interrupted. It has even been argued that existence is not interrupted by disassembly of an object if thereafter the object's recognizable parts have a continuous history – as when a clock is disassembled and later reassembled.[79]) The transitions do not effect any cessation or creation of a substance. Nor do we have any reason to think that the transitions are metamorphoses. The transitions are not transubstantiations defying the laws of nature; they occur in accordance with the laws of nature. The transitions are changes that things of humankind – here taking account of all kinds 'human' under different ontological categories – survive in accordance with the laws of nature. Thus we arrive at (PC). The transitions are phase changes. 'Cleaving ovum' is a phase sortal restricting the substance sortal 'human organism.' Every change during human embryogenesis is a phase change.

Scenarios in which substances appear and vanish, or change back and forth between ontological categories, show to the advantage of the simpler hypothesis that an embryo originates as an organism and remains such. The etymology of 'develop' suggests a kind of unfolding, an unfurling. It suggests phase changes, not changes in kind of substance or ontological category. I assumed this simpler hypothesis in §2.1 when applying the criterion for recognizing possible persons. If a substantial change were held to occur after oocyte activation, then no possible person would correspond to any entity preceding that change. The simpler hypothesis also draws empirical support, as I now mention in drawing attention to integration. Integration distinguishes a composite substance from an assemblage. J. S. Huxley suggested as a test for integration whether an entity loses functionality upon being cut in half. An early embryo passes that test. If a fertility clinician accidentally cuts across an embryo, the embryo will die. When clinicians remove blastomeres for testing, many embryos survive, but some perish, and we may not know the full effect on those that survive. That a worm survives being cut in half does not entail that the event had no effect.

Our concept of integration admits of vagueness.[80] If we understand integration in a strong sense of codependency of parts,[81] or as the condition that each part is requisite for development of the whole, we might take an embryo's survival of blastomere removal to indicate nonintegration. But

---

[78] Hoffman and Rosenkrantz 1997, p. 159.
[79] Lowe 1983, pp. 222–223, 228–230; Wiggins 2001, pp. 91–92.
[80] As observed in McMahan 2002, pp. 28–29.
[81] I have benefited from conversation with George Daley concerning the evidence that bears on this.

such survival may also evidence a compensatory mechanism. We might instead take integration to obtain when a boundary encloses parts and the parts affect each other. There must occur some significant integration in the embryo so as to explain why conjoined blastomeres so regularly develop into a single mature organism.[82] Evidence has been reported that by about the eight-cell stage, the embryo forms structures involved in intercellular communication. Tight junctions and desmosome-like structures have been observed at the six-cell stage.[83] Through such connections, developmental information might pass between cells so as to influence gene expression and eventual differentiation. The place at which a sperm inserts has been observed to affect the sorting of cells into those destined for embryoblast and those destined for trophoblast. This may indicate some interaction between cells. It appears that extent of integration increases over time – rapidly enough for a blastocyst to be integrated in the strong sense. By that stage, totipotency is no more, pluripotency obtains, and specialization has begun. Some cells have committed to the embryoblast, others to the trophoblast. Gap junctions have been observed connecting trophectoderm cells and the inner cell mass.[84]

Whatever extent of integration is demanded for an organism, or revealed by future research to be manifested by exemplars, *organisms* is not the only category within which there exist human individuals. There seems good reason to suppose that an embryo at all stages possesses the minimal extent of integration sufficient to render it a substance rather than an assemblage. We may join with this the fact that syngamy produces a distinctive new genome. Hence the early embryo is a substantial human genet. The same matter that constitutes the organism constitutes the genet. The embryo is also a develope. Because the germ line is terminally differentiated and access to the germ line is foreclosed – which entails that the universe of heritable allelic variations is already settled, save for mutation – the early embryo is also an interactor insofar as a human individual is such.

The embryo's status *ab initio* as a substantial human genet even reinforces its status as an organism, this as follows. The extensions of two kinds of substance can intersect only if the sortal persistence conditions governing the kinds are the same. To see this, suppose to the contrary that, taking the human as a representative example, the persistence conditions for the substance sortals 'human organism' and 'human substantial genet' were not the same. Then Socrates might persist as a human organism after ceasing to

---

[82] As argued in Haldane and Lee 2003, p. 274.
[83] Dale *et al.* 1991. A desmosome is a site of adhesion.   [84] *Ibid.*

be a human substantial genet, or vice versa, in which case, because substance sortals become inapplicable only when their referents cease, Socrates would both exist and not exist, which is impossible. The extensions of 'human organism' and 'human substantial genet' do intersect, as most developed humans (excepting mosaics and chimeras) belong to both kinds. Therefore the sortal persistence conditions of the two kinds are the same. We just noted that the embryo has become a human substantial genet by the time of the first cell division. We observe that there occurs no genetic change of significant scale during embryogenesis that would result in the embryo losing that status (although cells may vary within a genet by virtue of the normal incidence of mutation). We also have good reason to suppose that the zygote is an organism. We may thus deduce that, by virtue of the coincidence in sortal persistence conditions for 'human substantial genet' and 'human organism,' the fact that the embryo persists through the transitions as a human substantial genet entails that the embryo persists through the transitions as a human organism. A cogent argument obtains that identity is not sortal-relative,[85] and that the kinds 'human organism' and 'human substantial genet' are governed by a common criterion of identity supplied by the category *living substances*. From these premises follows this conditional: if a cleaving ovum is the same human substantial genet as the zygote, then the cleaving ovum is the same human organism as the zygote. It seems plain that the antecedent of this conditional is true – again because in the embryo there do not occur genetic changes beyond the normal incidence of mutation – and therefore the consequent is true. The embryo is the same organism continuously from formation onward.

Thus we have seen that an individual of a human kind falling under one or both of the categories *organisms* and *substantial genets*, and constituting a develope and interactor, exists from human oocyte activation onward. In the course of its organismic development, an individual of any such human kind may be an object of moral concern. It may coherently be thought to embody a person, or to be a person. We shall later see that the Roman Catholic Church's principal argument for Zygotic Personhood employs the premise that an embryo is a substantial genet.

(d) Other resources

Another objection to Zygotic Personhood consists in the claim that because cells that will become the placenta, amnion, and chorion intermingle during

---

[85] Wiggins 2001, ch. 1.

early development with cells that will become the embryo proper, individuation qua human cannot precede the assignment of cells to their embryo proper and trophoblast fates. That assignment is recognizable as of the blastocyst stage, when the embryoblast and trophoblast are distinguishable under the microscope. But the presence at any earlier stage of cells destined for supporting structures does not give reason to doubt whether there then exists a human individual. It suggests only that the developing individual will develop a part through which it will obtain nutrition during its gestational life.

David Wiggins characterizes the brain as the 'individuating nucleus' of a person, this while considering the hypothetical case in which Brown's brain is transplanted into Robinson's body. After the operation, it appears that the surviving human, Brownson, is – so far as one can tell by personality, memory, and all other behavioral traits – Brown.[86] With the brain goes the person. That a brain suffices for individuation as differentiation does not imply that a brain is necessary for individuation as discrete particularization. An embryo may be a human individual notwithstanding lack of a brain.

Religious traditions might bring an entirely different case against *NA*. It might be envisioned that twinning effects fission of a soul into two souls. In such case if a person is a soul, or partly a soul, a person is divisible. A fusion of twins could be a fusion of persons. Or it might be envisioned that inasmuch as God knows in advance, or decides, the course of an embryo's development, He creates two souls when twinning will occur, one when it will not. Any early embryo contains at least one human individual, and in an embryo that divides, two persons were cohabiting before the division.[87] For an analogous case, a Christian proponent of this view might cite the belief that there exist three persons in one God. Far from licensing experimentation, the foregoing views would pose the question whether an experimenter has sacrificed two persons or one. But we have seen how the refutation of *NA* proceeds without appeal to the metaphysical suppositions of theological or multiple occupancy views.

3.7 WHERE MATTERS REMAIN

Had *NA* succeeded, it would have prevented Zygotic Personhood from leaving the starting gate. But in its premise that no early embryo is an individual, *NA* has been tested and found wanting. Our analysis reveals

---

[86] Wiggins 1967, p. 51 (the Brownson case having first been posed by Sydney Shoemaker).
[87] Mills 1993.

that neither does divisibility preclude an embryo from being a person nor does there obtain any reason to deny that an early embryo satisfies any condition of human individuality requisite for personhood. If you and I are human individuals, so too are early embryos.

If *NA* slays no dragons, neither does its defeat win the day for Zygotic Personhood. The latter's proponents must still make their case. Meanwhile those who invoke concern for possible persons will remind us that even were the number of possible persons corresponding to an embryo contingent for the first fortnight, the possibility would obtain that such number will be resolved, and therefore that at the outset, at least one possible person corresponds to each embryo not already barred from the womb. The conversation has now returned to where it was before twinnability entered. We have completed an excursion resembling that of Wagner's audience, as whimsically depicted by Anna Russell, as of the moment in *Götterdämmerung* when the ring falls to the bottom of the Rhine, which happens to be where it lay when *Der Ring des Nibelungen* began. 'You could have skipped the first three nights and be as far ahead as you are now after sitting through this ordeal – and at these prices!'

We did acquire something valuable in the course of the journey, an understanding of human individuality in the most fundamental sense. This may prove useful in other contexts. On the morality of using some nascent human individuals as means, we are back to the argument from nonenablement. Having given that argument, in the next two chapters, I delve into the presumptive opposing views.

CHAPTER 4

Respect for specific life

We often hear it said that human life at all developmental stages is sacred. On this view, being an individual of *Homo sapiens* guarantees personhood for purposes of the duty not to kill and duty not to harm. Hence an embryo's progenitors may not permissibly implement their wishes – in bounding the size of their family, or in helping to advance research – at the cost of the embryo's life. In a parallel vein, it may be argued that it is virtuous, in view of the sacredness of human life, to treat an embryo with the same respect as one would accord a developed human. In such case, embryo use constitutes a loss in virtue.

Aristotle conceived plants and animals as existing for the sake of man.[1] Belief in human sacredness nests with the belief that humans rightfully hold dominion over the Earth and that they may permissibly exploit and consume nonsacred nonhuman life. While the concept of the sacerdotal is not exclusively religious, some religions hold that human sacredness originates outside *H. sapiens*, namely, with God. God has made humans, and only humans, in His image and likeness. There is something of the divine in us. God has granted to humans 'dominion over the fish of the sea, and over the fowl of the air, and over every living thing that moves upon the Earth.'[2] Christians believe that God so loved humankind that His only Son assumed human form so as to redeem humans from sin. Not all religions regard humanity as the pinnacle of creation, but many place it at or near the top. In the Great Chain of Being, long ago envisioned as the hierarchy of the universe, humankind is the third link – after God and angels. There also circulates the belief that procreation of humans is a divine–human collaboration. By virtue of this, it is often said that all developmental stages of humans are sacred.

Is it tenable that we should, or plausible that God does, hold the foregoing views? In the following, I enter into this topic at ground level. I first discuss

[1] *Politics* 1256b15–21. [2] *Genesis* 1:28, 9:2–7.

99

the concept of species, then the association of properties with species. I hope to overcome some unclarities, and in all events to show why we should take with a grain of salt invidious moral conclusions predicated upon inferences from species to properties. Toward the end of the analysis, I shall particularly draw our attention to the predication of duties concerning developmental stages on species membership. Study of that subject will confirm that respect for life does not alter the analysis, as given in §2.3, of the permissibility of epidosembryo use.

4.1 THE SPECIES PROBLEM

Biologists have put on offer a score or more notions of what constitutes a species. Proposed descriptions or criteria for recognition of a species include the following: a collection of populations of breeding individuals whose physical features are such that the populations are reproductively isolated from all and only populations except each other, a lineage, a segment on a phylogenetic tree, monophyly, phenetic similarities, morphological gaps, adaptive zones, evolution as a unit, a common fertilization system, genetic and demographic exchangeability, and cohesion. The respective species concepts advocated by systematists, ecologists, and evolutionary biologists yield taxonomies useful for their respective purposes but incompatible with one another.[3] For example, interbreeding (breeding within a population) is demanded for recognition of a species by Ernst Mayr's influential concept of a species as a collection of reproductively isolated populations. That concept issues in taxonomies that do not recognize any asexual species. By the lights of other species concepts, the history of Earth has seen more asexual species than sexual. Even when confining attention to sexual species, if one applies concepts predicated on evolutionary tendencies, then, to take another example, taxonomies will place the wolverine known as the mascot of The University of Michigan within the same species as the wolverine of Siberia, but if one applies concepts predicated on interbreeding, then insofar as the North American and Siberian wolverines differ in any feature such that they would not breed if they lived in the same place, the two populations will constitute distinct species. In view of the multiplicity of concepts, biologists have even been urged to abandon use of 'species,' to speak instead of 'phylospecies,' 'ecospecies,' and so on.[4] This suggestion

[3] Discussion of the concepts may be found in Ereshefsky 1992a, R. Wilson 1999, and Hull and Ruse 1998, part V.
[4] Ereshefsky 1992b.

resembles Quine's advice about knowledge – that we should 'give up the notion . . . as a bad job and make do rather with its separate ingredients.'[5]

During one or more past eras, the human species was ill-defined. From data yielded by the Human Genome Project, it has been inferred that subsequently to the emergence of separate human and chimpanzee lineages, members of the two lineages interbred, frequently giving birth to hybrids, and that such hybridization continued for more than a million years until the lineages fully separated.[6] Geneticists were led to this conclusion from the observation that the present day human and chimpanzee diverge in their X chromosomes very much less than they do in their other chromosomes. In respect of *H. habilis*, *H. ergaster*, *H. erectus*, and *H. neanderthalensis*, which preceded us in the line of descent from our common ancestor with the chimpanzee, the extensions of the various species concepts debated today would have notably diverged. Humans of our era are said to populate the subspecies *H. sapiens sapiens*. (I follow common practice in speaking of the species of shorter name.) A related subspecies, *H. sapiens idaltu*, is extinct. Evolution continues within our genus, as in every genus. The selection pressures include climate change, which, according to recent theories, has contributed to previous speciation within *Homo*.[7] Someday our subspecies could branch into more than one taxon that our descendants will call 'human.'

If biologists are 'drowning in a sea of species concepts,'[8] philosophers are not sure into which ocean the biologists have plunged. Philosophers disagree about what sort of entity a species is. This question is as fundamental as whether Mt. Everest is a physical object or an abstraction. In the next two sections of this chapter, I join in the effort to understand the ontological status of a species.

It happens to be the case – this is merely a contingent fact – that divergence in biological and ontological characterizations of a species do not give us pause about which individuals presently belong to *H. sapiens*. Without most of us recognizing it as such, in our common way of thinking many of us assume a version of the phylogenetic species concept according to which a species is the smallest diagnosable cluster of organisms within which there obtains a pattern of ancestry and descent from a common ancestor. Respecting genealogy, we acknowledge as human any individual in the lineage that we think of as the human lineage. But the conceptual struggle just noted leaves the following problem for morality. If we are to surpass mere prejudice in arriving at moral conclusions about how we should treat

---

[5] Quine 1987, p. 109.   [6] Patterson 2006.   [7] Behrensmeyer 2006.   [8] Hull 1999, p. 44.

various individuals, we must attend to their properties. (My references to individual living things are intended to encompass all stages of their development.) Classification according to a species concept, so we shall see, is an unreliable indicator of properties of moral importance.

4.2 SPECIES AS UNIVERSALS

As remarked in the previous chapter, if a kind is a type of thing, a natural kind is a type of naturally-occurring thing. The philosopher's standard example of a natural kind is a biological species. But to paraphrase Hilary Putnam, the concept of species, as a member of the natural kind family, has inherited the family's problems.

There are two plausible construals of a natural kind – as a universal and as a set. I begin with the species qua natural kind qua universal. I shall take *traditional essentialism* as to species to be the view that one or more properties, collectively an *essence*, are severally necessary and jointly sufficient for an individual to belong to a species, and are explanatory of an individual's other properties qua individual of its species.[9] The essence of being of a given species is possessed by all and only individuals of that species. In Aristotelian metaphysics, species are static, their essences fixed. Variation among individuals within a species arises from 'interfering forces' impinging on a 'natural state.' Do species have essences such as traditional essentialism claims? In Plato's Academy, there circulated the view that 'featherless biped' specifies man. Then Diogenes plucked a chicken. Being a featherless biped would not in any case explain much. Aristotle concluded that the essence of an individual of the human species is an *anima intellectiva* (a rational soul).[10]

If we want to inquire further into essences, we shall get no help from biologists' species concepts. Many of these concepts do not refer to intrinsic properties of individuals – such as ability to fly, swim, or reason – but instead

---

[9] Aristotle identified an essence as what it is to be of a kind, took a definition to be a true account of an essence, and envisioned constructing a definition of a substance in terms of genus and difference so as to specify the *infima species*, the lowest kind in a chain of kinds capturing the substance. Aristotle did not hold that an essence explains or causes accidental properties, but it has been argued that a more plausible Aristotelian view would depict essential properties as causing accidental (Copi 1954 as reprinted, p. 189). Locke suggests explanation or causation in speaking of real essences as the 'real constitutions' of things 'whereon their discoverable qualities depend' (*Essay*, III, iii, 15). Plantinga holds that the essence of a thing guarantees all the thing's necessary properties (1974, pp. 73–74). I am indebted to Sober 1980 for explanation of the role, in views deriving from Aristotle, of an essence as explaining other properties.

[10] *De Anima* 412b10–12, 415b10–14; *Politics* 1332b4–5.

refer to relations among individuals within populations (e.g., 'interbreeding with,' 'of common lineage with,' 'exhibiting genetic or demographic exchangeability with'), none of which explain individuals' intrinsic properties. In biologists' theorizing about species, population thinking has ousted traditional essentialism.

Suppose that we canvass the individuals of a species, over its history, for a putative essence. We discover that for any putatively essential allele, some individual of the species is found that lacks it. This is the legacy of the occurrence in meiosis of allelic segregation, independent assortment, and recombination, of the chance pairing of gametes, and of mutation and genetic drift. Even such alleles as are shared by conspecific individuals will vary in penetrance, their expression affected by epistasis and epigenetic mechanisms. For no species does there obtain a norm in the sense of an invariant. Variation is the norm. What is true for alleles is true for phenotypes. It is true for all properties, including 'rational animal,' 'having a large brain capable of abstract reasoning,' or 'user of language.' Within a polytypic species, individuals differ conspicuously. Mutation and genetic drift never cease. In consequence, advocates of traditional essentialism 'are forced to resort to embarrassing conceptual contortions to include retardates, dyslexics, and the like in our species, while keeping bees and computers out.'[11] Taking counsel from Wittgenstein's observation of family resemblance, we may have to say that humans have nothing in common apart from being humans.

As for uniqueness, many alleles are conserved across species descended from common ancestors. Parallel evolution occurs in multiple species encountering similar selection pressures. Hence a given property is likely to appear in multiple species. 'Rational animal' may characterize a chimpanzee. An individual may share so many properties with another of a sibling species as to seem almost indistinguishable from the other. The phenomenon that some one property is possessed by all and only members of a species is 'temporary, contingent, and relatively rare,'[12] and will not explain properties. To which Sober adds that 'our current theories of biological variation provide no more role for the idea of natural state than our current physical theories do for the notion of absolute simultaneity.'[13] Any phenotype within a genotype's norm of reaction – the range of phenotypes

---

[11] Hull 1986, p. 384.   [12] Hull 1986, p. 383.

[13] Sober 1980; Sober 1984b, pp. 155ff. A recent view echoes the Aristotelian in positing 'morphogenetic fields' as invariants from which perturbations occur. See Griffiths 1999, pp. 213–219. But the rationale for positing such fields seems to fade when an account is given, as in Boyd 1999 mentioned below, in which names of taxa become subjects of generalizations that support counterfactual conditionals.

resulting from interactions of the genotype with different environments –
is natural. Any variation in genotype by way of the aforementioned genetic
and epigenetic processes is natural.

Finding traditional essentialism in this much trouble on its claim that
all and only individuals of a given species possess a determinate essence, we
have reason to doubt the supposition that a species is a universal.

4.3 SPECIES AS STRUCTURES

A universal is an instantiable. Or as is sometimes said, a universal is a repeatable. Instantiation is infinitely repeatable. A species is not an instantiable.
A species consists of at most finitely many individuals extant during a temporal interval between spatiotemporal events recognized as speciation and
extinction. So we must look for a characterization of a species other than
as a universal. Any notion that properties map to individuals according to
species classifications will not gain much credence if one cannot say what
sort of entity a species is.

Philosophers who have rejected universals have conceived natural kinds,
and thereby species, as sets. (It might be ventured that a universal is a set,
but this view we may neglect. Sirius is not a star because it belongs to the
set of stars. Some property renders Sirius a star, and in virtue thereof, Sirius
belongs to the set of stars.) Natural kinds have been variously described as
'sets determined by their members,'[14] 'classes of things that we regard as of
explanatory importance; classes whose normal distinguishing characteristics are "held together" or even explained by deep-lying mechanisms,'[15] and
'sets corresponding to predicates that figure in our explanatory schemes.'[16]
('Class' is often used by metaphysicians as a synonym of 'set.' That usage
had become standard before John von Neumann's distinction between the
two terms in virtue of which some infinite classes, such as the class of all
sets, are too large to be sets. If natural kinds are classes, then because natural
kinds are finite, natural kinds are sets.) On the view that natural kinds are
sets, a species qua natural kind is a set of living individuals.[17]

The construal of a species qua set is not without its detractors. Some
philosophers of biology, followed by philosophically inclined biologists,
deny that species are natural kinds or sets.[18] They assert what I shall call
speciocompositism, the view that a species is a concrete composite. At first

---

[14] 'Natural Kinds' in Quine 1969.   [15] Putnam 1975, p. 139.   [16] Kitcher 1984a, p. 315, n. 11.
[17] Quine 1969, p. 136; Kitcher 1984a and 1984b. See also Kripke 1980, p. 121 (assimilating a species to
a natural kind having members).
[18] Ghiselin 1974, Hull 1978, Ghiselin 1997.

blush their reasoning seems to be the following. A species is not a universal; a species has no essence. A species, though comprising multiple individuals, is an individual. A set is not an individual. Hence a species is not a set. Since a species is nonatomic, a species must be a composite of which individual creatures are parts.

An apparent howler in the foregoing reasoning is the premise 'a set is not an individual.' A set *is* an individual – a discrete particular of the kind 'set.' But the speciocompositist is not using 'individual' in the metaphysical sense adduced in the last chapter. The speciocompositist takes 'individual' to signify what the set theorist calls a *urelement*. A urelement is a nonset, or more precisely, a thing that has no members, is a member of some set, and is not the null set.[19] When 'individual' and 'urelement' are synonymous, 'a set is not an individual' is tautologous. But the speciocompositist must defend the thesis that a species is a urelement.

To put more flesh on the bones of a set theoretic account of species, I offer the following.

A *biological species* is a structure $\mathbb{S} = \langle S, R_1, R_2, \ldots, R_i, \ldots, R_n \rangle$ where S, the *population*, is an underlying set of creatures, and each R_i is a relation, which may be time-indexed, on S. Where $\mathbb{R}$ is the set of real numbers, we define functions $f: S \to \mathbb{R}$ and $g: S \to \mathbb{R}$ such that for any $x \in S$, $f(x)$ is the time at which x's life begins and $g(x)$ is the time at which x's life ends. Let $\lhd$ be the weak linear ordering on S given for $x, y \in S$ by

$$x \lhd y \longleftrightarrow f(x) \leq f(y),$$

where $\leq$ is the natural ordering on $\mathbb{R}$. For any $j \in S$, we define the *segment* of $\mathbb{S}$ up to j as

$$\mathbb{S}^j = \langle \{x \in S \mid x \lhd j\}, R_1^{\,j}, R_2^{\,j}, \ldots, R_i^{\,j}, \ldots, R_n^{\,j} \rangle$$

where $R_i^{\,j} \subset R_i$ for $i = 1, 2, \ldots, n$.

$\mathbb{S}^j$ is a structure whose underlying set is a subset of S endowed with subsets of the R_i. The population of $\mathbb{S}^j$ consists of all members of S whose lives began before or at the same time as j's. To the history of the species, there corresponds a finite succession of segments $\mathbb{S}^a \subset \mathbb{S}^b \subset \ldots \mathbb{S}^j \ldots \subset$

---

[19] Other discussants join in the speciocompositist's usage of 'individual' (e.g., Ruse 1987, pp. 232–237; Sober 1984a, pp. 337ff.; Ereshefsky 1991 as reprinted, pp. 393–395; Kitcher 1984b, pp. 620ff.; Dupré 1993, pp. 20, 42–44). Use of 'urelement' is, to use a phrase of Leonard and Goodman 1940, p. 55, a way of 'divorcing the *logical* concept of an individual' from the metaphysical concept. I shall continue to reserve 'individual' for a discrete unit particular.

$S^N = S$, for $a \lhd b \lhd \ldots \lhd j \lhd \ldots \lhd N$, where N is the last member of the species to originate. The last of the segments is identical to the species. The population of the species is determined as of extinction.[20]

The *inhabitation* of S as of time t is

$$S_t = \langle \{x \in S \mid f(x) \le t < g(x)\}, R_{1t}, R_{2t}, \ldots, R_{it}, \ldots, R_{nt} \rangle$$

where $R_{it} \subset R_i$.

S_t is populated by all members of S alive at t. The lives of members of the population occur within one or more bounded regions of space and within a bounded time interval.

A *chain* is a set of creatures linearly ordered by 'descendant of.' A *lineage* is a set of chains originating at a common speciation event.

Starting from the foregoing understanding, we may refute the speciocompositist's animadversions against a set theoretic account of species. The speciocompositist contends that a species population differs from a set in that a set is expandable, at any time and place, by instantiation of the 'common characteristics' of members.[21] Here the speciocompositist mistakes a set for a universal. As a particular, a set is noninstantiable. A set also does not expand. When, in a loose way of speaking, someone says that a set S has expanded to include as members $x_1, x_2, \ldots, x_n$, they imply a different set $T = S \cup \{x_1, x_2, \ldots, x_n\}$. As for 'common characteristics,' a set is defined by its membership. For some sets, there may obtain a formulable membership criterion. Rival species concepts may be understood as rival sorts of population membership criteria and associated relations. But a membership criterion is not requisite for a set. {Ethelred, 2π, Geneva} is no less a set than is $\{x \mid x \text{ is a star}\}$.

The speciocompositist next claims that species evolve and that sets cannot evolve. Here we have what Kitcher calls 'the fallacy of incomplete translation.'[22] The untranslated expression 'a species evolves' is shorthand for 'the frequency distribution of properties across a later inhabitation will,

---

[20] So too a species qua composite would be determined only as of extinction, at the end of life of the last part. 'Whether an organism is in the same species as its parents,' writes Sober as a speciocompositist, 'is settled retrospectively' (1984a, p. 339).

[21] Hull 1978 as reprinted, pp. 294, 297, 305–306, describing a set as 'spatiotemporally unrestricted' such that new members can form intermittently, and Hull 1999, p. 34, characterizing a spatiotemporally unrestricted set as a universal. Sets and universals are mentioned interchangeably in Ghiselin 1974. Hull also says that sets are 'the sorts of things which can function in laws' (1978, p. 309). The subjects of laws are sometimes taken (as in Lowe 2006) to be natural kinds qua universals.

[22] Kitcher 1984a, pp. 310–311, and Kitcher 1984b, pp. 623–624.

in consequence of the process of natural selection, differ from the frequency distribution of properties across an earlier inhabitation.' The distributed properties may be genetic, epigenetic, or phenotypic. So also we translate 'the species branched into two species' and 'the species became extinct' respectively as 'two successions of segments began' and 'a segment of a species became its last.' In the case of selection for gene sequences, genomes, or developmental processes – to mention entities hypothesized as replicators – the foregoing expressions in terms of sets more accurately describe selection than does talk of species changing.

As for selection of species, if it occurs, 'only incomplete translation seduces one into thinking that sets . . . cannot be selected.'[23] Selection *of* an *object* is merely an effect of evolution. The speciocompositist might reply that selection *for* a *property* is a causal process in which only a concretum may participate. But we may observe that selection of one object may occur as an incidental consequence of selection for some other object's properties.[24] A process that appears to be selection of a species may be selection for heritable traits of creatures, with no causation occurring at the species level. Even so, suppose that there does occur selection for species properties (e.g., size or dispersal, if heritable). A set consisting of concreta – what Charles Parsons has called a 'quasi-concrete' set – may be understood as located in spacetime at the location of its members. This locus of a set, so Penelope Maddy has argued, is not 'any more surprising than that fifty-two cards can be located in the same place as a deck.'[25] A quasi-concrete set may participate in a causal process.

Hull also seeks to distinguish natural kinds and species on the ground that natural kinds are, while species are not, the subjects of laws of nature. We observe that some natural kinds are not such subjects (e.g., 'social animals' and 'plants of Peoria'), and some laws are not universal generalizations. A sentence that is not accidental may be lawlike despite admitting exceptions. 'The natural kinds that . . . are the subject of eternal, ahistorical, exceptionless laws,' writes Richard Boyd, 'are an unrepresentative minority of natural kinds.'[26] It is true, as Hull contends, that 'all swans are white' is not a law of nature. The explanation is not, as he urges, that the swan species is a urelement. The sentence is false, and even were the sentence true, it would be an accidental generalization.[27] There could obtain exceptionable lawlike generalizations about species.

[23] Kitcher 1984b, p. 624.   [24] Sober 1984b, pp. 258–259, 278–279, 360–368.
[25] Maddy 1990, p. 59.   [26] Boyd 1999, pp. 151ff., 169.
[27] Kitcher 1984a, pp. 311–313; Kitcher 1984b, pp. 621–623.

In stating their own ontological view, some speciocompositists declare that a species is a mereological *fusion*, or *sum*.[28] Others merely say that a species is a whole composed of parts. In either case, they usually leave the matter there. We first consider a species-sum.[29] According to the axioms of classical mereology, 'part of' is a reflexive, transitive, and antisymmetric relation, i.e., a weak partial ordering. Two things are said to overlap if and only if there exists at least one thing that is a part of each. A sum is a thing overlapping all and only those things overlapping at least one thing for which a specified well-formed formula is true.[30] 'The sum of all individuals satisfying a certain predicate,' Goodman explains, is 'the individual that exactly exhausts all such individuals. ... [T]he sum of all Dalmatians is that individual which overlaps all and only those individuals which overlap some Dalmatian.' By virtue of the classical axioms, a sum of specified summands is unique. The *fusionism* theorem states that every whole is identical to the sum of its parts.[31] The *extensionality* theorem states that x and y are identical if and only if x and y possess the same parts. The latter theorem's establishment of coextensiveness as a necessary condition of identity implies that a composite cannot without loss of identity undergo a change in parts. The contrary view that organisms and other substances persist through change motivates some philosophers to reject extensional mereology, others to embrace perdurantism. Perdurantism holds that change occurs in the succession of differing temporal parts of four-dimensional spacetime worms of which continuants consist.[32] The extensionality theorem's declaration that coextensiveness entails identity, which declaration is materially equivalent to antisymmetry for reflexive and transitive 'part of,' meets with counterexamples such as the clay statue of Goliath. This statue and the lump of clay composing it are coextensive yet arguably distinct. Their distinctness may arise because of a difference in historical properties – as when the lump originates first – although a perdurantist would in such case espy incomplete overlap of temporal parts precluding

---

[28] E.g., Brogaard 2004. Kitcher also interprets speciocompositism to equate a species with a mereological sum (1984b, p. 624).

[29] A full development of the analysis that follows is given in Guenin 2008.

[30] An ordering-relative sum is given by $\sigma_{\phi(u)} = \imath\sigma\forall x(\sigma \circ x \equiv \exists u[\phi(u) \wedge x \circ u])$ where '$\phi(u)$' is a well-formed formula, '$\circ$' denotes overlap, and '$\imath$' is the definite description operator signifying a unique σ. Speciocompositists, having rejected essentialism, are convinced that there is no nontrivial formula satisfied by exactly the creatures belonging to a species. This leaves a species qua sum to be defined (in the manner of Leśniewski 1983 and Leonard and Goodman 1940) by reference to a set of summands, here creatures.

[31] I.e., $w = \sigma_{u \preccurlyeq w}$ for a whole w, where '$\preccurlyeq$' is the 'part of' relation.

[32] As in Heller 1990, or in Sider 2001 (viewing a continuant as a stage with which are associated temporal counterparts).

coextensiveness. Even if the statue and lump originate simultaneously and are coextensive by all accounts, they may be distinct in virtue of one bearing a modal property (e.g., 'possibility of persisting through squashing and reshaping into a statue of David') that the other lacks. Establishing that coextensiveness does not entail identity will cut the props from underneath fusionism. Distinct coextensive objects could not be identical to a unique sum of their shared parts lest such composites be identical to each other. If, instead of distinct coextensive objects, one recognizes only one hunk of matter filling a given region of spacetime,[33] nothing would seem to be gained by supposing that there exists a sum rather than, say, a lump or statue.

Although it is therefore not plausible that *every* composite is a sum of its parts, might a species be a sum of creatures? Suppose that Molly is a sheep of the species *Ovis aries*, and that the species is identical to the sum of its sheep. At noon Tuesday, Molly burns some fat for energy. Because 'part of' is transitive, the species-sum thereby loses a part. By dint of extensionality, the sum that exists at noon Tuesday cannot be identical to what remains thereafter. The species-sum ceases at noon Tuesday. This result contravenes the common sense belief that *O. aries* has long persisted through changes in sheep. But so matters stand if persistence is governed by endurantism, the view that continuants do not atemporally possess temporal parts. Seeking to avoid this counterexample, a speciocompositist might embrace perdurantism so as to hold that the species-sum worm's temporal cross-sections before the fat is burned are succeeded by temporal cross-sections not containing the fat. Or the speciocompositist might cling to endurantism while adopting a nonextensional mereology in which time-specific 'part of' is nonsymmetric, and thus a weak partial tiering.[34] Lacking an extensionality theorem, this mereology recognizes continuants, including sums,[35] that persist through changes in parts. It also recognizes distinct coextensive things. But the following implausibilities attend both ordering- and tiering-relative species-sums. A sum accords no special status to creatures or demes: from the atomic level up through arbitrary intermediate sums, all parts of a sum are on a par. What is more, a sum will not at a given time incorporate as parts any then past creatures.[36] Within perdurantism, there might be conjured an ordering-relative aggregate worm, or tiering-relative

[33] A view presented in Heller 1990, pp. x, 32.
[34] A tiering is defined in Guenin 2001c as a transitive nonsymmetric relation.
[35] Such as $\xi_{\phi(u)} = \xi \forall x \forall t (\xi \circ_t x \equiv \exists u [\phi_t(u) \wedge x \circ_t u])$, after Simons 1987, p. 185, CTD18.
[36] This by virtue of an axiom that if two things overlap at a time, they must both then exist. See Simons 1987, pp. 179, 257; Sider 2001, pp. 57–58.

cumulative sum worm, that does have concrete past things as parts, but the speciocompositist would be hard put to cite any familiar example of such a thing. Whereas the underlying set of a species may contain creatures whose lives occur during an interval spanning millions of years. A species, whatever else it may be, is or corresponds to a lineage.[37] The roster of creatures within the transitive closure of a lineage is cumulative. Socrates still belongs to *H. sapiens*.

Might a species instead be an *integrate*, a composite not identical to any sum of its parts? The least demanding category of integrate is *scattered colligation*.[38] A colligation of creature constituents will cease when any creature originates or dies. A successor colligation will not contain any deceased creature. A substance too does not contain past creatures. The parts inventory of a substance is not strictly cumulative. A substance replaces and discards parts.

To propose on behalf of speciocompositism a type of entity that is neither ephemeral nor underinclusive, there might be posited what I shall call a *cumulative corpus*, or *corps*. A corps would be a concretum that expands as new creatures originate, and of which creatures remain parts after they die. If a species were a corps, then for a perdurantist, a creature would be a part of a temporal segment (the region between two hyperplanes each of constant time) of the species-corps worm. Because a worm is conceived as spread over time, its temporal parts cannot all exist at once, but it may be said that a worm atemporally has as parts all things that at any time are parts of it. Hence past creatures could atemporally be parts of a species-corps worm. Opposing this we have endurantism, which has already pronounced atemporal parthood *hors de combat* as endurantism recognizes change in 'wholly present' continuants.[39]

Alas, there is no evident example of a corps. Suppose we nominate 'the Long Gray Line,' as the cadets and alumni of the U. S. Military Academy are known. If a concretum presently exists in this case, it would more plausibly be a present colligation than a corps. It would be a colligation constituted by the present cadets and soldiers, the latest in a sequence of such colligations. Even when a long-lived family is said to exert influence – we might think of the Medici – deceased people do not seem to accumulate as parts of a concrete object. They populate a lineage, which is a set. A lineage's present members constitute a segment in a succession of segments

---

[37] So argued not only for phylogenetic but for all species concepts in de Queiroz 1999, pp. 50–54, 63, and Ereshefsky 1992b, pp. 351, 353.
[38] As defined in §3.6(b).   [39] Assuming rejection of extensionality.

ordered by inclusion. If the category *corps* is nonempty, species may have to be the sole occupants.

Even that prospect begins to look dim when we ask whether the often farflung creatures of a species are sufficiently tied together to constitute an integrate of any sort. Integration is an elusive concept. Peter van Inwagen illustrates this as he canvasses conditions such as contact, fastening, cohesion, and fusion as candidates for the sorts of conditions that objects must satisfy in order to compose another object.[40] Two sorts of ties would be demanded for an integrate of creatures: ties among contemporaries, and transtemporal ties. Interbreeding might seem a candidate for the former insofar as interbreeding results in gene flow. But there obtains contrary evidence that demes of conspecifics exist among which no gene flow occurs.[41] Although a species has been likened to a firm in commerce,[42] absence of gene flow seems more significant than any ligature suggested by analogy to a firm. Interbreedability, as a dispositional property, would not in any event be a ligation. What else might integrate creatures into a composite? Conspecifics fall within the field of a 'codescendant with' relation. But a reason would have to be given why the members of that field, a set, form an integrate. A deme might qualify as what Peter Simons describes as a dependence system, which he exemplifies by a closed gravitational system,[43] but if creatures are unaffected by far distant conspecifics, their species would not so qualify; in any case, a dependence system is not a composite but a structure. Where mereology lacks the resources to account for configuration and connectedness, mereotopology may offer an account,[44] but the scattered creatures of many species seem insufficiently connected to constitute an integral whole. Lack of contemporaneous integration seems to preclude a colligation, substance, or corps. If things linked as tenuously as are conspecifics compose a concrete object, it would seem that every natural kind is a concrete object. That understanding would obliterate any categorial difference between kinds and the things that belong to them.

For a species to be a concretum in spacetime, some account would also be needed of persistence, this for as long as millions of years. Perdurantism occupies itself with accounting for relations among temporal parts of a given whole,[45] but here we do not have a given whole. Rather we have the question of what might transtemporally tie together multiple creatures

[40] van Inwagen 1990, pp. 56–71.
[41] A familiar observation discussed in Ereshefsky 1991, and Ruse 1987, pp. 232–237.
[42] Ghiselin 1974.   [43] Simons 1987, pp. 342–349.   [44] See Casati and Varzi 1999.
[45] As in Sider 2001, pp. 5, 8, 194, 217, 224, describing a worm as a sum of temporal parts and adducing other relations among parts.

into a persisting concretum. Transtemporal interbreedability? This putative property, disclaimed by Mayr, seems on its terms to lie beyond empirical observation. After describing 'descendant of' as a characteristic relation of an integral whole, Simons observes that such a relation may characterize either a composite or a set.[46] The 'descendant of' relation seems insufficient as an integrating ligature across the centuries, this for the same reason that we do not think of the Medici, or of the kings and queens of England, even if all of one recent lineage, as a concrete object. Even if contemporary conspecifics were integrated enough to form some contemporary concretum, there would not seem to exist the same concretum after some of them die. The cadets currently enrolled at West Point form a different colligation than the colligation formed by the cadets enrolled last year.

Thus a species is not plausibly a composite identical to a sum, nor a composite not identical to a sum. The mereological ramifications of speciocompositism refute it. In the species qua structure, we have a simpler, plausible categorization. The members of the population of a species are creatures. Once a member, always a member. Demes are subsets of the population endowed with subsets of the structure's relations. Various of those relations capture, *inter alia*, the geographical distribution of members. Proper parts of creatures are not members. A species segment as of any time prior to extinction will not capture any future beings. The population will be complete at extinction, which is soon enough.

Sober poses the following as a *reductio* of a set theoretic account of species: if one creature belonging to a set were not to exist, the set would not exist.[47] This argument does not dent the construal of a species qua set or structure. Given that I belong to *H. sapiens* in the actual world, a possible world in which there exists each *H. sapiens* member (or its counterpart) other than me is a world in which '*H. sapiens*' names a species constituted by a structure different from, but corresponding to, the structure constituting the species named '*H. sapiens*' in the actual world.[48] The speciocompositist must have recourse to a like reply when met with the claim that if a creature belonging to a sum, colligation, or corps purportedly constituting a species were not to exist, the species would not exist. That claim does not assert mereological essentialism (i.e., 'for any composite x, if x has y as one of its

---

[46] Simons 1987, pp. 330–331.   [47] Sober 1984a, pp. 337–338.

[48] Kitcher 1984a, p. 310, n. 5, and 1984b, pp. 616–620. Another reply might invoke the view offered by David Lewis, as brought to bear in Armstrong 1989, p. 27, that k-kind includes all k in all possible worlds. This view also preserves a distinction between kinds named by a pair of contingently coextensive terms such as 'renate' and 'cordate.' There are possible worlds in which such terms are not coextensive.

parts then *y* is part of *x* in every possible world in which x exists'[49]), rather it invokes the definitions of such entities and axioms governing them.

When biologists first encountered the notion that species are ethereal universals, they embraced the alternative that species are individuals in the sense opposed to universals. I suspect that few biologists advanced unbidden from that alternative to the notion of a composite or mereological sum. Biologists heard the latter metaphysical categories from philosophers who, in flight from realism about universals, overlooked the species qua structure as a refuge.

We have seen the reasoning why a species is a structure. Now we observe the following. Some sets are fuzzy. Nothing in the concept of structure requires a precise formula determining membership in the population of a species. A creature's membership value as to a population may fall anywhere within [0, 1]. Even were a species a composite, a perdurantist will say that what we recognize as concreta are the relatively few worms that we select for attention from among the infinitely many worms definable in spacetime, and that concreta may, as constructs of our conventions, be vague for lack of precise persistence conditions.[50] An endurantist such as van Inwagen, defining parthood as 'being caught up in the life of an organism,' may observe that parthood is vague, a matter of degree.[51]

Fuzziness may be a consequence of the intrinsic properties of objects, our conventions, or both. In any case, the prospect of fuzziness should give pause to anyone who contemplates reading off properties of creatures from their taxonomic classifications. To consider such inferences, I now turn to contemporary views that ascribe essences and property clusters.

4.4 PROPERTIES

Several 'essentialist' theories furnish what I take to be the most robust accounts on offer by which one might attempt to map properties to members of species as such. I shall provide a hearing for each account, then try to say how we should respond to views that associate morally significant properties with, and predicate moral verdicts upon, species membership.

(a) Kripke's causal theory of reference

For many sets of which we are aware, including the taxa of the Linnean binomial system that partitions and subpartitions the set of living things, we have not reckoned necessary and sufficient membership conditions. Saul

[49] Chisholm 1976, p. 145.   [50] Heller 1990, p. 48.   [51] van Inwagen 1990, pp. 94, 217ff.

Kripke's causal theory of reference describes the following phenomenon. A speaker originates a name by 'baptism,' by ostensively assigning a name to some referent or referents. If the name is a proper name (e.g., 'Socrates') or natural kind term (e.g., 'water'), the name often will stick so well that it becomes a *rigid designator*, a name that designates the same referent in every possible world in which that referent exists.[52] For Kripke, a possible world is not a region that we might observe as in observing a planet through a telescope. Rather a possible world is a counterfactual situation. Against philosophers who hold that a thing in the actual world cannot also exist in another world, or who follow Lewis in speaking of a thing's counterparts in other possible worlds, Kripke insists that we may just 'point to' a thing under possible counterfactual conditions.

Frege and Russell characterize proper names and natural kind terms as placeholders for conjunctions or clusters of descriptions. Against this view, Kripke maintains that names designate rigidly while descriptions do not.[53] A baptizer assigning a natural kind term k may have in mind some description of the referents, but that description is not taken as a synonym of k. A description serves only to fix k's reference initially. The initial designation is passed on by the baptizer to another speaker, by that speaker to someone else, and so on in a causal chain of usage. Rigid designation by k will soon capture more objects. Successive speakers will apply k to other things exhibiting properties thought 'at least roughly characteristic' of k-kind and believed to be possessed by the things first baptized.[54] Speakers will seize upon sundry contingent properties as defeasible markers for distinguishing things of k-kind. Some properties of the initial referents may later prove to be peculiar to those referents, other properties not espied initially may later be thought requisite for being k. An animal could be a horse even if born with only three legs. The process of resolving designation is hit and miss. The process could lead to rejecting k-kind as such. For example, the Greeks took water to be one of the four elements of all matter. In the eighteenth century it became known that water is not a chemical element. Speakers have sometimes used different names for what their successors see as one thing (e.g., 'Hesperus' and 'Phosphorus' for the planet Venus). But rigid

---

[52] Kripke 1971, pp. 78–79; Kripke 1980, p. 48. On most accounts, 'water' is a bulk term, not a sortal, but still a natural kind term. An account that treats both bulk terms and count nouns as sortals is given in Lowe 1989, pp. 30, 32–33, 37.

[53] *Contra* Kripke, Plantinga argues that many a proper name designates different things in different worlds, and that what is notable about a proper name is that it expresses an essence consisting in a property or properties instantiated by the same object in every world in which the property is instantiated (1974, p. 80).

[54] Kripke 1980, p. 137.

designation somehow leads us to say that a horse-like animal possessed of a spiral horn, cloven hoofs, and the tail of a lion is not a horse but a unicorn. Rigid designation seems to operate in virtue of something that lies beneath markers.

As speakers, we surefootedly use and understand natural kind terms without pausing for formalization of kinds. Our credulity is no doubt a valuable economy facilitating communication. Kripke offers a deeper explanation. Kripke's ontology includes necessary properties of things and necessary properties for belonging to natural kinds.[55] A *necessary property*, if such there be, *for belonging to a kind K* is a property *P* possessed by all members of *K* in all possible worlds in which *K* is nonempty.[56] A *necessary property of a particular thing* is a property possessed by the thing (or its counterpart) in every possible world in which the thing (or a counterpart) exists. That a thing lacks a necessary property for belonging to a given kind does not entail that the thing cannot exist. To illustrate a necessary property for belonging to a natural kind, suppose a possible world in which, in place of the horses of the actual world, there appear nonanimal robots. This does not entail that horses are not animals; we could conclude that the robots are not horses. If horses are animals in every possible world in which horses exist, then being an animal is a necessary property for belonging to horsekind.

A statement is necessary, in the metaphysical sense used by Kripke, if true in all possible worlds. In respect of stuffs designated rigidly, Kripke asserts that 'statements representing scientific discoveries about what this stuff *is*' are necessary truths. Scientists sometimes discover the 'internal structure' of a member of a natural kind. Lavoisier inferred that water, long recognized by markers such as 'odorless' and 'fills lakes,' consists of H_2O. Kripke holds that 'water is H_2O,' if true in the actual world, is true in all possible worlds and is therefore a necessary truth. Concomitantly he asserts that the 'internal structure' of a kind member constitutes a necessary property for belonging to the kind. Consisting of H_2O is a necessary property for belonging to the kind 'water.' If water consists of H_2O in the actual world, and if, in a possible world, some substance possesses all properties of water except that of consisting of H_2O, this will not be taken to show that water is not H_2O. Instead it will be concluded that the substance in that possible world is not water.

---

[55] On things, see Kripke 1971, p. 86, and Kripke 1980, pp. 39–41, 53.
[56] One who holds that a kind is a universal may read 'belonging to' as 'being an instance of.'

'Science can discover empirically,' Kripke adds, 'that certain properties are necessary of cows, or of tigers.'[57] This is not to suggest that science searches only for necessary properties. Rather science seeks to find 'the essence (in the philosophical sense) of the kind,' i.e., a set of properties that are severally necessary and jointly sufficient for belonging to the kind.[58] An essence may be understood as the smallest set of properties that guarantees all necessary properties.[59] For belonging to 'water,' consisting of H_2O is not only necessary but sufficient, as water has no isomers. Similarly, being an element of atomic number 79 is necessary and sufficient for belonging to 'gold.' Necessity and sufficiency in this context are metaphysical, not logical.

From our point of view, the foregoing picture presents two flaws. The first is that the account adumbrates essences of biological kinds but does not adduce a compelling reason to believe in them. Kripke gives as examples of essences only water's molecular formula and gold's atomic number. Those properties do not vary from one mass of those chemical species to another. What obtains for chemical species may not obtain for biological. Is there a set of jointly sufficient properties for belonging to the population of a biological species? If N_K is putatively the set of all necessary properties for belonging to K, then an individual's possession of all members of N_K will be sufficient in the metaphysical sense for the individual to belong to K, since there could be no non-N_K property that an individual must possess in order to be of K.[60] To ascertain the membership of N_K for an individual, one might turn to the genome, an 'internal structure.' Mayr once remarked that 'there is a species-specific unity to the genetic program (DNA) of nearly every species.'[61] In debate about universals and particulars,

---

[57] Kripke 1980, p. 128.

[58] For Kripke, the contrasting sense to this 'philosophical sense' in respect of a kind is the sense in which an essential property is a necessary property of a thing (Kripke 1980, pp. 39, 138; Plantinga 1974, pp. 55–56). For the latter case, essentialism is the view that things possess *de re* necessary properties. The *essence of a thing* is taken to be the thing's unique concatenation of necessary properties, the set E of properties such that (a) the thing (or its counterpart) possesses all members of E in every possible world in which the thing (or a counterpart) exists, and (b) there is no possible world in which something other than the thing (or its counterpart) possesses all members of E. One imagined essence of a given thing is a primitive 'thisness,' an all-inclusive property of being this very particular (a property called by Scotus a '*haecceitas* '). But the target of our present discussion remains properties for belonging to a kind.

[59] Dupré 1993, p. 66.

[60] Kripke observes that for the different case of being a particular thing, it is questionable whether there exists a set of jointly sufficient properties that do not refer to the thing by name – that do not fail to be 'purely qualitative' (Kripke 1971, p. 86, n. 12; Kripke 1980, p. 46). A purely qualitative property is a property not predicated on an individual. See Salmon 2005, p. 20. For discussion of this, I thank James Van Cleve.

[61] Mayr 1982, p. 297.

it is sometimes said that types are marked off by sets exhibiting a 'distributive unity' not found in other sets.[62] What 'DNA unity' suffices for a species? Genome will vary, from one individual to another within K, at every gene locus. Gene expression will vary by virtue of epigenetic mechanisms distinct from DNA. Environment and the gene-environment interaction will affect phenotypes. Genes do not tell the whole story. Macrostructural properties not determined entirely by genes may be part of the fabric that knits species and other taxa together. After whales were observed to breathe air and to suckle their young, 'fish' ceased to be a rigid designator of whales. Various proponents of species concepts have urged nongenetic criteria as pivotal, though we are not sure which of the proposals deserves credence. Attempts to characterize human nature – as rational, political, linguistic, good, selfish, evil, sympathetic, or social – will surely fail if they leave out of account the effects of reason, environment, society, and other influences not encoded in genes. All of which makes N_K elusive. Suppose a set S_K of putatively sufficient properties numerous enough to distinguish K from species to whose members the members of K bear a high degree of genetic homology. S_K could be so large as to exclude some members of K. If there is no determinate N_K, it is unclear how one could winnow S_K to an essence. Nor is it clear how one could ascertain an essence by starting with an indeterminate N_K, which by definition is too bloated to be an essence.[63]

The second and more fundamental concern about Kripke's account is that necessity of a proposition (e.g., 'water is H_2O') and a necessary property of a thing (e.g., consisting of H_2O) are two different matters. The former is necessity *de dicto* (of what is said), the latter necessity *de re* (of a property of a thing). Necessity *de re*, if it obtains, is a feature of the physical world. Belief in necessity *de re* coheres with Aristotle's notion that definitions are of things, not of words. Since Hobbes, empiricists have denied necessity *de re*. Kripke asserts necessity *de re*. But because Kripke speaks alternately of what seem *de re* and *de dicto* modalities,[64] he leaves the impression that in the guise of necessity *de re*, he has adduced only necessity *de dicto*. If 'P is possessed by all members of K in all possible worlds in which K is nonempty' is understood as '$\Box(\forall x)(Kx \rightarrow Px)$,' we have only a case of *de dicto* necessity.[65]

Plantinga holds that 'one can explain the *de re* by the *de dicto*.'[66] But it may be replied that one cannot derive a claim that things possess necessary

---

[62] Armstrong 1989, pp. 21–25, 119–120.   [63] See Fine 1994, pp. 4–5.   [64] Kripke 1980, pp. 123–125.
[65] This because the only variable within the scope of the necessity operator is bound. I owe this example to Van Cleve 1995, p. 137.
[66] Plantinga 1974, pp. 29–43.

properties from a theory of how words rigidly designate.[67] Reporting *de dicto* necessity is only reporting use of language. Of course any thing possesses trivial necessary properties (e.g., being identical to itself). In the case of things that populate species, it is not obvious that necessity *de re* obtains as to any nontrivial properties. When we turn to properties for belonging to species, we cannot even seem to agree on definitions that would ground necessity *de dicto*.

We have not heard a compelling reason to think that there exist well-defined mappings of properties to individuals as members of species. We have no reason to assume that whether a thing possesses properties of moral significance can be read off from its belonging to a particular species.

(b) Putnam's theory of reference

Like Kripke's, Putnam's account of natural kinds is predicated on rigid designation.[68] Putnam holds that there is associated with each natural kind term a theory describing a normal member possessing characteristic properties. What constitutes normality is unclear, but the idea of a normal member's characteristic properties is said to form a stereotype of a kind. When speakers apprehend the extension of a natural kind term and the stereotype, they acquire linguistic competence in use of the term.[69] For a definition of the term, they defer to experts. This 'linguistic division of labor' helps to explain our credulity in using rigid designators.

Putnam goes on to say that to belong to a natural kind is to stand in a similarity relation to a normal member of a set of 'local examples' in the actual world. '"Water" is stuff that bears a certain similarity relation to the water *around here*.' The relevant similarity is said to obtain in respect of 'important physical properties.'[70] (This conception is vulnerable to a charge of circularity if each of 'kind' and 'similar' depends for its definition on the other.[71]) But in virtue of similarity, a natural kind term rigidly

---

[67] An argument developed in Salmon 2005.
[68] For which Putnam's term is 'indexicality' (Putnam 1975, pp. 233–234), rendered by Plantinga thus: 'A sentence in which a proper name is used ordinarily expresses the same proposition as is expressed by the result of replacing it by a demonstrative ("this", "that") when the latter is used to demonstrate or refer to the appropriate bearer of the name' (1974, p. 41).
[69] *Ibid.*, pp. 148–152.   [70] Putnam 1975, pp. 234, 239.
[71] Quine 1969. It is also objected in Mellor 1977 that the archetypes nominated by biologists to demarcate plant and animal kinds 'are chosen to fit botanical and genetic knowledge, not the other way round.' But we observe that some kinds (e.g., the Higgs boson) are recognized on the basis of predictions even if no members have yet been observed.

designates 'whatever has the same nature as the normal examples.'[72] This 'nature,' also called the 'essential nature' of a thing of a kind, 'accounts for' the thing's other properties. It specifies the thing's components and how they 'produce the superficial characteristics.' The nature consists in the thing's 'microstructure' or 'hidden structure.'[73] Water's nature is H_2O. And necessarily so. 'Once we have discovered the nature of water, nothing counts as a possible world in which water doesn't have that nature.' But this is only necessity 'in a loose sense.' Evidently this last remark is directed against a claim that 'water's nature is H_2O' is analytic, but Putnam also writes, 'It isn't logically possible that water isn't H_2O.'[74] The latter claim seems plausible only as an assertion of a *de dicto* modality.

For members of biological kinds, 'chromosome structure' or 'genetic code' are said to constitute the essential nature. We have already observed in reviewing Kripke's account why a genetic essence is implausible. Putnam acknowledges (though not for biological species) that in the case of some natural kinds, members do not possess a common microstructure. But he thinks that for these kinds there still obtains a necessary and sufficient condition for belonging, namely, 'possession of sufficiently many of the superficial characteristics.'[75] This reiterates the notion, rejected by Kripke, of possessing 'enough' properties of a cluster. Hull also speaks of property clusters.

Nathan Salmon replies that as Putnam purports to show that rigid designation leads to *de dicto* necessary truths concerning properties of natural kinds,[76] Putnam begs the question of essentialism by relying on an enthymematic essentialist premise. Putnam's reasoning to the conclusion that 'water is H_2O' is a necessary truth relies on the premise that 'consubstantiality consists in having the same chemical structure.' Putnam does not demonstrate essentialism, he assumes it.[77] The only sort of essentialist claim sustained by the Kripke–Putnam causal theory of reference, insists Salmon, is of the form 'Mark Twain could not fail to have the property of being Samuel Clemens.' But ascribing a haecceity to a thing 'is little more than a boring truism' that 'can hardly begin to stir the emotions of foes of Aristotelian essentialism.'[78]

Thus Putnam's account, like Kripke's, supposes genetic essences in virtue of which individuals belong to a species, but it does not present a convincing

---

[72] Putnam 1975, p. 243. Supposing some description that assists in picking out things of a kind, the corresponding natural kind term will rigidly designate 'whatever things share the *nature* that things satisfying the description normally possess' (p. 238).
[73] *Ibid.*, pp. 140–141, 239.   [74] *Ibid.*, pp. 230, 233.   [75] *Ibid.*, pp. 140–141, 233, 240–241, 244.
[76] *Ibid.*, pp. 232–233.   [77] Salmon 2005, pp. 161–192.
[78] Salmon 2005, p. 84. Mellor 1977 offers further criticisms of Kripke–Putnam essentialism.

reason to believe in genetic essences. Most of the species concepts of biologists say nothing of genetic essences. Nor does the Kripke–Putnam theory of reference give us reason to believe that members of species uniquely possess nontrivial necessary properties *de re*. Or even that sentences ascribing nontrivial properties are necessary *de dicto*.

Quine poses this question: if a mathematician is necessarily rational and not necessarily bipedal, and a cyclist is necessarily bipedal and not necessarily rational, what is a mathematician cyclist? The root of bewilderment here, for Quine, is that 'necessity resides in the way we talk about things, not in the things we talk about.'[79] A distinction *de re* between necessary and contingent properties of things, 'however venerable,' is 'surely indefensible.'[80] The taxonomist's inability to specify necessary properties for belonging to a species counts as but one of the 'sorrows of modality.' Things look no more promising for the specification of sufficient properties.

(c) Homeostatic property cluster natural kinds

When we assume that to a given predicate there corresponds a property, we may be encountering 'another example of the way in which the structure of language can prejudice our thoughts about ontology.'[81] Were we to apply Wittgenstein's insight to say that horses have nothing in common apart from being horses, we would strike a blow against essentialism in respect of kinds. Family resemblance may elude explanation. Enter now Boyd to put more flesh on the notion of a cluster of properties. Boyd defines a *homeostatic property cluster* as a set of properties, including dispositional properties, none of which is necessary for being a member of a natural kind, but many combinations of which, as brought about by various *homeostatic mechanisms* in nature, suffice. Such mechanisms include gene exchange, inheritance, reproductive isolation, and similarity of environment. By virtue of homeostatic mechanisms, operating interdependently in complex ways not fully understood, contingently clustered properties tend to be exemplified together. Homeostasis affects the statistical distribution of phenotypes. A cluster of properties and associated homeostatic mechanisms define a term whose extension is a natural kind. Species are

---

[79] Quine 1976, pp. 174–176. See also Quine 1961, pp. 155–156. Plantinga disputes the pertinence of Quine's example, saying that 'there is less than a ghost of a chance' that defenders of *de re* necessity think bipedality a necessary property of cyclists (Plantinga 1974, p. 25).

[80] Quine 1960, pp. 199–200. Kitcher too is 'agnostic' on essences (1984a, p. 315, n. 11).

[81] Lowe 2006, p. 183.

'historically delimited' homeostatic property cluster natural kinds. Subpopulations and demes are members of species.

Boyd adverts to a homeostatic property cluster as the essence of a species.[82] This is a far cry from what others have called an essence. Members of a kind share in a homeostatic property cluster variably and imperfectly. Through succeeding generations of a species over the course of evolution, the clustered properties and the mechanisms impinging upon them also change, the roster of each not closing till extinction.[83] How many properties in combination, or how much of each, suffice for belonging to a given natural kind? Sometimes 'no rational considerations' will answer the question whether things belong to a given species.[84] Natural kinds could be fuzzy sets. Boyd warns that 'any "refinement" of classification which artificially eliminated . . . indeterminacy in classification would obscure the central fact about heritable variations in phenotype upon which biological evolution depends. More determinate species would be scientifically inappropriate and misleading.'[85]

Our talk about natural kinds passes the test of scientific usefulness. It allows us to frame lawlike generalizations. One way to define a natural kind is to say that it is a kind by reference to which it is possible to make better than chance predictions about the properties of its instances or members.[86] But, asserts Boyd, 'natural kinds are social artifacts. . . . No natural kinds exist independently of practice.' 'A natural kind just is the implementation – in language and in conceptual, experimental, and inferential practice – of a (component of) a way of satisfying the accommodation demands of a disciplinary matrix.'[87] Here we have an echo of Locke's view that 'the boundaries of the species, whereby men sort them, are made by men.'[88] In Locke's ontology, 'all things that exist being particular,' a thing has a real but unknowable 'constitution' or 'essence.' Locke opposes to a real essence the 'nominal' essence of a thing of a kind. The nominal essence 'comes to nothing but the abstract idea which the . . . name stands for.' Nominal essences are 'ideas established in the mind, with names affixed to them.'[89] Observing 'so near a connection' between names and nominal essences, Locke anticipated the theory of rigid designation. But he held that we have no direct access to real essences. Hence 'essential and nonessential relate only to our abstract ideas and the names annexed to them.'[90] About species,

---

[82] Boyd 1999, p. 142. [83] On this point I have benefited from Hull 1965, p. 326.
[84] Boyd 1999, pp. 143–144. [85] Boyd 1988, p. 198. [86] Thus in Griffiths 1999, p. 216.
[87] Boyd 1999, pp. 174–175. [88] *Essay*, III, vi, 37. [89] *Essay*, III, iii, 1, 12, 15, 19; III, vi, 7.
[90] *Essay*, III, vi, 4.

Locke envisioned disagreements.[91] He would have doubted that scientists will discover real essences.

(d) Essentialism for species-corresponding kinds

The last view that I shall mention is that of Lowe, who holds that, where 'thing' stands for 'any sort of entity whatever,' there is for every thing both its essence as a thing ('that in virtue of which it is the very entity that it is')[92] and one or more 'general' essences in virtue of the thing's exemplifying the essential characterizing universals of a kind. In this account, Lowe countenances the essence of a species as a thing. Whether a species be a structure or composite, this essence will be lightweight, consisting in being a structure or composite, and having the members and relations, or parts, that it has. The account also recognizes the essence of the natural kind that corresponds to the species. Essence constitutes the ground of metaphysical necessity and possibility, not vice versa.[93] This revives the notion that an essence explains or guarantees nonessential properties. Essence-grounded modalities are *de re*, but an essence itself is not an entity. To say that it is part of the essence of water that water is composed of H_2O, or of an organism that it includes DNA, is not to say that an essence *consists in* a molecular constitution, or consists in any entity. If an essence were so to consist, presumably the essence would have an essence, and an infinite regress would follow.

For Lowe, the essence of a kind, what it is to be of the kind, consists of some – usually not all – of the property and relation universals that characterize the kind.[94] The essence of dogkind includes warmbloodedness and carnivorousness. Not all necessary properties are essential. While all of electronkind's characterizing universals may be essential, it will not be part of water's essence that it dissolves salt, since the laws of physics in other possible worlds may differ from those in the actual world.[95] For the same reasons that impel Putnam and Boyd to speak of things exemplifying

---

[91] As noted in Copi 1954, pp. 184–185.

[92] For Aristotle, the essence of a thing is what it is *kath hauto*, in virtue of itself (*Metaphysics* 1029b13–15). Locke's phrase is 'the very being of any thing, whereby it is, what it is' (*Essay*, III, iii, 15). Lowe harkens to what he takes to be Aristotle's view that 'real essences of material substances are known to those who talk or think comprehendingly about such substances' (Lowe 2008).

[93] Lowe agrees with the view that 'assimilation of essence to modality is fundamentally misguided' (Fine 1994).

[94] Lowe 2006, pp. 62, 132, 152, 165, 173.

[95] Notwithstanding this in Lowe 2006, it is argued in Lowe 2008 that because essence is the ground of possibility, it puts the cart before the horse to predicate essentiality of a property on possession thereof in every possible world.

some but not all properties of a cluster, this account seems to require that things of a kind variably coexemplify a cluster of universals. As Boyd suggests, coexemplification of clustered properties by members of kinds is contingent, only dimly understood, and varies so much between individuals that species populations may only be fuzzy sets. Lowe construes a kind as a sortal universal denoted '*k*-kind' for some sortal *k*. Sortals can be vague. Lowe suggests variable coexemplification in the following manner. A law 'consists in a kind's possessing . . . a property.' So a law about *K* takes the form '*Ks* are *P*.' This, he says, is not materially equivalent to '$(\forall x)(Kx \rightarrow Px)$,' a generalization about particulars, because lawlike characterization of a kind by a property universal admits of exceptions. 'Dogs are carnivorous' will continue to support counterfactual conditionals even if Spot shuns meat. Creatures resemble one another, hence conform to lawlike generalizations, in consequence of reproduction and exposure to similar environments. But exceptions arise because the copying process is imperfect, environments differ, and boundaries of kinds may be vague.[96] A discussant would be hard pressed to define, from generalizations or otherwise, mappings from species into a codomain of properties so as to warrant ignoring the actual properties of particular living things – especially for purposes of life and death decisions.

4.5 TAXA

Biologists' attempts to classify living things by properties have issued in the recognition not only of species, but of genera, families, orders, classes, phyla, and kingdoms. It has occasionally been argued that higher taxa are onto-logically different from, and perhaps less real than, species. Linnaeus saw species and genera as more real than higher taxa insofar as the former have essences.[97] More recently, speciocompositism has issued in the claim that species are evolving urelements while higher taxa are not. Boyd's account suggests that taxa in general are homeostatic property cluster natural kinds. The notion that there obtain ontological differences among species and higher taxa is beginning to vanish. Distinctions among taxonomic cate-gories are as blurred in practice as in theory. Ducks are classified as a family, owls as an order. The lily family includes onions. There is no taxon coex-tensive with 'tree.'[98] As successive generations of biologists observe nature, taxonomists move populations up and down, and shift populations across

---

[96] Millikan 1999, pp. 54–56.   [97] As pointed out in Ereshefsky 1999.
[98] I owe these examples to Dupré 1981.

limbs, of their taxonomic trees. The biologist Brent Mishler comments that 'we have no and are unlikely to have any criterion for distinguishing species from other ranks in the Linnean hierarchy. . . . The species rank is a human judgment. . . .'[99] The hierarchy of categories, he reasons, is 'a meaningless formality' that biologists would do well to abandon. 'The species rank,' he says, 'must disappear along with all the other ranks.'

I suggest how we may generalize to one category, the taxon. We first say that where X is a set partially ordered by the superset relation $\supset$,[100] an element M is a *minimal element* of X if and only if M is not a superset of any element of X. A structure is a superset of another structure if the former's underlying set is a superset of the latter's underlying set. Now we say that

> A *biological taxonomic tree* Λ is a finite set such that
> (i) each $\mathbb{T} \in \Lambda$ is a structure of the form $\langle T, R_1, R_2, \ldots, R_i, \ldots, R_n \rangle$,
> (ii) in each $\mathbb{T} \in \Lambda$, T is an underlying set of creatures, and each R_i is a relation on T,
> (iii) Λ is partially ordered by $\supset$,
> (iv) for any $\mathbb{T} \in \Lambda$, the set of $\mathbb{T}$'s predecessors under $\supset$ (i.e., $\{X \in \Lambda \mid X \supset \mathbb{T}\}$ is well-ordered by $\supset$, and
> (v) Λ contains two or more minimal elements.
>   An element $\mathbb{T}$ of Λ is a *taxon*. A linearly ordered subset of Λ is a *branch*. A minimal element of Λ is a *leaf.*

That a set of predecessors is well-ordered entails that every nonempty subset thereof has a least element. This assures that every taxon has at most one direct predecessor (or *parent*) in a tree. Species will be minimal elements except insofar as they have substructures such as races, varieties, or subspecies recognized as elements of a tree. The extent to which higher taxa are endowed with relations may be significantly less than in the case of species. The universe of taxa may be represented as a stand of trees – or, as biologists construct taxonomies, as a single tree of life. We may proceed to define a segment and inhabitation of a taxon as we did those of a species, observing that the last segment is the taxon. We may translate talk about taxa evolving as we translated talk of species evolving. There seems no conceptual reason why a taxon cannot be selected in evolution. A taxon may be viewed by a nominalist as a structure whose underlying set is a natural kind. Goodman acknowledges that there exist concreta whose aggregation it is more useful to characterize as a set than as a sum. For example, 'we

---

[99] Mishler 1999, pp. 308–309, 313.   [100] $A \supset B \equiv B \subset A$.

are normally concerned with the members of a squad.'[101] Trope theory also
has the resources to recognize taxa as structures. An immanent realist may
hold that there corresponds to the underlying set of a taxon a natural kind
understood as a universal of which that set's members are instances.[102]

There are other mathematical ways to describe taxa, especially in computational phylogenetics, but the foregoing will serve to suggest the set
theoretic generality within which species are subsumed. We are curious
about sets such as $\{x \mid x \text{ is a tiger}\}$, sets that seem to mark off biological
types, in contrast with sets such as {your chin, DNA, Hume}, which do
not. The taxonomist will publish a brief official list of properties chosen
as membership criteria for a taxon, but the taxonomist has no illusion
that the listed properties constitute an essence. Insofar as each taxon is
built up from organisms or other creatures that are real, no taxon is more
real than another. Types in general, as Armstrong says, 'are rough-and-
ready. . . . [E]ven when the ordinary types do carve the beast of reality
along its true joints, they may still not expose those joints for the things
that they are.'[103] We are reminded of 'the grounds for accepting a taxonomic
scheme: not that it is the right one, since there is none such; but that it
serves some significant purpose better than the available alternatives.'[104] As
taxonomists shoehorn creatures into places within their schemes, they help
us put together a comprehensible picture of nature. Their classifications
facilitate reliable inductive inferences.

We may now take stock of the consequences of what we have learned
about properties, essentialist accounts, and taxa. Because people are the
authors of taxonomies, we have reason to take taxonomies with a grain of
salt. In the improbable event that there exists a set of properties possessed
by all and only members of some inhabitation of a species, it is likely that
the properties are neither possessed by all and only members of multigen-
erational segments, nor possessed uniquely by every species member in all
possible worlds in which the species (or counterpart) is nonempty, nor
explanatory of other properties. Rigid designation may explain our use of
names for taxa, but rigid designation cannot be cashed out to obtain *de
re* genetic or other microstructural essences of organisms. The plausible
hypothesis of homeostatic property clustering suggests that the underlying
sets of taxa are fuzzy sets, their memberships dependent on variable coexemplification of contingently clustered properties. Generalizations about

---

[101] Goodman 1977, p. 43.
[102] This realist view derives its inspiration from the view that a natural kind corresponds to a species
qua colligation (Lowe 1998, pp. 53, 187).
[103] Armstrong 1989, p. 87.   [104] Dupré 1993, pp. 50–52.

properties possessed by members of those sets appear tenable only insofar as the generalizations admit exceptions. As Russell once said, all generalizations are false, including this one. Because variability is the norm, even generalizations cum exceptions seem to elude us. In making life and death decisions, we ought to look through and beyond taxonomic classifications. We need to do so in order to take fair account of actual properties of living things.

4.6 BEARERS OF MORALLY CRUCIAL PROPERTIES

Our universe of moral concern intersects branches from various taxonomic limbs, and we have reason for concern about kinds other than taxa. Consider properties of living things in virtue of which it may be wrong for us to harm them. We associate sentience with the taxon 'vertebrate' (a subphylum). But a creature could experience pain by means other than a spinal column. We need to be concerned about {all sentient beings}. Or again, there is no taxon even approximating {all self-conscious beings} or {all rational beings}. We must ascribe self-consciousness and rationality on the basis of behavioral observations. Sets of things that are objects of moral concern may be fuzzy.

About living things, we humans, or at least some of us, seem to have painted a montage of moral standards. The following are some of the components. We may hunt and eat animals and plants, but not what we classify as endangered species. We may kill humans in self-defense, but not otherwise. We abhor suffering and oppose torture, but in quest of gains in our nutrition and health, we may raise sentient animals in cages before slaughter for food. We may experiment upon self-conscious animals. When we summon the resolve not to buy meat from animals raised in miserable conditions, we increase our consumption of other animals. Notwithstanding how captivity adversely affects animals, we condone trapping and presenting animals in zoos in the belief that we benefit from seeing them. For sport, we may kill deer, but not dogs. Unlike our ancestors, we condemn killing of animals for fur. We may trap tuna in nets, but not dolphins. We are urged to manifest respect for human life at all stages but to impose the death penalty and curtail welfare programs. Notwithstanding whatever modest constraints we may impose, we think it permissible to consume trees and pollute the atmosphere so as to alter Earth in ways that will adversely affect flora, fauna, and our descendants. The foregoing abridged litany understates the confusion. Its use of 'we' masks many disagreements.

We are predators, as are nonhuman animals that we favor. 'Most of us,' adds Singer, 'are speciesists.'[105] Species partiality seems embedded in common sense morality. So our ideal of respect for life wants for clarification. Hare would have us resolve some of our confusion by commanding that we maximize the number of quality-adjusted life years of sentient beings. He would thereby justify raising a sentient animal for food if the animal were given a good life, killed painlessly, and replaced by another equally happy animal that would not have existed were the first animal not sacrificed.[106] Hare goes on to venture that collective demand for meat, poultry, and diary products serves to increase aggregate quality-adjusted life years insofar as it induces raising more animals who receive better nourishment. Optimistic assumptions must hold for this result to obtain – painless killing, that animals live happy lives on farms now run like factories, that having more animals boosts aggregate welfare more than would other uses of the resources that animals consume. Singer starts from a similar principle – that we owe equal consideration of interests of all sentient beings – but opposes killing self-conscious animals who will be harmed by loss of a future.[107] He allows that sentient but not self-conscious animals may be killed if a farmer replaces them, or if, in general, their deaths bring about increases in aggregate utility. Such accounts raise the hackles of those who do not conceive morality as maximizing a maximand.

From our montage of moral verdicts, I take instruction that respect for life is not a well-formed principle resident in our prereflective thinking such that we need only call it up when we encounter a new situation. Rather we are continually challenged to construct norms of respect. Doing so requires careful thought about properties.

Biologists have observed advanced cognition among nonhuman great apes. Chimpanzees, gorillas, and orangutans can learn sign language. They joke and teach one another. Orangutans, known as the escape artists of zoos, show cleverness in using tools. They evidently can hold existence of themselves and others as a mental representation. Chimps sometimes sign to themselves. Orangutans and gorillas can recognize themselves in mirrors, as can dolphins.[108] Indications even appear of the ability of nonhuman apes to reflect on their thoughts. Great apes appear to be self-conscious, to be aware of themselves as what we would call continuing subjects of experiences. It is plausible that nonhuman apes have preferences, that they adopt ends. They hide food, then eat it in order of perishability. They

[105] Singer 2002, p. 93. See also Arneson 1999, p. 123.   [106] Hare 1993, pp. 219–235.
[107] Singer 2002, pp. 119, 121, 224; Singer in Jamieson 1999, pp. 310, 325–326.
[108] As noted by various writers in Cavalieri and Singer 1993, pp. 19–77, 241.

observe unripe fruit, then return to it after a few sunny days. They plan. That they sometimes lie suggests an ability to see things from another's point of view (though it is unclear whether they can detect another's having a false belief, which children cannot do until about age 4). They can solve problems. They display remarkable immediate memory. In extent of intelligence, adult nonhuman apes resemble human children. It has even been contended that conscious animals are 'essentially minds.'[109] They have emotions, they suffer, they feel the loss of a loved one or member of their community. Years after her favorite kitten had died, a gorilla communicated in sign language her sadness over the loss.[110] After learning sign language in a comfortable environment provided by human caretakers, chimps transferred to laboratories have communicated their fear and anguish.

From homology of more than 98% between human and chimpanzee DNA sequences, biologists have inferred that the two taxa have descended from a common ancestor that lived as recently as half a million generations ago (about five million years, a short time on the evolutionary scale).[111] As knowledge has grown of genetic homologies and other comparisons, designers of taxonomic trees have gradually demoted the human from a one-species limb to a twig on a branch. According to a tree that is recent as of this writing, the genus of *H. sapiens* is *Homo*, which, with *Pan*, the genus of the two species of chimpanzee (common and bonobo), forms the tribe *Hominini* (the hominins), which, with *Gorillini* (the tribe of gorillas), forms the subfamily *Homininae* (the African apes or hominines), which, with *Ponginae* (the subfamily of the orangutan), forms the family *Hominidae* (the great apes or hominids), which, with *Hylobatidae* (the family of the gibbons, the lesser apes), forms the superfamily *Hominoidea* (the hominoids). Taxonomists have been tripping over themselves in sketching all these taxa and coining all these names. Any notion of a definitive taxonomic scheme is belied by the taxonomists' unceasing process of redrawing their trees. As biologists accumulate observations, taxonomists rearrange the branches, move populations around, and recharacterize the memberships.

A ring species is a sequence of populations each of which interbreeds with its predecessor and successor except that the first and last in the sequence are geographical neighbors that do not interbreed. *Hominini* might nowadays appear to us as a ring species were it not the case, *per accidens*, that many intermediates in the sequence beginning with humans and ending with

---

[109] McMahan 2002, p. 321.   [110] Cavalieri and Singer 1993, pp. 67–68.
[111] The hypothesis in Patterson 2006 of hybridization following the beginning of speciation suggests another common ancestor that lived about a million years earlier.

chimpanzees are now extinct.[112] If there were still living such intermediates as *H. habilis*, *H. ergaster*, *H. erectus*, and *H. neanderthalensis*, it would be salient that there is no discontinuity between human and chimp. So extensive are the present similarities of their members that it has been suggested that taxonomists should place the human and the two chimp species in the same genus. The human, it is said, is 'the third chimpanzee.'[113]

Of the taxa just mentioned, is there a reason why one should be more an object of moral concern than another? Donald Davidson holds that 'to be a rational animal is just to have propositional attitudes.' He expresses doubt that a creature could satisfy this condition without spoken language.[114] But rationality is arguably not a requisite of personhood for purposes of the duty not to kill. One could argue that in virtue of self-consciousness and other attributes, nonhuman apes are persons according to the definitions of Locke and Boethius. Kant, who too associates personhood with a being's ability to 'have the representation "I",'[115] does not confine personhood to one species. Kant imagines as rational beings both angels and inhabitants of other planets. As Kant did not know, some nonhuman animals can think of a self. Christine Korsgaard notes that a nonhuman animal may have a sense of a self even if it is not self-conscious to the extent that humans are. Such an animal may experience what is good for it from its point of view. Humans enjoy some of the same sorts of experiences and things that are good for nonhumans. We may prize our ability to comprehend quantum mechanics or to act morally, but we also value food, sunshine, and reproduction. 'Animal nature,' Korsgaard argues, 'is an end-in-itself, because our own legislation makes it so.'[116]

It would pose a false dichotomy to say that we must either treat nonhumans as we now treat humans (ceasing to eat and experiment upon self-conscious animals), or treat humans as we now treat nonhumans (practicing cannibalism and experimenting on humans against their will). We could choose some practice other than those alternatives.[117] We might carefully take account of observed differences in creatures as grounds for different treatments. It has been urged that we recognize all apes as persons in a community of equals.[118] That could entail that there extends to them our duty not to infringe, as Rawls would say, a scheme of liberties compatible with a similar scheme of liberties for others.

---

[112] Richard Dawkins in Cavalieri and Singer 1993, pp. 82–87.
[113] Jared Diamond in Cavalieri and Singer 1993, observing that 'the chimpanzee's closest relative is not the gorilla but the human' (p. 95).
[114] Davidson 2001. For an account supporting rationality of apes, see Glock 2000.
[115] As noted in Wood 1998, pp. 189–190, 210, n. 16.   [116] Korsgaard 2005, pp. 100–106.
[117] As suggested in Singer 2002, p. 224.   [118] Cavalieri and Singer 1993, pp. 4–7.

Consider the conjunction of carnivory and Zygotic Personhood, under-stood as the stance that (1) we may exploit self-conscious nonhumans at the dinner table and in the laboratory, and (2) we may never sacri-fice a human embryo. Those who adopt this stance may believe that we should favor human life because human life is sacred at all stages, and because being human is overriding. The potential to develop into sentient or self-conscious beings may also be possessed by embryos of other species, but as they are not human, their lives are not sacred. Let us scrutinize this view.

4.7 SPECIES PARTIALITY

Isaiah Berlin once wrote, 'Unless men are held to possess some *attribute* over and above those which they have in common with other natural objects – animals, plants, things, etc. – . . . , the moral command not to treat men as animals or things has no rational foundation' (emphasis added).[119] Suppose then

> *Property-Based Partiality* ('*PBP*'). It is permissible in all circumstances to favor, over members of all other species, members of a species whose developed normal members possess property ϕ.[120]

As a moral principle, *PBP* is addressed only to such creatures as are capable of moral choices. We may think of ϕ as one property, though it could be an n-tuple of properties.

What we have learned concerning variability and essentialism reveals *PBP*'s insecure footing. *PBP* presupposes, but does not justify, the premise that possession of ϕ by some number of species members to some extent allows it to be said that the 'normal' members possess ϕ. *PBP* does not provide for cases in which there is more than one ϕ-associated species. Similar problems would arise if *PBP*, instead of referring to normal members possessing ϕ, referred to a kind characterized by ϕ.

It is difficult to say whether partiality is defensible without knowing what ϕ is. If *PBP* is to justify partiality toward humans, then ϕ must be a relatively advanced cognitive capacity. In such case, *PBP* would undermine the case for moral equality amongst humans. Following Richard Arneson,[121] let us define the following.

---

[119] Berlin 1969, introd., p. xxiv.
[120] I am led to distinguish between property-based and other partiality by Graft 1997, p. 108.
[121] Arneson 1999.

Γ Property. A Γ property is a property such that

(1) possession of the property by humans to a greater extent than its possession by nonhumans qualifies humans for the superior moral status of persons, yet

(2) the moral importance thereby established for the property does not furnish a reason for according unequal moral status to human individuals correlatively with each individual's extent of possession of the property.

Viewed from the perspective of humans, a Γ property would be a nonrivalrous preeminence, a badge of humanity that is not a basis for invidiousness among humans. Arneson argues persuasively that none of the properties usually associated with personhood – rational agency, second-order volitions, an arbitrary minimum of cognitive ability, autonomy, capacity to set ends, complex interests – is a cognitive Γ property. To which he adds that it seems unlikely that there exists an affective Γ property. Even the 'range properties' envisioned by Rawls fail to qualify as Γ properties. A range property is such that all people possessed of at least some minimum thereof are entitled to equal justice regardless by how much the extent of their possession ranges above the minimum. Rawls envisions two such properties, the capacity for a sense of justice and the capacity to form, pursue, and revise a conception of rational advantage or good.[122] Rawls imagines that his difference principle will treat the extent of either capacity above some minimum not as a basis for invidiousness, but as a common asset. Rawls is content to say that 'we cannot go far wrong' in granting that all humans, including infants, possess whatever is the minimum of the two capacities. Granting this for humans does not vindicate – instead it presupposes – the permissibility of partiality toward humans.[123] Inasmuch as Rawls does not specify a minimum – he says that a minimum as a 'vague' parameter is 'troublesome' and 'best discussed in the context of definite problems' – the two capacities do not reliably mark off humans from nonhumans. There is no evident Γ property.

PBP is objectionable because even if 'members of a species' were ascertained without regard to ϕ, *PBP* assigns great importance to ϕ. *PBP* inexorably puts forth the extent of possession of ϕ, which for a cognitive ϕ will vary, as a ground for inequalities in moral status among humans. In the case

---

[122] Rawls 1971a, pp. 506, 509, 512; Rawls 1993, pp. 19, 80.

[123] Rawls prescinds from interspecies justice. He observes that an account of right conduct toward animals will require from metaphysics 'a theory of the natural order and our place in it' (1971a, p. 512).

of prenatal humans, *PBP* furnishes a reason for inequalities in moral status according to the extent of ϕ for which potential is possessed. Since *PBP* is only a permission, this precept even allows an agent to treat some humans less well than nonhumans. One could rewrite *PBP* as an obligation, but that would exacerbate the invidiousness of ϕ's importance. Beyond this, there is the need for an argument why possession of ϕ warrants partiality. Predicating partiality on contingent properties of individuals risks neglecting moral persons who lack those properties, thereby failing the requirement of universality.[124]

Mary Warnock argues that

[T]he concept of 'speciesism' as a form of prejudice is absurd. Far from being arbitrary, it is a supremely important moral principle. If someone did *not* prefer to save a human rather than a dog or a fly, we would think him in need of justification. It is not prejudice to work for the survival of one's own species; nor is it culpable injustice to accord to one's own species a privileged position with regard to resources and care. . . . I do not, therefore, regard a preference for humanity as 'arbitrary,' nor do I see it as standing in need of any other justification than that we ourselves are human.[125]

In this vein, Robert Nozick offers

the general principle that the members of any species may legitimately give their fellows more weight than they give members of other species.[126]

This principle too affirms a permission rather than an obligation. It allows if not invites unequal treatment of one's fellows. A permission to favor affords leeway to seize upon a non-Γ property in selecting whom to favor. Only a partiality *obligation* can establish a Γ property.[127] Nozick's principle may be revised to state a general obligation.

> *Species Self-Partiality* ('*SSP*'). The members of a species must give their fellows more weight than they give members of other species.

Membership in the set of 'fellows' is a Γ property. To illustrate for the case of human agents, all and only members of *H. sapiens* are fellows of human agents, thus persons entitled to the benefit of *SSP*, and, insofar as membership in *H. sapiens* does not admit of degrees, fellowship cannot ground inequalities among humans.

But the set of human fellows would be fuzzy if fellowship were acquired gradually, as is personhood on some accounts. The value of a fuzzy set's membership function μ may vary within $[0, 1]$ correlatively with the extent of possession of some property. For *SSP* to endorse partiality toward human

---

[124] Here I follow Rawls 1971a, p. 132.   [125] Warnock 1983, p. 242.   [126] Nozick 1997, p. 308.
[127] As pointed out in Arneson 1999, p. 124.

fellows, there must be some μ minimum attained only by humans. We, upon positing some minimum, cannot merely assume that humans attain it. That would beg the question of the permissibility of partiality toward humans. For a minimum μ to exclude nonhuman African apes from the set of fellows, μ must be predicated on some relatively advanced cognitive property, one that doubtless will exclude from personhood human infants and mentally-impaired adults. Whereupon *SSP*, having rested personhood on that property, will have established a reason for varying the extent of personhood according to variation in extent of possession of that property. Why not, some will ask, recognize as persons for some purposes only exceptionally intelligent people? It is untenable that by appeal to species partiality one would partition a human population so as to corrode moral principles affirming equality.

For *SSP* to be grounded on a Γ property and to avoid undermining the equality of humans, the set of fellows must be interpreted to be crisp (i.e., nonfuzzy). If we interpret fellowship as membership in *H. sapiens*, the set of fellows will be crisp at least in the present epoch. Notice that this entails that the set of fellows includes every developmental stage of the species.[128] Whereupon *SSP* becomes

> *SSP′*. The members of a species must give their conspecifics, of all developmental stages, more weight than they give members of other species.

To appraise *SSP′*, let us generalize the Rawlsian original position. The convening parties represent a set of creatures that includes members of more than one species, and of more than one higher taxon, living amongst each other. Each of those represented is self-conscious and possessed of sufficient cognitive and other capacities to have a sense of justice and to appreciate the strains of commitment. The parties seek to foster cooperation for mutual advantage among those represented. By virtue of the veil of ignorance, the parties do not know to which taxa they respectively belong. Just as Rawls's parties imagine the lot of the least advantaged humans, our parties imagine the lot of the weakest represented taxon. They reject force as a means of resolving claims. They license use of force against a represented being only in self-defense. Free to fashion terms of cooperation rather than rules of species partiality, the parties are not motivated to deny fuzziness of species, or to eschew fuzziness in sets of persons. The parties know that because reproductive communities are single-species structures, they have reason to distinguish interspecies from intraspecies justice, and to

---

[128] This would also hold for *PBP* if converted to an obligation.

render them consistent. The parties will know that nutrition will motivate preying on nonrepresented taxa. Survival will require defense, especially of the young, against nonrepresented predators. Neither circumstance will determine whether agents may treat embryos of their own species as means for benefit of conspecifics. 'We ought not allow pathogens to harm *in vitro* embryos' does not entail 'we ought not sacrifice an embryo for benefit of our fellows.' On intraspecies morality, the argument from nonenablement will draw their attention.

Our parties will face complexities similar to those that arise in fashioning the law of nations. Much more may be theorized about how they would reason. But I infer from the foregoing that rational beings would not, if they had the power to govern, adopt *SSP* or *SSP'*. Such a rule does not provide for an ordering of claims, even amongst those rational and capable of agreement, by any means other than cunning and force.[129] It instead rests morality on luck. We humans happen to have larger brains. We dominate our planet. *SSP'* would justify our dominance. But suppose that Martians invade the Earth. They are more intelligent than humans. They enslave humans and wantonly consume humans for food and in experiments. 'The members of a species,' the Martians explain, 'are duty bound to give their conspecifics, of all developmental stages, more weight than they give members of other species.' *SSP'*, it now seems to us, is a travesty of morality.

Which is not to say that all species partiality is mere prejudice. Warnock's view and Nozick's principle seem to capture a moral intuition that many of us share. Human interests may be more complex than those of many other animals, and we may, and perhaps must, take account of complexity of interests. But given our exploitation of animals, there is more reason for concern about the danger of species partiality than about its defense.

Absence of property mappings does not leave us completely in the dark. We surely can reason that if an animal is a robin, it is highly likely that it flies. But we cannot ignore the likelihood of multiple realizability of properties by virtue of variety in mechanisms. If we are thinking of properties such as self-consciousness and rationality to which humans assign moral significance, we should be cognizant of chimps as well as ourselves. When someone in the grip of species partiality infers properties from species membership, they may be recognizing only properties included in the stereotypes by which, as Putnam's account describes, species are posited. Species stereotyping may neglect properties of moral significance. Nowhere in the official taxonomic

---

[129] Here I apply the argument against general egoism in Rawls 1971a, p. 136.

description of apes, dolphins, or pigs will we find 'self-conscious.' Favoring one's species regardless of properties possessed by nonmembers has been assimilated to favoring one's race regardless of properties possessed by nonmembers.[130]

In *SSP'*, 'give more weight' is vague. The scope of what one could justify under Warnock's standard of working for survival of one's species is narrow. Neither *SSP'* nor Warnock's standard explicitly licenses killing. No one has successfully reduced interspecies justice to a prescription, nor to an internally consistent list of situations in which, and the extent to which, species partiality is justified. Hare envisions that we would navigate by maximizing quality-adjusted life years of sentient beings; Singer urges the rule of according equal consideration to sentient beings' interests. Both schemes will stumble in executing their computations, not to mention opposition thereto in principle. Kantian morality issues in a duty to respect rational nature, which, as interpreted by Allen Wood, commands respect not only for rational beings, but also for nonhuman animals insofar as the latter possess 'fragments' and 'the infrastructure' of rational nature. But Wood concludes that 'I do not know how in general to decide' when animal welfare should prevail over the ends of humans. We are bound by 'wide rather than strict duties, and . . . we can never find a mechanical procedure for deciding between the claims they make on us and the claims made by human ends.'[131]

The notion of respect for life as often invoked against embryo use relies on a covert appeal to species partiality. According to one who conjoins Zygotic Personhood and carnivory, we may never sacrifice those early humans whose potential is so bounded that they cannot become self-conscious, but we may exploit nonhumans that *are* self-conscious. We should not use any human embryos in the relief of suffering of self-conscious humans, but we may inflict suffering on chimps and other self-conscious nonhumans as research subjects. A similar double standard is applied by a vegetarian adherent of Zygotic Personhood who condones human consumption of fertilized chicken eggs, a practice that exploits chicken reproduction, but who condemns use of fertilized human eggs after the progenitors have declined intrauterine transfer.

Of species partiality, no clear permission or duty has been established. Operating by a double standard calls for a justification. We also have no reason to allow candidate permissions or duties that foist species partiality to dictate *intra*species morality about developmental stages. *SSP'* does

---

[130] Singer 2002, p. 315; Wood 1998, p. 199.
[131] Wood 1998, pp. 200, 202, 210. Kant uses the notion of 'analogues' in referring to nonhuman animals in respect of humanity (*Lectures on Ethics* 27: 459).

not even say what weight conspecifics must give one developmental stage relative to another. All that *SSP'* may be taken to imply about creatures in early stages is their undifferentiated inclusion as fellows. That inclusion, the lumping of all stages together, has originated in a strategy to avert invidiousness in the treatment of developed humans. It has not issued from any thought given to early human stages themselves. Species partiality in what I take to be its most plausible form, *SSP'*, provides no reason against using human embryos for benefit of other humans.

4.8 INFERENCES WITHIN THEISTIC ETHICS

Let us return to the religious fount from which the ideal of respect for life emanates. This source advances another reason for holding that duties concerning developmental stages should differ by species. It adduces a belief in God's special affection for humans. From this affection, Zygotic Personhood is said to follow. In opening this subject here, I assume, for reasons given in the next chapter, that we should accord religious views a wide berth.

The decisive consideration in theistic ethics is what God wants. The challenge is to learn what God wants. In the work of Robert M. Adams, we are given a carefully constructed theistic framework for ethics. This account does not purport to answer directly the ethical questions left unanswered by ancient religious texts, but instead shows how a theist may insightfully tackle questions. Adams argues that excellences of things 'must consist, not in God's attitude toward them, but in something in them that grounds God's attitude, or provides God a reason for it. Excellence should have grounds in the nature or condition of the excellent thing.'[132] In particular, the excellence of a thing consists in those properties in virtue of which it resembles God. The ground of reverence for life is respect for such an excellence. Of course it may be believed that God has caused things to possess the properties that they do. But Adams effectively argues that it is not plausible to believe that God loves a thing on no grounds in particular. Adams rejects Ronald Dworkin's view that things become sacred to the extent of God's or our investment of effort in creating them.[133] If Dworkin's investment theory were correct, everything would be sacred to an extent correlative with its complexity alone. A galaxy might be more sacred than a human. Adams holds that God does not value a being solely by virtue

---

[132] Adams 1999, pp. 35, 114, echoing Plato in the *Euthythro* on whether something is good because the gods love it, or the gods love something because it is good.
[133] Adams 1999, pp. 122–124, replying to Dworkin 1993, pp. 73ff.

of how it came to be. So if one wishes to govern one's conduct by a view of how God values a being, one inquires into all that being's properties. If humans can resemble God, there seems no reason that other things cannot.

The relative minority in the Judeo-Christian tradition who interpret *Genesis* literally would interject that therein only man is said to be made 'in the image and likeness of' God. But a literal reading would also say that the universe was created fewer than 10,000 years ago in a six-day process that formed Earth and placed upon it 'every kind' of animal and plant. Our scientific evidence contradicts that account. An alternative reading of *Genesis*, as allegorical and figurative, is as old as Augustine.

> The Bible itself speaks to us of the origin of the universe and its make-up, not in order to provide us with a scientific treatise, but in order to state the correct relationships of man with God and with the universe. . . . [I]t expresses itself in the terms of the cosmology in use at the time of the writer. [T]he Bible . . . does not wish to teach how heaven was made but how one goes to heaven.[134]

Consider how an omniscient, all-loving, and all-merciful supreme being might view our predecessors. In a lineage, individuals resemble those immediately before and after them. This obtains even during speciation. Speciation does not happen fast enough so that parents belong to one species and their offspring to another. Members of the earliest human and chimp segments would have closely resembled each other. As earlier indicated, some of their members may have hybridized over a span of more than a million years after speciation began. Their resemblances could be salient today across a hominin ring species were it not for the accident of extinctions. Why would God select some but not all closely resembling beings as resembling Him more than others, and make them supreme in His affection? It might be suggested that mental attributes would motivate such discrimination. But we have noted mental attributes found in multiple taxa. Perhaps surpassing divine affection extends up the taxonomist's tree to a more inclusive taxon than our species. This point may be easier to see as to the future than the past. Suppose that speciation occurs within our subspecies when a subpopulation becomes reproductively isolated from the rest. If our subspecies today is sacred and supreme in God's affection, why would not both resultant subspecies be so? On the evolutionary time scale, the duration of a species is short. Our subspecies for long did not exist, may branch, and someday will become extinct. Is it plausible that divine affection attaches singularly to something that comes and goes?

---

[134] Pope John Paul II 1981.

It is said that humans are capable of thinking of God and of living so as to relate to God. They can identify the principles on which they are inclined to act, assess those principles, and engage in normative self-government.[135] Still it seems that the affection of an all-loving God, even supreme affection, would embrace more creatures than us. If so, any creature's dominion over others could be taken to imply not merely use, but stewardship. God may not be as invidious as the very brief passage in *Genesis* on dominion may seem to suggest. Were invading Martians to cite dominion granted them by God as a justification for exploiting us, we might doubt whether they had got God's will right.

'The image and likeness of God' is introduced in *Genesis* to describe a sort of being that God chose to create as master over earthly life. Like species partiality, dominion over *non*humans does not illuminate morality *among* humans about human embryos. The authors of the Bible and other ancient religious texts provide no guidance about extracorporeal embryos, whose existence they did not foresee. Since God is capable of regarding all developed humans as equal in any respect He chooses, He has no need of a Γ property. No pressure of theoretical consistency compels Him to separate humans from others, or to regard all human developmental stages as equal in every respect.

Since divine will is the arbiter of theistic morality, let us reason as one must within such a moral view. Imagine that we could have a conversation with God. We mention techniques with which we believe it likely that we can alleviate human suffering, techniques in which we would use donated extracorporeal embryos. We ask God's wishes. He knows the bounded developmental potential of an extracorporeal embryo, the vagaries of compelled remote parenthood, and all the other considerations adduced in the argument from nonenablement. I do not know a cogent argument for the conclusion that when humans are motivated to use their rational faculties to relieve human suffering by means of epidosembryos that cannot suffer and would not otherwise mature, an all-merciful and all-loving God would prefer that they refrain from such practice. The belief that God allows suffering to occur, or expects His children to endure suffering with patience, does not imply that He disfavors collective efforts to relieve suffering. The biblical accounts of Christ's ministering to the sick suggest just the opposite.

A crucial point is that for one who believes that God loves every human, it is implausible to impute to God the wish that the more humans, the better. A commitment to maximizing aggregate human well-being leads to

---

[135] This is the Kantian conception of rationality articulated in Korsgaard 2005, pp. 85–87.

the Repugnant Conclusion, namely, that it will always be better to increase aggregate well-being even if that action reduces average well-being to the extent that lives become barely worth living. Parfit's sensible response is that we are obliged to make people happy, not to make happy people. God could wish a lesser extent of suffering rather than a larger population. It seems implausible that an all-loving supreme being would wish that we adopt the rule that we shall gestate all human embryos regardless of the cost in well-being of other humans. This consideration, joined with the burdens that the Duty of Intrauterine Transfer would impose, suggest it implausible that such duty would be God's command. While affection for human life surely seems to include regard for human procreation, there seems no reason to think that the latter exhausts the former.

Thus neither an appeal to species partiality nor inferences concerning divine affection provide a cogent rationale for imposing the Duty of Intrauterine Transfer or for insisting on Zygotic Personhood as to epidosembryos. Embryos do not become persons for purposes of the duty not to kill merely because of the species to which they belong. The foregoing redeems the promissory note given in §2.3(e) for the premise that respect for life does not alter the analysis there given. Whereupon the argument from nonenablement proceeds. Mindful of symbolic, indirect effects, we observe that by definition, epidosembryo use may occur only in medicine, only in service of a humanitarian end. We observe the fresh voice given to respect for life by those who donate epidosembryos to the welfare of the living, and by scientists who labor to turn those gifts into the relief of suffering. The symbolic effects of their actions may be ennobling. Rather than it being the case that respect for life furnishes a reason to resist the argument from nonenablement, such argument helps us shape our understanding of virtuous respect for life.

CHAPTER 5

Consensus

The argument from nonenablement does not employ premises peculiar to any comprehensive moral or religious view, this because I have attempted to construct the argument to serve as the foundation of a moral consensus. As the next step toward attaining a consensus, in this chapter I turn to comprehensive views. I consider two views that constitute the source of the most significant opposition to embryo use other than the objections that I have already posed and discussed. The first is a view sometimes thought to oppose, and the second a view usually interpreted to oppose, all embryo use. I shall in due course offer an interpretation of each view, an interpretation that will issue in approval of epidosembryo use as permissible, virtuous, and a fulfillment of a collective duty.

As some would have it, our society's moral conversation about embryo use is already complete. Views on embryo use polarize correlatively with views on abortion, those views are incorrigible, and it remains only for citizens to vote. Although voting is inevitable, I want to urge that we not rest when we have merely found a position that some of us, or even a majority, find compelling. I do not take the matter at hand to be an instance in which managing conflict is better than trying to eliminate it. Should it come to pass that embryo use is installed by majoritarian rule in the absence of a moral consensus, that could leave a principled minority to chafe under what it regards as the yoke of immorality. In the alternative, if public policy prohibits or constrains embryo use so as to leave ameliorable suffering unrelieved, that outcome could bring deep regret by and for many left to suffer. Neither outcome would be harmonious or stable. Circumstances therefore present a compelling reason to strive for a consensus. Only cold comfort can be gotten from the prediction by commentators that consensus will form when embryo use first issues in a cure. Such talk may strike an opponent of embryo use as betraying a willingness to bring about embryo use *per fas et nefas*. The first cure might also be long in coming, or its use might be suspended because of side effects. In all events, the fact of achieving an end will not constitute a cogent reply to the objection that the means are impermissible.

We may take encouragement from the discovery, which I hope that this chapter will reveal, that we have not yet explored every conceptual opportunity for a consensus. We may also take instruction from the precept *'audi alteram partem'* ('hear the other side'). By framing questions from an opponent's point of view, by walking in the shoes of others, one can learn much about the struggles and unclarities within moral views that have led discussants to their verdicts. Sometimes we may wish to challenge another view at its roots, contesting one or more of its fundamental commitments. On other occasions on which we do not question any of a view's fundamental commitments, our analysis may reveal a position that, so it appears, is more faithful to those commitments, taken as a whole, than are conclusions previously offered by some of the view's adherents. The study of the morality of embryo use is an occasion of the latter sort. I propose to show how the argument from nonenablement compels assent within presumptive opposing views, sympathetically interpreted. If I am correct, then despair about prospects for consensus may yield to optimism as heretofore undeveloped and unaccentuated interpretations come to light. Given that the argument from nonenablement yet more easily finds favor within less strict views, we shall end with good reason to believe that the leading moral views of our time intersect in support for the humanitarian use of epidosembryos.

5.1 PUBLIC REASON

Let us consider the proposal that citizens and policymakers, when engaged in a public political forum in a discussion of embryo use, should refrain from appealing to religion or to any nonconsensus moral view. They should conform to what Rawls describes as 'public reason.' This constraint immediately appeals to some defenders of embryo experimentation. They have come to rue the influence of what they call 'insular' religious views. On the other hand, some religious believers complain that the constraint of public reason 'emasculates legitimate forms of democratic activity that are motivated by religious or private ethical considerations.'[1] I devote the first section hereof to the development of Rawls's revised view of public reason as it applies to the matter in controversy. I explain that such view is much less restrictive than might be supposed. Public reason furnishes a framework within which moral and religious views about embryo use should gain

---

[1] As described in Macleod 2001, p. 155.

expression. Understanding this may help well-meaning people mold their approach to hearing the other side. In my own account, I shall continue to consider pertinent views regardless whether they fall within public reason.

By a 'comprehensive doctrine,' Rawls understands a view of morality in general that includes an account of value, virtue, and character. Drawing on moral psychology and plausible conjectures about political dynamics, Rawls offers an account of how citizens may be induced to develop political conceptions of justice – conceptions that others can share – such that, across reasonable comprehensive doctrines, there develops not merely a compromise or *modus vivendi*, but an overlapping consensus on justice. Since justice is a moral matter, a 'political' conception of justice is intrinsically moral, not a slant on politics.[2] When competing interests preclude agreement on any one political conception of justice, the consensus will consist of more than one conception. In a democracy, all component conceptions will be liberal political conceptions.[3] A conception is said to be liberal if, first, it specifies and gives special priority to basic rights, liberties, and opportunities typical in a democracy, and second, it includes 'measures assuring to all citizens adequate all-purpose means to make effective use of their liberties and opportunities,' the latter a minimal condition for citizens taking part in society.[4]

As Rawls originally presented them, the requirements of public reason are twofold, one a general precept, the other a rule of exclusion said to follow from the precept. The precept is that

[C]itizens are to conduct their public political discussion of constitutional essentials and matters of basic justice within the framework of what each sincerely regards as a reasonable political conception of justice.[5]

Matters of basic justice and constitutional essentials are together 'fundamental questions.' The implication is that a conception will be reasonable just in case it is among those of which the overlapping consensus consists. Since a consensus will contain more than one such conception, 'to engage in public reason is to appeal to one of these conceptions. . . .'[6] The rule of exclusion is that public reason excludes all content of comprehensive doctrines other than components lying within the overlapping consensus:

[I]n discussing constitutional essentials and matters of basic justice, we are not to appeal to comprehensive religious and philosophical doctrines – to what we as individuals or members of associations see as the whole truth. . . .[7]

---

[2] Rawls 1996, pp. 147, 175; Rawls 1997, p. 610n.   [3] Rawls 1996, pp. 6, 134, 158–171, 164–171, 226.
[4] Rawls 1996, pp. 6, 156–157, 223.   [5] Rawls 1996, p. l.
[6] Rawls 1997, p. 584.   [7] Rawls 1996, pp. 224–225.

Public reason is a creature of reciprocity. Reciprocity 'requires of a practice that it satisfy those principles which the persons who participate in it could reasonably propose for mutual acceptance. . . . '[8] As I join with others in accepting the requirements of public reason, I refrain from insisting that the state implement my comprehensive doctrine. In the bargain, I gain the comfort that no one else's comprehensive doctrine will be imposed on me. Thus do I accept the wisdom of separating church and state – and the folly of merging them for short-term gain.

When citizens indirectly exercise state power through their votes, that exercise is legitimate only 'in accordance with a constitution the essentials of which all citizens may reasonably be expected to endorse. . . .'

Since the exercise of political power itself must be legitimate, the ideal of citizenship imposes a moral, not a legal, duty – the duty of civility – to be able to explain to one another on those fundamental questions how the principles and policies they advocate and vote for can be supported by the political values of public reason.

Like the political conceptions of justice from which they emanate, 'political values' are intrinsically moral.[9]

No one flouts public reason by harkening in their thoughts to their comprehensive doctrines – any more than they flout theorems of geometry by harkening to axioms – but all of us must discipline ourselves, when confronting fundamental questions, to think and advocate in accordance with public reason.

Justification is argument addressed to those who disagree with us, or to ourselves when we are of two minds. . . . Being designed to reconcile by reason, justification proceeds from what all parties to the discussion hold in common.[10]

For example,

If we argue that the religious liberty of some citizens is to be denied, we must give them reasons that they can not only understand – as Servetus could understand why Calvin wanted to burn him at the stake – but reasons we might reasonably expect that they, as free and equal citizens, might reasonably accept. The criterion of reciprocity is normally violated whenever basic liberties are denied.[11]

Imposing a comprehensive doctrine would illegitimately exercise state coercive power.[12]

The duty of civility, for Rawls, binds citizens in political advocacy and in voting when fundamental questions are at stake. It also binds legislators, government officers, and judges. For guidance in choosing how to vote,

---

[8] Rawls 1971b, p. 208; Rawls 1997, p. 579.
[9] Rawls 1996, p. 217; Rawls 1997, p. 583, with examples of political values given at p. 584.
[10] Rawls 1971a, p. 580.   [11] Rawls 1996, p. 217; Rawls 1997, p. 579.   [12] Rawls 1996, pp. 61, 247.

citizens would best imagine themselves legislators, envisioning enactments to which public reason leads them. 'Understanding how to conduct oneself as a democratic citizen,' Rawls holds, 'includes understanding an ideal of public reason.' The duty of civility also requires citizens to listen to others, and, when they have heard a compelling reason, to change their minds.[13] Openness to criticism, Bernard Williams once said, is the homage that candor pays to truth.

For Rawls, the extent of personal liberties is a fundamental question. So too, it would seem, is the matter of who possesses liberties, and who receives 'the protections of the rule of law.'[14] The legitimacy of sacrificing an embryo is a fundamental question.

What public reason asks is that citizens be able to explain their vote to one another in terms of a reasonable balance of public political values, it being understood by everyone that of course the plurality of comprehensive doctrines held by citizens is thought by them to provide further and often transcendent backing for those values.[15]

To illustrate balancing, Rawls supposes that among values that come to bear on whether to recognize the right to an abortion within the first trimester (which he plausibly classifies as a fundamental question), 'the equality of women is overriding.'[16] Or, we are to suppose, there obtains a cogent argument in public reason for recognizing such right. No reasonable balancing of values denies that putative right. In this situation, a comprehensive doctrine that strikes a balance of values denying such right will 'run afoul of public reason.' If a citizen follows such a doctrine to a voting decision against recognizing that right, the citizen violates the duty of civility.

In his original account of public reason, Rawls added the qualification that in some situations, it would be constructive for adherents to adduce their comprehensive doctrines as they bear on fundamental questions.[17] If doubt lingers whether an advocate subscribes to an overlapping consensus, the advocate may dispel that doubt, may reinforce the ideal of public reason, by explaining the roots of the advocate's allegiance to the overlapping consensus. A bishop might explain his church's rationale for separation of church and state. The Abolitionists who invoked religious considerations against slavery in the US spoke consistently with public reason inasmuch as a solid case against slavery already obtained within public reason. Their advocacy boosted that urgent case in the eyes of the public.

---

[13] Rawls 1996, pp. 217–219, 236; Rawls 1997, pp. 577, 605–606.   [14] Rawls 1996, p. 227.
[15] *Ibid.*, p. 243. Because 'political values' arise from an intrinsically moral political conception of justice, they too are intrinsically moral (Rawls 1997, p. 583).
[16] Rawls 1996, pp. 243–244; Rawls 1997, pp. 605–606.   [17] Rawls 1996, pp. 248–251.

In his revised account, Rawls takes the 'wide view' of public reason. According to this,

[R]easonable comprehensive doctrines, religious or nonreligious, may be introduced in public political discussion *at any time, provided that* in due course proper political reasons – and not reasons given solely by comprehensive doctrines – are presented that are sufficient to support whatever the comprehensive doctrines introduced are said to support (emphasis added).[18]

Public reason will exclude appeals to religious or other comprehensive doctrines if such appeals are unaccompanied by nondoctrinal reasons. But one can always urge the claims of one's comprehensive doctrine if one can find support for their conclusions in the overlapping consensus. Listeners may appreciate hearing how a discussant's religion or moral theory supports a consensus conclusion. Sharing the reasoning may enhance stability. In his revised account, Rawls even says that comprehensive doctrines furnish the 'vital social basis' of the conceptions of justice forming the overlapping consensus. For instance, the social teachings of the Roman Catholic Church support a safety net.[19] Religion may motivate moral action.

Fidelity to public reason will not work magic. It will not so much eliminate disagreement as legitimate it. 'The ideal of public reason does not often lead to general agreement of views, nor should it.'[20] It requires no apology that we must resolve matters by majority rule.[21] Holders of reasonable comprehensive doctrines who have made their case within public reason, but who have lost in the voting – Rawls uses the example of Catholics on abortion – will acknowledge the legitimacy of outcomes issuing from a democratic political process. They will not resort to force so as to oppose an outcome or to impose their comprehensive doctrine. They may continue to profess their view.

Rawls's valuable legacy for our understanding consists in his insightful account of how religions should accept majoritarian democratic rule, the separation of church and state, and the constraint of public reason. This account follows as an answer to the question,

How is it possible – or is it – for those of faith, as well as the nonreligious (secular), to endorse a constitutional regime even when their comprehensive doctrines may not prosper under it, and indeed may decline?

Under the regime of public reason, 'discourse may seem shallow because it does not set out the most basic grounds on which we believe our view rests. . . .'[22] Rawls responds that

---

[18] Rawls 1997, p. 591; Rawls 1996, p. lii.   [19] Rawls 1997, pp. 592–594.   [20] Rawls 1996, p. lvii.
[21] *Ibid.*, p. lv, and p. 241; Rawls 1997, p. 605.   [22] Rawls 1997, p. 590; Rawls 1996, pp. 242–243.

[T]he answer lies in the religious or nonreligious doctrine's understanding and accepting that, except by endorsing a reasonable constitutional democracy, there is no other way fairly to ensure the liberty of its adherents consistent with the equal liberties of other free and equal citizens.

He adds that

[I]t is only in this way, and by accepting that politics in a democratic society can never be guided by what we see as the whole truth, that we can realize the ideal expressed by the principle of legitimacy: to live politically with others in the light of reasons all might reasonably be expected to endorse.

Rawls supplies for a religious tradition the following justification of the foregoing bounds:

In endorsing a constitutional democratic regime, a religious doctrine may say that such are the limits God sets to our liberty. . . .

If anyone insists on enacting their version of 'the whole truth' – Rawls mentions fundamentalist religious believers and those who reject democracy in favor of autocracy or dictatorship – political liberalism as Rawls conceives it will reply that insistence on the whole truth in politics is 'incompatible with democratic citizenship and the idea of legitimate law.' It is 'politically unreasonable.' But Rawls believes that 'all the main historical religions' are reasonable doctrines. All will intersect an overlapping consensus on justice. Proponents of reasonable doctrines appreciate that public reason 'does not trespass on citizens' comprehensive doctrines so long as those doctrines are consistent with a democratic polity.'[23]

I began by mentioning a stricture, occasionally broached by scientists and others, that no one should interpose their 'insular' religious views as an obstacle to progress. One version of this stricture says that public advocacy should appeal to 'fact-based reasoning' alone, and that religious objections therefore must yield to progress in biomedical science. Of course we should insist on facts and reject falsehoods. But given facts, moral discussion remains. A controversy about whether we may kill something seems an unlikely occasion for categorical exclusion of religious espousals. In any case, the notion that a scientific endeavor should proceed without obstruction by a moral view is itself a moral view.

We are now able to see the import of public reason for epidosembryo use. Consider first opposition to such use. A religious believer could not, within public reason, merely assert Zygotic Personhood as an article of faith and leave the matter there. But as we shall see later in this chapter, there exist

[23] Rawls 1997, pp. 579, 613–615; Rawls 1996, p. 170.

religious proponents of Zygotic Personhood who have not taken that tack. They have argued for Zygotic Personhood. They have argued from genome to personhood, from respect for life to the classification of every embryo as a person, and from the effect of symbolism to the value of forbearance. While I shall contend that their arguments fail as to epidosembryos, still the arguments may be offered. They may be stated within a reasonable liberal political conception of justice; they appear to include no appeal to any part of a comprehensive doctrine lying outside an overlapping consensus of such conceptions. Sending forth those arguments, opponents of embryo use may adduce such of their comprehensive doctrines' teachings as yield the same conclusions. The wide view of public reason allows such discussants to present effectively their whole view on the issue. The duty of civility will also compel them to forbear, in public deliberations, from advocating teachings for whose conclusions they cannot find support in a reasonable conception lying within an overlapping consensus.

The argument from nonenablement also qualifies for inclusion within public reason. The argument may be stated within a reasonable liberal political conception of justice. The argument includes no appeal to any part of a comprehensive doctrine lying outside an overlapping consensus of such conceptions. It may even constitute an exemplar of argument within an overlapping consensus. Within public reason, proponents of the argument from nonenablement may go on to adduce such teachings of their religious or other comprehensive doctrines as yield the same conclusions as that argument. A Christian may invoke the duty of charity and support it by the argument from nonenablement's invocation of the Duty of Beneficence. A utilitarian who deduces that an epidosembryo should not be treated as a person for purposes of a pertinent duty may offer that conclusion, then adduce independent support from the argument from nonenablement. It might be rejoined that my account, while not invoking any premise peculiar to one moral or religious view over another, comes to a conclusion that takes sides in a dispute among religious views. What I have said does choose sides as to the conclusion – any stance for or against embryo use will choose sides in that sense – but does not choose among religious premises.

The 'wide view' allows introduction of a religious or secular *doctrine* – even if it is illogical – provided that for its conclusion, independent support obtains within an overlapping consensus.[24] A doctrine is a comprehensive moral, philosophical, or religious view that includes an account of value, virtue, and character.[25] The Nonindividuation Argument Against Zygotic

[24] Rawls 1997, p. 592.   [25] *Ibid.*, p. 573, n. 2; Rawls 1996, pp. 13, 175.

Personhood (again, '*NA*') is not a doctrine. Hence to *NA* applies the requirement that public reason conform to guidelines of inquiry chosen in the
original position, guidelines that include 'principles of reasoning and rules
of evidence.'[26] If my analysis is correct, *NA* departs from public reason
by deploying unsound reasoning. Thus *NA* fails the least demanding
requirement of public reason.

If unsound reasoning must be sent by the board, there is no room for
reactive attitudes unsupported by reasoning. Yet it has occasionally been
urged that we proceed by the rule, 'Any act or practice that strikes me as
repugnant ought not be allowed.' To be sure, there is much to be said for
moral intuitions, as well as for back and forth consideration of intuitions
against principles, this in progression toward an equilibrium. Repugnance
alone is an unreliable guide. In a moral discussion, when someone urges
us to reject an alternative because it repulses them but they do not offer
a convincing argument for rejecting it, we should continue to insist on
moral reasoning. An appeal to repugnance without argument is an appeal
to bare prejudice. Any view 'that proves resistant to explication may turn
out to be a prejudice that should be discarded.'[27] Imagine the shame if, as a
matter of public policy, felt repugnance constituted a basis for legislation.
The majority might legislate against religions, races, opinions, or conduct
on no grounds other than intense dislike.

I mention a sometimes broached, and, in comparison with public reason, rather crude rule about debate. This is the rule that when religious
views concerning a policy choice conflict, a government should abstain
from choosing sides. Whatever merits this rule may hold for the general
case, we are considering an issue that is intrinsically moral. Government
funding of research that uses embryos is a matter of policy and law, but the
permissibility of embryo use is a moral issue. Opponents may point out
that government has long since interdicted murder. The premise that we
ought not commit murder is not solely religious. It is a public reason. Religious proponents of epidosembryo use, asserting that charity and love of
neighbor are collective moral duties conformably with the consensus Duty
of Beneficence, may argue that a government that hampers the fulfillment
of those duties deserves collective morality; such a government relegates
citizens to suffering from which they might be relieved by morally com-
mendable collective action. As Rawls saw, it will be offensive to religious
believers of all stripes to exclude from public debate the views that lead
them to conclusions for which support already obtains within a consensus

[26] Rawls 1996, pp. 223–226, 243–244, n. 32.   [27] Arneson 1999, p. 124.

understanding of justice. Such exclusion would needlessly suppress the story of their motivation.

It has been argued that the 'wide view' of public reason is too indulgent as to official decisionmaking, and that in legislative halls, appeals to religious views 'cannot but be out of place.'[28] In theory, the separation of church and state disqualifies religious views as official bases for public policy. But in some local settings, no rule on separating church from policy obtains. Imagine a private secular institution – a university, research institute, or hospital – deliberating about whether to perform biomedical research that will use or create embryos. No consensus norm on the morality of that research seems apparent within the community served. It seems that the institution lacks an anchor to windward. I suggest that the institution should aim to follow such reasoning as lies within such consensus as there is, this by confining its analysis analogously to the way in which a citizen, in public debate, would conform to public reason. I say 'analogously' because insofar as a private institution is classified by Rawls as a private association, the constraint of public reason applicable in the public arena may not bind its deliberations.[29] But fundamental principles of justice penetrate into private associations. Officers of an institution deliberating about embryo research will inexorably take a stand on an applicable rule concerning sacrifice of early human individuals. That deliberation will place them in the virtual public arena. There public reason may serve as both beacon and constraint. For such an institution, moral justification obtains for use of epidosembryos.

To the extent that a religious doctrine cannot be adduced within public reason, its adherents may resent the ideal of public reason. Importuning a collective moral decision, they may regard insistence on public reason as dismissive.[30] We might respond by beckoning them to be reasonable, in Rawls's sense, concerning any of their contentions that evidently fall outside public reason. Our chances of persuading them will be better still if, on the merits, we provide a good reason for reexamining their view. Hence in §4.8, we considered some familiar claims about respect for specific life, regardless whether they fell outside public reason. I shall consider a theological view again in §5.3.

5.2 KANTIAN MORALITY

May we treat an embryo solely as a means? Some who have taken on board the second form of Kant's categorical imperative, including religious

---

[28] Larmore 2003, p. 387.   [29] I am grateful to Rawls for conversation concerning this.
[30] I owe this point to Stephen Darwall.

believers who may not attribute the precept to Kant, have thought that this question answers itself. They understand that it is never permissible to use a human being solely as a means. But the precept that they have imbued, the Formula of Humanity, reads thus:

So act that you use humanity, whether in your own person or in the person of any other, always at the same time as an end, never merely as a means.

By 'humanity,' Kant understands 'rational nature.' By 'person,' he refers to an autonomous rational being capable of legislating the moral law for itself.[31] Embryos are not rational beings.

What then of the treatment of embryos in Kantian ethics? Kant himself does not provide an account of the morality of abortion,[32] and he doubtless never imagined an extracorporeal embryo. But we may construct the following account faithful to his principles. The ground of the dignity of rational nature, which is above price, is autonomy.[33] Rational nature's characteristic feature is the capacity to set ends through reason. An injunction against using a rational being solely as a means may be understood, *inter alia*, as a command not to override another rational being's pursuit of ends of that being's own choosing. Beings that possess the capacity rationally to decide for themselves should be allowed to decide for themselves. In the case of a *non*autonomous being, use solely as a means cannot be said to override an autonomous will. But the Formula of Humanity is not merely an injunction against use of rational nature solely as a means. Neither it nor the other formulae of the categorical imperative constitute a decision procedure for ethics. The Formula of Humanity enunciates a *value* that is one of the most fundamental in Kantian morality, namely, respect for rational nature as an end in itself. Kant invokes this value in deriving duties to persons.

Within Kant's architecture, any duty that one has about how one should treat nonrational beings must be a duty to oneself, in particular a subcommand of the duty to promote one's own moral perfection. This obtains because Kant operates on the premise that every duty is owed to a person, either to self or to another. Wood argues for abandoning that premise. 'To treat humanity (or rational nature) as an end in itself requires more than treating humanity *in persons* as an end in itself.'[34] Wood continues, 'a reasonable interpretation of the principle of humanity as an end in itself requires us to respect the value of rational nature even in human beings who are literally nonpersons,' including conceptuses who have the potential to

---

[31] *Groundwork of the Metaphysics of Morals* 4:428–429, 4:435. As noted in Rawls 2000, pp. 187–190, Kant in various places also associates 'humanity' with understanding and moral feeling.
[32] Wood 1999, p. 370, n. 31.   [33] *Groundwork* 4:435–436.   [34] Wood 1999, p. 144.

become rational.[35] '[W]e surely would dishonor rational nature if we did not cherish its development. . . .' We shall lack a good will unless we show concern for the welfare of the potentially rational. 'It would show contempt for rational nature,' Wood says, 'to be indifferent to its potentiality. . . .'

As with respect for life, respect for rational nature is a concept that we must shape. How should we express respect for rational nature in our actions toward humans who are not full-fledged rational beings? What acts would or would not treat rational nature as an end in itself? A Kantian view could assert a duty not to use any enabled embryo or infant solely as a means. That duty could also encompass mentally incompetent adults as well as developed humans who happen to be asleep or anesthetized. Each such human has an unbounded potential to become rational, has been rational, or has the capacity to resume being rational.[36]

What of respect for rational nature in the case of extracorporeal embryos? The argument from nonenablement serves to shape a Kantian view. That argument comports with, and may draw support from, Kantian reasoning. It will be recalled that the argument rejects the Duty of Intrauterine Transfer on the ground that whether to undergo an invasive medical procedure or to initiate a pregnancy is reserved to a person's autonomous discretion. To this a Kantian might add that to oblige a woman to undergo transfer of an embryo into her when she does not want to bear a child is to oblige her to dishonor dignity in her own person. It may also oblige her to risk disserving the happiness of others. As to whether there obtains a duty to allow adoption, Kant states no duty to rescue as such. A duty to rescue must be inferred in 'transition' to particular situations.[37] The analysis given in §2.3(b) considers the scope of mandatory aid and the burden of rescue in the situation of an extracorporeal embryo that can develop further only via intrauterine transfer. That analysis leaves no reason by which a Kantian view should command surrender of an embryo for adoption after autonomous discretion has been exercised against transfer into self. The argument from nonenablement showed the reasonableness of the maxim 'I shall decide as I wish, in view of my situation, about whether to undergo intrauterine transfer or to allow adoption of an extracorporeal embryo of which I am a progenitor.' It may be argued that within a harmonious system of legislation in a kingdom of ends, a rational being expressing respect for the dignity of a rational will as an end in itself

---

[35] Wood 1998, pp. 197–199.

[36] Insofar as this duty applies only to use of a being without killing it, it should not be mistaken for a verdict on abortion, whose more complicated analysis would consider respect for the mother's autonomy as well as for the potential of the conceptus.

[37] *The Metaphysics of Morals* 6:468–469.

would will the universalization of that maxim. Thus does Kantian reasoning support the conclusion that intrauterine transfer into self or other lies within a progenitor's discretion. From this follows the permissible boundedness of an epidosembryo's developmental potential.

On the question whether the state should take custody of extracorporeal embryos that would not otherwise begin gestation, Kant's view supports the same conclusion yielded by Mill's harm principle. Kant would reject any notion that the state, or citizens against citizens, may enforce ethical duties.

Now enters the duty of beneficence of which Kant was a leading proponent. To establish that duty, Kant argues that treating humanity an end in itself, as well as consistency in what from self-love we will as to ourselves, require that we further the ends of others, that we take their ends as our own, and that we assist them when in need.[38] We must imagine ourselves standing seriatim in the shoes of our fellows who suffer from maladies that we might cure. We must imagine ourselves in the shoes of those generous people willing to donate embryos of permissibly bounded developmental potential. We owe respect to the autonomous choices of such people as fellow originators of the laws of a moral commonwealth.

Wood observes that 'cultural advancement in the interpretation of what it means to respect rational nature in persons is something that moves slowly, often in fits and starts.' Intrauterine transfer of an unwanted embryo, he holds, is an 'extraordinary measure.' In a cogent Kantian defense of embryonic stem cell research, he writes,

> If preserving the life of an embryo would require extraordinary measures, and also stand in the way of scientific research that promises to extend the lives and protect the rational capacities of many, many persons in the strict sense, then preserving the life of that embryo expresses, on the whole, a gross disrespect for rational nature.[39]

While acknowledging that multiple Kantian lines of reasoning sometimes arise concerning a given moral practice, we have learned through the foregoing analysis of a Kantian justification for epidosembryo use – a justification that may contribute to an overlapping consensus.

---

[38] *The Metaphysics of Morals* 6:393, 453. In the more well-known argument of the *Groundwork* 4:423, 431, Kant contends that we cannot universalize a maxim of nonbeneficence. Wood points out (1999, pp. 100–102, 358–359) that the nonuniversalizability of a maxim, while establishing that we sometimes may not take the action set forth in the maxim, does not entail that we must adopt the maxim's contradictory, and hence that this argument depends on the premise that for all rational beings, one's own happiness is an end.

[39] Wood 2005, pp. 319–320.

5.3 THE CATHOLIC MAGISTERIUM

One cannot expect to grasp the deliverances of any well-developed moral view if, in judging a practice, one consults only aphorisms or fails to secure an understanding of that view's deepest commitments. This caution bears particularly on the interpretation of Catholicism. Believers have often heard that 'life begins at conception,' that 'every human being has a right to life.' We need to ask on what ground those declarations rest, and how they should be interpreted. I shall be concerned in the balance of this chapter to probe the pertinent beliefs of Catholicism to their roots. Of course there are many other religions, some of which have been interpreted to support what I have defined as epidosembryo use,[40] and others of which have been interpreted to oppose it. In discussing the teachings of the Roman Catholic Church (hereafter 'the church'), I shall be neglecting direct discussion of other religious views. I believe that this is an appropriate economy for the following reason. In respect of embryo use, I endeavor to consider opposition in its strongest form. Hence I travel the path of most resistance. I take the magisterium of the Holy See, as set forth in the instructions of the Sacred Congregation for the Doctrine of the Faith, to be the most fully developed religious stance against embryo use. Within its instructions, one finds the principal objections to embryo use that one hears advanced by members of other denominations. Even nonreligious moralists have sometimes asserted the magisterium's claim that human life is sacred. Inasmuch as the magisterium's instructions were originally issued in Latin, and are lengthy and in some places recondite, the details of their arguments may not be widely known, even among Catholics.

I undertake to show that, all things considered, the verdict that most faithfully fulfills the principles of Catholicism supports epidosembryo use.

(a) Two doctrines

According to the mores of ancient Greece and Rome, it was permissible to kill slaves and barbarians. The Spartans abandoned deformed infants to

---

[40] E.g., these words of an Anglican theologian: '[T]he view to which I find myself drawn is that embryos at a developmental stage prior to the formation of a brain, a necessary condition of conscious life, are not human persons. It is thus morally permissible to conduct experiments which promise a great and otherwise unobtainable good for persons, since there is no possibility of causing pain or distress to the organism. Further, I would regard this as part of the proper exercise of human responsibility for eliminating suffering and gross malfunction. . . .' (Ward 1990, pp. 117–118). Or again, 'The Judeo-biblical tradition does not grant moral status to an embryo before 40 days of gestation. Such an embryo has the same moral status as male and female gametes, and its destruction prior to implantation is of the same import as the "wasting of human seed." . . . [T]he moral obligation to save human life, the paramount ethical principle in biblical law, supersedes any concern for lowering the barrier to abortion by making the sin less heinous' (Tendler 2000, p. H3).

the elements. Aristotle and Seneca endorsed infanticide of the deformed.[41] Infanticide is still practiced in some modern societies, often as a means of sex selection. Against these and other assaults, the church has long championed human life. Against abortion, the current magisterium asserts two doctrines, Zygotic Personhood (as defined in §2.1) and the following.

> *Respect for Human Life.* Human life is a sacred gift of God that we must respect.

Invoking Respect for Human Life, the magisterium does not oppose technology in general, but it issues a condemnation extending across the broad sweep of artificial interventions in human reproduction. Other people may fall into inconsistency as they approve the practice of assisted reproduction, in which surplus embryos perish in vain, while condemning use of embryos for humanitarian purposes. The magisterium does not fall into any such inconsistency. The magisterium condemns *in vitro* fertilization (again 'IVF'), intrauterine embryo transfer, embryo cryopreservation, reprocloning, and all other methods of assisted reproduction, as well as all forms of embryo experimentation not therapeutic for the embryo, including nonreprocloning.[42] The only artificial reproductive technique that the magisterium approves is artificial insemination that 'facilitates' intercourse. The magisterium explains its position as follows. Assisted reproduction achieves conception by nonconjugal means, thereby departing from God's manner of giving life. Nonconjugal conception deprives children of emotional bonding with their parents. Assisted reproduction may lead to eugenics. Assisted reproduction casts aside surplus embryos. It is wrong to destroy a surplus embryo, yet wrong to transfer it to a uterus. Artificial conception, observes Pope John Paul II,[43] poses risks for the conceptus.

In its consistent stance against taking human life, the magisterium also condemns capital punishment. 'The motive,' writes the theologian G. R. Dunstan, 'is admirable: to resist the erosion of the value of human life, already savagely assailed. . . .' Dunstan continues,

There are compelling reasons, theological, philosophical, and practical, why moralists should affirm the sacredness of human life. The task is the more urgent when every day brings news of assassinations, murder by terrorists, secret police and soldiery under the command of despotic governments; of wars, invasions, and insurrections; of widespread death from starvation; of torture and unjust imprisonment as instruments of political oppression. . . . It is to be expected,

[41] Aristotle, *Politics* 1335b20–27; Seneca, *De Ira* I 15. It should be added that in his *Medea*, Seneca apparently does not condone Medea's killing of her children.
[42] Sacred Congregation for the Doctrine of the Faith, *Donum Vitae*.   [43] *Evangelium Vitae*.

therefore, that those who feel most strongly that the sacredness of human life is under new threat should stake their claim at the highest conceivable point. . . . Unless a stand is made, no life is safe. . . . Desperate situations evoke desperate remedies; but not always the right remedies.[44]

In Chapter 4, we studied respect for specific life. From that analysis, it will be plain that Respect for Human Life alone is too nebulous to resolve the obligations of well-meaning people toward conceptuses in all loci. As to extracorporeal embryos, the analysis of Chapter 4 reveals how the argument from nonenablement contributes to shaping an understanding of Respect for Human Life and kindred precepts. To oppose epidosembryo use, the magisterium must rely on Zygotic Personhood. I therefore concentrate on Zygotic Personhood here. I first relate some pertinent history.[45]

(b) The first nineteen centuries

Aristotle held that all living things possess a nutritive or vegetative soul. All animals also possess a sensitive soul.[46] Only humans possess an *anima intellectiva*, a rational or intellectual soul. Insofar as it was Christian belief that only a soul enjoyed eternal life, early Christians were concerned whether a recently deceased conceptus or infant possessed a soul and might enter heaven. When does a human acquire an *anima intellectiva*? Throughout the first nineteen centuries after Christ, the magisterium, guided by leading theologians, adhered to the following Aristotelian view. Soul and body constitute a single substance standing to each other in the relation of form to matter. In Aristotle's theory of hylomorphism, form and matter correspond. This led Aristotle to the conclusion that an embryo cannot acquire an *anima intellectiva* any earlier than about day 40 in the male, or day 90 in the female – when, according to his observations, the conceptus first acquires a form distinguishing it from nonhuman possessors of sensitive souls. Morphologically, 'about this period the embryo begins to resolve into distinct parts, it having hitherto consisted of a fleshlike substance without distinction of parts.'[47]

Though time of ensoulment may have interested theologians as a purely theoretical question, from early on, as today, Christians were concerned with the question of what is the developmental stage after which abortion is homicide. The fifth commandment given to Moses declared, 'Thou shall

---

[44] Dunstan 1988, pp. 39, 56.
[45] At various places in this history I draw on Dunstan 1988, Ford 1988, and Engelhardt 1974.
[46] *De Anima* 434a22–434b8, *Politics* 1332b4–5.   [47] *Historia Animalium* 583b10–11.

not kill.' Kill whom? It was not doubted that one may kill nonhuman animals for food. Another rendering of that commandment, adopted in some Protestant traditions, is 'Thou shall not commit murder.' Murder consists in the unlawful killing of a person with malice aforethought. Who is a person for this purpose? Aristotle's framework – ensoulment – served Catholicism in answering these questions.[48] Aristotle condoned abortion of a conceptus not possessed of an *anima intellectiva*. Augustine declared that 'it lacks all sense' to think of a soul associated with a body 'not yet endowed with its senses.'[49] Augustine therefore distinguished an abortion in which 'the baby was already living' from an abortion in which the offspring 'dies before having lived.' Augustine's view, we may note *en passant*, would not recognize embryos as 'unborn children.'

In a definition quoted so often through the centuries as to become a standard, the Roman patrician and Catholic theologian Boethius (c. 480–524) defined a person as 'an individual substance of rational nature' (*naturae rationalis individua substantia*). Aquinas later wrote, 'The "individual substance," which is included in the definition of a person, implies a complete substance subsisting of itself and separate from all else (*substantia completa per se subsistens separata ab aliia*); otherwise, a man's hand might be called a person. . . .'[50] Adoption of the Aristotelian view by Aquinas secured its influence for many more centuries. Aquinas held that the intellectual soul is 'the formative principle of the body.' Until an embryo acquires an intellectual soul, the embryo is an animal.[51] Until then, *conceptio non perficitur* ('conception is not completed').[52] Upon the advent of an intellectual soul, the conceptus becomes *formatus et animatus*. Formation (acquisition of human shape) and animation (ensoulment) coincide. Aquinas settled upon day 40 in the male and day 90 in the female as the time of rational ensoulment. We may leave to one side this distinction between the sexes, which in 1753 was repudiated by Liguori.

The Aristotelian–Thomistic view was understood to preclude recognition of embryos as persons. A conceptus cannot be a person before formation of that soul that separates humans from beasts. Because context invariably made clear that it was an *anima intellectiva* with which they

---

[48] The predicates 'person' and 'ensouled' may have different intensions and extensions, but writers discussing abortion have not always been clear about this.
[49] *De Nuptiis et Concupiscentiis*, c. 15, as quoted in *Declaration on Procured Abortion*, n. 10. One reading of this view attributes it to Augustine struggling with a mistranslation in the Septuagint of the original Hebrew of *Exodus* 21: 22–23 (Jones 2005). But the Aristotelian view independently buttresses Augustine's.
[50] *Summa Theologiae* III, q. 16, art. 12.   [51] *Summa Theologiae* I, q. 76.
[52] *Scriptum Super Libros Sententiarum*, Lib III, d. III, q. 5, art 2.

were concerned, Catholic thinkers did not write 'intellectual ensoulment,' but instead simply referred to 'ensoulment' or 'animation.' Animation has also been called 'hominization.'[53] 'It has always been accepted Catholic teaching,' writes one commentator, 'that the presence of the human soul conferred human status. As its departure marked death of the human being, so its assumption into the body marked the beginning of the life of the human being.'[54] Proponents of 'delayed animation,' as the Aristotelian–Thomistic view of ensoulment no earlier than day 40 has become known, also call it 'delayed hominization.'

The present magisterium takes pains to say that none of the church fathers condoned abortion. Some thinkers in early Christianity and during the Reformation have been read to suppose 'immediate animation,' the infusion of a soul at fertilization.[55] But the church fathers who followed Aristotle and Aquinas in the thesis of delayed animation spoke of the severity of wrong as graduated by stage of development.[56] Pope Innocent III (serving from 1198 to 1216) settled on the view that the most grievous wrong was an abortion performed after quickening. Quickening (*vivificatus*) occurs between 12 and 16 weeks – roughly the time of ensoulment in the female according to Aristotle. Neither Aristotle nor Aquinas realized, as now appears to us, that sentience begins later. Had they the benefit of modern knowledge of when there develops a cortex and the neural connections necessary for sensation, would Aristotle and Aquinas have placed infusion of the sensitive soul in the late second trimester? It has been argued that since Aquinas must have known that no functioning brain has formed as early as day 40, he should be read to have believed that a soul can infuse when merely 'the *primordium* of the brain' has developed.[57] In any case, to kill flesh *and* soul (*carnis et animae*) was homicide. Abortion of an unensouled fetus was not as severe a wrong. Canon law solidified this view, declaring it fetal homicide to kill a pregnant mother whose fetus has formed. If her fetus has not formed, the wrong is less.

Early common law also fixed on ensoulment – no compunctions here about separation of church and state – as the critical event, taking quickening to evidence it. If anyone killed a fetus by striking or giving poison to

---

[53] Donceel 1970.   [54] Tauer 1984, p. 8.

[55] In Jones 2005, this reading is given of Tertullian, Basil the Great, Bonaventure, and the Eastern churches.

[56] As noted in *Declaration on Procured Abortion* ¶7.

[57] Haldane and Lee 2003, pp. 266–268. The authors go on to suggest that, given the biological facts now known, Thomistic principles could support immediate animation. Whatever view might now thus be constructed, there remains the historical fact that the Aristotelian–Thomistic view described in the text long held sway.

a pregnant woman, the question of homicide would turn on whether the fetus was formed and animated. Even at birth, a badly deformed fetus was, for lack of formation, not a person at law.[58] A brief departure from this doctrine occurred when Pope Sixtus V in 1588 extended the penalties for homicide to every abortion. But in 1591, Pope Gregory XIV reinstated the distinction between formed and unformed conceptuses. Notwithstanding discussion of contrary views, delayed animation held sway within Catholic teaching until late in the church's second millennium.

(c) Assertion of immediate animation

Formal adoption of the view that a soul infuses at conception dates from 1869. In that year Pope Pius IX issued a bull that added *procurantes abortum effectu secuto* ('those who procure a successful abortion') to the list of the excommunicated.[59] Pius IX did not accompany this insertion with any explanation. His decision could be accounted for by saying that abortion at any time is a serious wrong regardless whether there exists a soul. Or he could be read to have believed that if one does not know whether there exists a soul, one should not risk murder. Because the phrase that Pius IX inserted does not refer to any developmental age of the conceptus, observers interpreted Pius IX to imply immediate animation. In support of this interpretation, it was noted that in 1708 there had arisen for Pope Clement XI the question of what day shall be the feast day of the Immaculate Conception of the Blessed Virgin Mary. The church had already fixed September 8 as the feast of her birthday. The doctrine of the Immaculate Conception states that Mary's soul was created without taint of sin. Clement XI chose December 8 as the feast day of the Immaculate Conception. This implied immediate animation. The actions of Pius IX and Clement XI have since been taken as epochal. What is striking about them from our vantage point is the absence of an accompanying argument, theological or moral.

Dworkin suggests that Pius IX was executing a strategy. The incidence of abortion was rising in the late nineteenth century, and as Dworkin would have it, the church decided that, in legislative and other political deliberations on abortion wherever there prevailed the separation of church and state, immediate animation would serve as a more compelling ground of opposition than would the sanctity of God-given life.[60] But in 1859, people did not oppose the use of religious arguments in legislative debate

---

[58] As explained by Lord Bracton in passages quoted in Dunstan 1988, p. 46.
[59] Pius IX 1869.   [60] Dworkin 1993, pp. 39–50.

as they do today. No constraint such as public reason held sway. Whatever heed was paid to political circumstances, Pius IX was in any case taken to define the moment of ensoulment, transparently a theological construct. As we have just seen, this doctrine took effect only by inference from an entry on a list of the excommunicated.

(d) Prescinding from the timing of animation

The magisterium's writings eschew mention of the views of non-Catholic thinkers, although occasionally they allow that some philosophical discussion has occurred. By the twentieth century, there circulated among philosophers the Lockean view that self-consciousness is requisite for personhood, at least in the ontological sense. Meanwhile some Catholic theologians held to the Aristotelian–Thomistic teaching of delayed animation. The magisterium, seemingly aware of this, announced in an instruction published in 1974 that the proponents of immediate animation and delayed animation had argued to a draw. Whence the magisterium declared that ensoulment is 'a philosophical problem' and that the magisterium will prescind from it. 'For the matter will not ever be established' (*non enim de re unquam constabit*).[61] In a later instruction concerning reproductive technologies, the magisterium repeated its abstention thus: 'The Magisterium has not expressly committed itself to an affirmation of a philosophical nature.'[62] Though this statement might seem to indicate that the magisterium has prescinded from sundry philosophical questions, on scrutiny it appears that the intended referent of 'philosophical' is only the metaphysical question of ensoulment. The magisterium does intend to answer 'questions that are properly philosophical and moral such as the moment when a human person is constituted. . . .' To the question of when a person 'is constituted,' the magisterium's response is 'our moral affirmation,' to wit, Zygotic Personhood.

5.4 ARGUMENTS CONCERNING PERSONHOOD

In Chapter 2, I argued that the assertion of Zygotic Personhood as to epidosembryos permissibly barred from the womb cannot accomplish anything for anyone. But to assure a full hearing, I now consider the magisterium's case for Zygotic Personhood.

---

[61] *Declaration on Procured Abortion*, n. 19.   [62] *Donum Vitae* § I(1).

It is open to any religious tradition to declare its beliefs. The church could declare that its 'moral affirmation' of Zygotic Personhood is Catholic belief and that anyone who does not accept it is not Catholic. But the magisterium has not said that. It has acknowledged that personhood is a 'properly philosophical' question. For a religious institution, such acknowledgment is not the platitude that it might be for others. This acknowledgment concedes that there may be more than one answer worthy of consideration.

So we search the church's texts for an argument. Scripture is silent. This the magisterium effectively concedes after canvassing the oblique scriptural references to nascent life.[63] In biblical times, no one understood how reproduction occurs. They had no reason to muse about oocyte activation in a culture dish; they did not know of the existence of oocytes. The magisterium's rationale for Zygotic Personhood appears in the instruction in which it prescinds from the timing of ensoulment. The magisterium argues that because fertilization forms a new genome, a zygote is a new person. It writes as follows:

> 12. . . . From the time that the ovum is fertilized, a life is begun which is neither that of the father nor of the mother, it is rather the life of a new human being with his own growth. It would never be made human if it were not human already.
>
> 13. To this perpetual evidence – perfectly independent of the discussions on the moment of animation – modern genetic science brings valuable confirmation. It has demonstrated that, from the first instant, there is established the program of what this living being will be: a man, this individual man with his characteristic aspects already well determined. Right from fertilization is begun the adventure of a human life, and each of its capacities requires time – a rather lengthy time – to find its place and to be in a position to act. The least that can be said is that present science, in its most evolved state, does not give any substantial support to those who defend abortion. Moreover, it is not up to biological sciences to make a definitive judgment on questions which are properly philosophical and moral such as the moment when a human person is constituted or the legitimacy of abortion. From a moral point of view this is certain: even if a doubt existed concerning whether the fruit of conception is already a human person, it is objectively a grave sin to risk murder.[64]

Appended to the above text's phrase 'perfectly independent of the discussions on the moment of animation' is this footnote:

---

[63] *Declaration on Procured Abortion*, n. 5.

[64] *Declaration on Procured Abortion* ¶¶12–13 (a translation of which also appears in Ford 1988, pp. 60–61), as reaffirmed in *Donum Vitae*, § I(1).

This declaration expressly leaves aside the question of the moment when the spiritual soul is infused. There is not a unanimous tradition on this point and authors are as yet in disagreement. . . . It is not within the competence of science to decide. . . . It is a philosophical problem from which our moral affirmation remains independent for two reasons: (1) supposing a belated animation, there is still nothing less than a human life, preparing for and calling for a soul in which the nature received from parents is complete, (2) on the other hand, it suffices that this presence of the soul be probable (for the matter will never be established) in order that the taking of life involve accepting the risk of killing a man, not only waiting for, but already in possession of his soul.[65]

The foregoing is the full passage earlier quoted in which the magisterium prescinds from the timing of animation. Later in reiterating the above argument, the magisterium adds,

[R]ecent findings of human biological science . . . recognize that in the zygote . . . the biological identity of a new human individual is already constituted.

Certainly no experimental datum can be in itself sufficient to bring us to the recognition of a spiritual soul; nevertheless, the conclusions of science regarding the human embryo provide a valuable indication for discerning by the use of reason a personal presence at the moment of this first appearance of a human life: how could a human individual not be a human person?[66]

Using 'human being' and 'person' interchangeably, the magisterium goes on to evoke 'the personal dignity of the human being' and 'the dignity of the person.' It holds that respect for human dignity precludes experimentation with embryos:

No objective, even though noble in itself, such as a foreseeable advantage to science, to other human beings or to society, can in any way justify experimentation on living human embryos or foetuses, whether viable or not, either inside or outside the mother's womb.[67]

In addition to the argument that the church thus offers by reference to a new genome, two other lines of argument are discernible in its teaching as set forth above. I shall argue that, as viewed sympathetically from within Christian belief, each argument fails.

---

[65] *Declaration on Procured Abortion*, n. 19.

[66] *Donum Vitae*, § I(1), as also translated in Ford 1988, p. 63. A reiteration of this occurs in *Evangelium Vitae* ¶ 60, where John Paul II quotes approvingly its mention of 'discerning by the use of reason a personal presence at the moment of the first appearance of human life: how could a human individual not be a human person?'

[67] *Donum Vitae*, § I(4)–(6).

(a) From genome to person

In the magisterial instructions, two versions may be found of an argument from genome to person. The first version asserts that

(1) The genome of a new human being forms during fertilization.
(2) Formation of the genome of a new human being determines the characteristic aspects of that human being.
(3) Therefore, a zygote and any developmental successor is a human being for purposes of the duty not to kill.

Fertilization does produce a new human genome. Since the process is not instantaneous, premise (1) would plausibly be read to say that in fertilization, there occurs a pairing of haploid gametic genomes, and that by the two-cell stage, the genome of a new human being has formed. There has formed what we defined in §3.6(b) as a substantial genet. Let us so interpret (1).

Premise (2) paraphrases 'there is established the program of what this living being will be: a man, this individual man with his characteristic aspects already well determined.'[68] Even if a genome never were to change after formation, (2) delivers a dosage of genetic determinism that not even the most enthusiastic devotee of genetics could swallow. As for the implication of the new genome's uniqueness, to borrow a remark from Ayer, 'it is a contingent fact that the conditions of unique instantiation are ever fulfilled.'[69] What may be said is that, by virtue of the number of possible mating pairs and the occurrence in meiosis of allelic segregation, independent assortment, and recombination – in consequence of which the set of gametic genomes that each human is capable of producing is astronomically large – it is highly improbable that the complete DNA sequences of any two zygotes will be the same. If we interpret (2) sympathetically, reading 'characteristic aspects' narrowly, we could take (2) merely to assert that a two-cell embryo's genome is sufficiently formed to serve as such, subject to mutation, throughout life.

Even assuming that (1) and (2) when thus interpreted are true, the argument is invalid by reason of equivocation. A human zygote is a human being if 'human being' is understood in the sense in which biology can

---

[68] The following counterexample has been posed to suggest that genome fixation might occur too early to be plausible as the commencement of personhood. Engelhardt assumes (in 1974, p. 225) that removal of a donor skin cell in anticipation of somatic cell nuclear transfer establishes the clone's genome. Surely, he says, we do not recognize a new person merely upon removal of a skin cell. But this overlooks that a clone genome includes not only the donor cell's nuclear DNA but the enucleated ovum's mitochondrial DNA. Hence the clone genome does not originate prior to embryo formation.

[69] Ayer 1954, p. 22.

establish (1) and (2): the zygote is a being, and by virtue of association with humankind and with the species *H. sapiens*, 'human' is predicable of the zygote. That does not say much, since in that weak biological sense, any human body part is a human being. We know that people often use 'human being' in the stronger sense of an individual of humankind. So let us suppose that stronger sense here, and grant that, as concluded in Chapter 3, fertilization produces an individual of humankind. It is another matter to say that something is a human being if by that is meant a person. To say that a being is a person is to express a conclusion about the extension of a normative predicate. Biological premises cannot alone establish that an embryo is a person; one needs some moral reason. The magisterium remarks that at fertilization, the adventure of life begins. But that remark neither adduces any property peculiar to persons, nor conveys any explanation of how an unconscious life constitutes an adventure. 'Person' is the sense of 'human being' used in (3). The argument from genome to person slides from one sense of 'human being' in (1) and (2) to another in (3).

Our collective discourse is littered with the wrecks of arguments that thus equivocate.[70] 'Human being' and 'life,' because their extensions are larger than some discussants imagine, are not decisive classifications. Life has begun *before* conception. If gametes were not already alive, conception could not occur. Each part of us is a being of which 'human' is predicable, and it cannot be gainsaid that either in the weak biological sense or in the sense of a human individual, 'human being' applies to an embryo. 'Once a philosophical statement has been shown to be harmless,' Ayer also remarked, 'there is seldom much point in making it.'[71] The locutions 'human being' and 'life' breed equivocation. In my account, I refer to 'persons' because an assertion of personhood has the least chance of being mistaken for an exclusively empirical report. When we hear claims about whether an embryo is a human being or when life begins, we may say, 'These are pseudoquestions. Our genuine question is, "All things considered, how ought we to treat this being?"' That question calls for a decision rather than an answer.

To avoid equivocation, a second construal of the magisterium's presentation would have it advancing this argument.

(1) The genome of a new human being forms during fertilization.

(4) A genome suffices for a person.

(3′) Therefore, a zygote and any developmental successor is a person for purposes of the duty not to kill.

---

[70] For example, Kuhse and Singer 1990 points to this argument: every human being has a right to life, a human embryo is a human being, and therefore every human embryo has a right to life.

[71] Ayer 1954, p. 4.

The rhetorical question 'How could a human individual not be a person?' supports this interpretation of the text.

The magisterium cautions, in the same breath as it first makes its case, that it does not fall to the sciences to establish 'the moment when a human person is constituted.' The magisterium nods in the direction of Hume's dictum that we cannot derive an 'ought' from an 'is.' Yet the magisterium later contends that scientific observations suggest Zygotic Personhood. I leave aside the question of what science can show.

What is being asserted in (4) is that a being is a person in virtue of or by identity with a genome, regardless whether ensouled. This assertion foists what is, from the Catholic point of view, a radical version of materialism. It also commits to genetic reductionism with a vengeance. Materialism collides with the bedrock Christian doctrine that a person is a unity of body and soul, a *corpore et anima unus*.[72] Person and soul are inextricable. On this view, a being cannot be a person in virtue of having chromosomes if it does not have a soul. A Catholic must reject (4) on pain of self-contradiction. Or more. The Council of Vienne in 1312 declared that one who denies that the intellectual soul is the form of the body is a heretic.[73] To which the Lateran Council of 1513 added, '[W]e . . . condemn and reprobate all those who assert that the intellectual soul is mortal.' The heretics that Dante places in circle VI lie there by virtue of the latter assertion (*Inferno* 10.15). Of course mere matter such as chromosomes cannot be immortal. Spinoza's denial of the immortality of the soul brought about his excommunication from the Jewish community of Amsterdam, which evidently perceived belief in the soul's immortality as so fundamental that it was common to Judaism and Christianity. Thus the second version of the argument from genome to person does not square with Christian teaching. By dint of contradiction of a bedrock belief, the argument cannot stand.

The magisterium's equivocal use of 'human being' may have caused it to miss this self-contradiction. Suppose that, in an effort to escape the corner into which the magisterium by means of (4) has painted itself, the magisterium revises its position. The notion that it could have specified the timing of personhood while prescinding *tout court* from the timing of animation now seems self-beguiling. So the magisterium asserts immediate animation. It now characterizes genome formation as an indicator of ensoulment. It replaces (4) with two premises:

(5) Animation coincides with syngamy.

(6) A *corpore et anima unus* is a person for purposes of the duty not to kill.

---

[72] This concept of a unity stands opposed to any other notion of soul as separate from body rather than being the form of body. Among places in which the concept is articulated is *Donum Vitae* itself.

[73] Ford 1988, p. 59.

For the church, (6) is the definition of a person, hence a tautology. In (5) we have only the claim that a soul arrives simultaneously with a genome, not the claim that a genome is a soul. Since it is easily granted that fertilization initiates body, the burden in establishing that there exists a *corpore et anima unus*, and hence (3), is to establish soul. That burden must be borne by (5). But (5) is a bare assertion. It leaves the matter as Pius IX left it – immediate animation has been asserted, but without plausible explanation. When the magisterium chose to prescind from the timing of animation, it evidently recognized that there was no plausible account according to which syngamy, or any other biological event, evidences infusion of a soul. How and when a soul infuses is 'not within the competence of science to decide.' It is consistent with the Christian understanding of person and soul as inextricable, as eventuating simultaneously if ever, that person and soul would simultaneously eventuate at some time *after* syngamy.

Construing the argument from genome to person so as to avoid equivocation thus only brings into relief a contradiction of a fundamental belief. In retreat from that contradiction, a stance on timing of ensoulment cannot plausibly be resuscitated when it has been declared that *non enim de re unquam constabit*.

(b) Lack of a nonarbitrary beginning

A fertilized egg 'would never be made human,' the magisterium writes, 'if it were not human already.' Let us interpret this remark in its strongest form as advancing the claim that a zygote would never develop into the body of a person if a zygote were not such already, and as advancing the following familiar argument. There occurs no biologically significant event after conception and before birth that could plausibly be said to begin personhood. Hence the only nonarbitrary position on the advent of personhood is that personhood begins at conception. Of this, 'modern genetic science brings valuable confirmation.' A genome is either fully formed in syngamy, in which case 'characteristic aspects' of a human are 'well determined,' or the conceptus does not survive.

The following three considerations refute this argument. First, personhood in the normative sense is not an empirical fact ascertained by observation, as in recognizing a particle by streaks in a bubble chamber. Personhood is conferred when someone chooses to accord a being some treatment. A religious believer may envision a divine choice. Any choice is arbitrary in some sense. When Bernard Williams had occasion to defend the Warnock Committee's decision to settle on day 14 as the oldest developmental age of an embryo eligible for experimental use, he put forth a view that bears as well on this point:

It may be said that a line . . . cannot possibly be reasonable since it has to be drawn between two cases that are not different enough to distinguish. The answer is that they are indeed not different enough to distinguish if that means that their characteristics, unsupported by anything else, would have led one to draw a line there. But though the line is not, in this sense, uniquely reasonable, it is nevertheless reasonable to draw a line there. . . . [I]t cannot be an objection to drawing the line just here that it would have been no worse to draw it somewhere else – if that were an objection, then one could conclude that one had no reason to draw it anywhere, and that is a style of argument that led to the death of Buridan's ass, who (it will be remembered) died of starvation between two piles of hay because neither pile had any characteristic that drew him to it rather than to the other.[74]

We establish arbitrary thresholds for many roles (e.g., eligibility to drive a car or to hold public office). We seem confident that some time must pass after birth before the qualifications that we deem important for various roles have solidified, but we recognize that our rules are arbitrary in that there doubtless is no uniform age at which the qualifications are first possessed.

Second, the argument helps itself to the assumption that personhood can only be attained instantaneously. There arises the following contrary view. Nerves, the brain, and connective mechanisms that effect sentience develop over a period of months. According to Parfit's view, a human's continued existence involves nonbranching psychological and physical continuity and connectedness. One consequence of the degradation of connections over time would seem to be that personhood is not all-or-nothing. The extension of 'person' might have no sharp borderline.[75] Some may reckon personhood by family resemblance, or by discerning characteristics each satisfied to a degree. As Williams further remarks,

'Person' looks like a sortal or classificatory notion while in fact it signals characteristics that almost all come in degrees – responsibility, self-consciousness, capacity for reflection, and so on. It thus makes it seem as if we were dealing with a certain class or type of creature, when in fact we are vaguely considering those human beings who pass some mark on a scale.[76]

'Person' may be a phase sortal. We may conceive of the set of persons for a given purpose as a fuzzy set. A being could belong to the set more or less, with a membership value in the interval $[0, 1]$. Over the course of a being's development, its membership value may change. We may think

---

[74] Williams 1986, p. 190.   [75] Parfit 1984, pp. 322–323.   [76] Williams 1995, p. 114.

of the heterochrony of personhood.[77] To affirm equality, we may assign to all adults and children the same nonzero membership value. Catholic doctrine seems already to contain an instance in which a fuzzy set of persons is implied. It is held that only after a child acquires the faculty of reason is the child capable of sin. Although the age of seven is ordained for sacramental purposes as that at which reason is acquired, it is not supposed that reason is acquired instantaneously. The contrary view may also be taken that 'person' denotes an unanalyzably primitive kind of substance – persons can recognize persons even if unable to say exactly how.[78] That will not save the magisterium's argument at hand, which purports to establish Zygotic Personhood.

Third, a being developing from a zygote would not be classifiable as human if the zygote had not been human. Mutation does not occur to an extent sufficient to transform a nonhuman into a human. This does not establish the proposition that a being developing from a zygote could not become a person if the zygote had not been a person. Assuming delayed animation, which the magisterium in prescinding allows to be a tenable belief, a zygote could fail to be a person (or have a very low membership value as such) and thereafter in virtue of properties acquired in gestation and growth, its developmental successor could be a person.

(c) Possibility of a soul

The magisterium characterizes two propositions in its quoted footnote as reasons for the independence of Zygotic Personhood from a stance on timing of animation. We have seen that such independence is implausible. Let us consider instead what support those propositions might offer for Zygotic Personhood.

According to the first proposition, an embryo, if not ensouled, is at least 'preparing for and calling for a soul.' If 'preparing for a soul' describes an embryo, it would seem to describe oocyte development in the ovary. Yet we could not, without violence to common sense, classify all immature oocytes as persons. If we did, we ought to bar physicians from removing ovaries. Neither does a conceptus literally 'call.' Nor is it clear how it can be claimed that an embryo metaphorically calls without the claimant's begging the question of what moral demands an embryo places upon us. In any case,

[77] 'Heterochrony' is introduced in Gould 1977 for the timing of emergent features in the course of development.
[78] As in Lowe 1989, pp. 115–118, by which 'person' becomes one of those few sortals that do not embed an identity criterion.

when, as supposed here, an embryo is not yet ensouled, the embryo cannot be a human *corpore et anima unus*, hence cannot be a person. Nothing has been shown about how we are obliged to act toward an embryo.

Another proposition warns that because there obtains a nonzero probability of immediate animation or immediate personhood, anyone who kills a conceptus risks killing an ensouled human or person. While no one will ever prove immediate animation, no one will ever prove delayed animation either. Thus the magisterium admonishes against risking murder. This way of putting the matter as to personhood suggests that the question is, 'How should we act toward a being when unsure whether it is a person?' Outside theistic circles, this would be thought to betray a misconception of personhood. It does not make sense to say that we do not know whether something is a person; it is our choice whether to regard it as one. But for one who believes that morality consists in following divine will, there arises the question whether God's view may fairly be described as regarding a given being as a person for some purpose, or as having ensouled it. The medieval church developed an approach to answering a question such as that. *Tutiorism* (after L. *tutior* for 'safer') counseled that when in doubt about what moral verdict to render as to a contemplated act, one should forego the act.[79] This imprecise precept was given various formulations. The general notion was that one should follow the safer course.

In its admonition to avoid risk of murder, the magisterium appeals to tutiorism. The following considerations militate against applying tutiorism in this case. Seventeenth century theologians waged a protracted and polemical debate concerning tutiorism and casuistry. After Pascal's *Les Lettres Provinciales* satirically exposed casuistry as lacking an analytical foundation, and as rife with inconsistency, the influence of casuistry declined precipitously. Tutiorism succumbed to the criticism that it stifled liberty and unreasonably vexed individual consciences. '[A] tutiorist casuistry,' according to a recent retrospective, 'will not allow your conscience to be easy unless you avoid all actions *against* which any case whatever can be made. . . .'[80] Tutiorism offered no criterion for deciding which of two verdicts is safer. Nor did tutiorism become the church's teaching on the duty not to kill in general. Tenable arguments obtain for just war and killing in self-defense, but a religious believer cannot know for sure that those arguments comport with divine will. For all one knows, God does not allow exceptions to 'Thou shall not kill,' or may allow exceptions different from those that a given believer surmises. Notwithstanding this uncertainty, the

[79] Soane 1988, p. 83.   [80] Jonsen and Toulmin 1988, p. 260.

magisterium approves just war and killing in self-defense. The magisterium does not say that one ought not risk murder. Tutiorism is not its rule.

If consideration is to be given to casuistical notions of decisionmaking, one would have to consider the later and influential notion of *probabilism*. This term was predicated on 'probable' not in the sense of 'likely' but when taken to be a synonym of 'arguable' or 'tenable.' Probabilism holds that in a situation in which there seems to obtain more than one tenable verdict, one should adopt some tenable verdict that, after careful reflection, one thinks right. An approved method of reflection is to rest on how many wise doctors favor one verdict over another. This reduction of justification to headcounting became another easy target for Pascal. Probabilism has survived in the form of Liguori's 'equiprobabilism.'[81] Liguori, whom Pius IX called 'the helmsman of the safest course between laxism and rigorism,' held that 'where there is doubt whether the fetus is animate, there is doubt also about the fact of homicide.' Stripped of deference to wise doctors, probabilism nowadays seems understood within Catholic thinking as the precept that when considering whether an available act or practice is moral, one should reflect on known analyses and verdicts, then resolve one's conscience on some tenable verdict, then govern one's conduct in accordance with that verdict. Seventeenth century probabilists imagined an ordering headed by undisputed verdicts in paradigm cases, though they did not provide a rigorous criterion by which to compare verdicts in tenability. Probabilism does not suppose that one ascertains the most tenable of verdicts.

It has cogently been argued that Catholic theology installs probabilism over tutiorism as the appropriate precept with respect to an embryo.[82] For a probabilist, the magisterium's view that one may not sacrifice embryos in research constitutes only one candidate verdict. That one may use epidosembryos in research constitutes a tenable alternative. The magisterium's admonition against risking murder comes down to an admonition to apply tutiorism without considering the permissibly bounded developmental potential of an epidosembryo. Probabilism does not command agents to stand down in deference to possibilities that they conscientiously believe to have been permissibly foreclosed. So long as conscientious conviction precedes action, probabilism holds that one should act. Just as theists believe in God and govern themselves accordingly notwithstanding Hume's argument that of no being is existence demonstrable, lack of proof need not restrain one from reasoning to a belief and governing oneself accordingly.

---

[81] Not to be confused with the principle of equiprobability (Laplace's principle of insufficient reason) applicable as to future events.

[82] Tauer 1984.

Must a Catholic refrain from action when unsure what moral verdict to render on the action? Or must a Catholic follow that precept judged in good conscience to be more, or the most, tenable? We can imagine tutiorism and probabilism invoked in the choice of themselves. To say that a Catholic's choice lies between tutiorism and probabilism is to pose a false dichotomy. These are but two of theologians' inventions concerning moral doubts. The probabilist precept is a fancy way of saying that one should use one's wits to think through what is right. The authors of the magisterium have done that. They have reasoned concerning morals in light of faith. Since the questions with which they concern themselves are professedly philosophical, their reasoning lies open for scrutiny and debate. What we have learned about that reasoning is that the magisterium has not given a compelling argument for Zygotic Personhood. The magisterium seems to contradict Zygotic Personhood when, echoing Boethius on 'what a human person is and should be,' it writes as follows: 'Constituted by a rational nature, man is a personal subject capable of reflecting on himself and of determining his acts. . . .'[83] Embryos are not rational, self-conscious, or autonomous.

A claim of species partiality will not establish that unenabled embryos are persons for purposes of some duty, because as shown in the previous chapter, species partiality does not resolve intraspecies morality about developmental stages. Failing the establishment of Zygotic Personhood, a moral view may invoke the potential of embryos, but the magisterium does not mention potential. As we earlier saw, developmental potential varies with situation, and the argument from nonenablement shows why an epidosembryo becomes an eligible research subject by virtue of a permissible exercise of discretion that bounds developmental potential.

5.5 SUPPORT FOR EPIDOSEMBRYO USE

(a) The social duties

The church is a leading proponent of the Duty of Beneficence, known in Christianity as the duty or law of charity. In imitation of Christ, who showed great concern for healing the sick, the church exhorts its faithful to works of charity and mercy. In one of the instructions that we have been considering, the magisterium writes,

---

[83] *Declaration on Procured Abortion* ¶8.

To measure happiness by the absence of sorrow and misery in this world is to turn one's back on the Gospel.

But this does not mean that one can remain indifferent to these sorrows and miseries. Every man and woman with feeling, and certainly every Christian, must be ready to do what he can to remedy them. This is the law of charity. . . . Considerable progress in the service of life has been accomplished by medicine. One can hope that such progress will continue, in accordance with the vocation of doctors, which is not to suppress life but to care for it and favor it as much as possible. . . . [I]n the outpouring of Christian generosity and charity every form of assistance should be developed.[84]

The second greatest of the commandments, said Christ, is to love thy neighbor as thyself. The magisterium would not ordinarily look for illumination to Kant, but the following passage admirably explains love of neighbor:

Beneficence is a duty. If someone practices it often and succeeds in realizing his beneficent intention, he eventually comes actually to love the person he has helped. So the saying 'you ought to *love* your neighbor as yourself' does not mean that you ought immediately (first) to love him and (afterwards) by means of this love do good to him. It means, rather, *do good* to your fellow human beings, and beneficence will produce love of them in you. . . .[85]

As Hare points out, the command to love thy neighbor as thyself is of like effect as the Golden Rule. That command also comports with Kant's explanation of why we should further the ends of other's as if they were our own.[86] The Golden Rule, in various formulations, has appeared in virtually every moral view since Confucius, from 'Do unto others as you would have them do unto you,' to Hare's 'We are to do to the others affected, taken together, what we wish were done to us if we had to be all of them by turns in random order.'[87] In applying the Golden Rule, I must imagine myself seriatim as the possible persons corresponding to lives in development. I must also imagine myself as progenitors who wish to help others by donating embryos, and as each of the millions of people now or hereafter afflicted with diseases and disabilities that embryo use might alleviate.

If Zygotic Personhood obtained and embryo use were therefore wrong, it would not matter how many millions might be helped. We may not rob

---

[84] *Declaration on Procured Abortion* ¶¶25–26.   [85] *The Metaphysics of Morals* 6:402.

[86] Hare 1993, pp. 61, 107, 178, 221–222, and Hare 1997, pp. 149–151, 157; Kant, *Groundwork* 4:430 and *Metaphysics of Morals* 6:451–452, the latter of which discusses the principle of loving another as oneself. This principle is not to be confused with a 'trivial' negative version of the Golden Rule that Kant pulls no punches in rejecting (*Groundwork* 4:430n.).

[87] Hare 1993, pp. 10, 107, 153, 158, 221–222; Hare 1981, p. 129, following C. I. Lewis.

the bank to aid the poor. But the magisterium's arguments do not establish Zygotic Personhood against the argument from nonenablement, which has shown that the assertion of Zygotic Personhood as to epidosembryos could not gain anything for anybody. Meanwhile donations of embryos to research draw our attention to the love of children manifested by women who undergo fertility treatment and who only by statistical accident possess surplus embryos. Contributors of oocytes for use in embryo creation display exceptional generosity as they undergo the considerable burden and discomfort of ovarian stimulation and oocyte retrieval solely for benefit of others. Devoting the gifts of all these generous people to the relief of human suffering would express respect for the dignity of human life. I suspect that the solution to our present struggle lies not in asking anyone to compromise, but in asking others to look deeply into their respective views.

(b) Inferring divine will

A related Christian belief is that life belongs to God. Since human life is lived by humans, how should a believer act in deference to divine ownership of life? In theistic ethics, everything comes down to what God would want. The question whether as of any moment a soul has infused is the question whether God has chosen to infuse one. No one could plausibly claim to know divine will about embryo use from ancient texts, since they do not discuss extracorporeal embryos. But the following seems a plausible inference from within traditional Catholic belief. In Catholicism, it has been taught that only the souls of the baptized enter heaven, that the souls of unbaptized infants pass into limbo. If the thesis of immediate animation were true, limbo would swell with the souls of those many embryos that die *in vivo* or are miscarried. In such case, limbo's population would vastly exceed that of heaven and hell combined. According to Christian belief, God is all-kind and all-merciful. It would not seem that He would allow the vast majority of the objects of His affection to languish eternally outside His presence. This has led the church to consider abandoning the belief in limbo in favor of the belief that the souls of all innocents go to heaven. There is another plausible conclusion, namely, that ensoulment is not immediate. There is no soul that lives on when an embryo dies in the earliest stages of development. This seems assumed in Catholic ritual. When a miscarriage occurs, no funeral occurs.

We have seen how Christian theology has tied itself in knots over the timing of ensoulment. The very concepts of soul, of the time at which such a soul comes into existence – for all a religious believer knows, these notions are but primitive conceptual machinery cobbled together by humans in hopes of fathoming an ontology of a world that is quite otherwise as God omnisciently sees it. So if a believer can infer anything about divine will, whether by reflection on the divine attributes or otherwise, that furnishes a reason for action, regardless whether the reasoning is couched in the language of souls. Imagine again that we could have a conversation with God. We present to Him all the circumstances supposed in the argument from nonenablement, which I need not recount here. We explain our hopes of helping our fellow humans. He would know that if we refrain from research and therapy using extant surplus embryos and embryos formed from the surfeit of oocytes, no greater number of babies would likely be born. He would know that embryos as to which progenitors do not wish to begin gestation cannot suffer. As I suggested in the last chapter, it does not seem plausible that, all considered, an all-merciful, all-loving, omniscient God would wish us to forbear from epidosembryo use for humanitarian ends.

(c) Charity and assisted reproduction

One objection that Catholic doctrine might still lodge against epidosembryo use asserts that because agents use putatively illicit artificial means such as IVF to create epidosembryos, anyone experimenting with epidosembryos or their derivatives is complicitous in wrongdoing. It was wrong to create the embryos by nonconjugal means in the first place, and a good end will not justify a wrongful means. I propose to answer this objection first by broaching the possibility that the church could conclude that assisted reproduction is not wrong. I shall then argue that even if the church insists that assisted reproduction is wrong, epidosembryo donation is not wrong, nor does epidosembryo use render donee scientists, or any entity funding their research, complicit in wrongdoing.

The magisterium predicts that assisted reproduction in any of its non-conjugal varieties will deprive offspring of the bonding that usually occurs between parents and children conceived naturally. The magisterium holds that children are a divine gift. Parents fortunate to receive the gift are not entitled to it, and those not so fortunate should not complain. The magisterium also warns that assisted reproduction could lead to eugenics. Many theologians and believers, observing the happy lives of children conceived by artificial means, have reached opposite conclusions, enough so that many sincere Catholics have brought forth children by means of assisted reproduction. There seems no reason to think that bonding with the mother is any less for an artificially conceived child than for one conceived naturally.

In either case, a pregnancy occurs. There also seems no reason to suppose, in the general case, that parents who have resort to assisted reproduction will not enjoy a conjugal life. Hence it is unclear what detriment could follow from the fact that an embryo was not conceived conjugally. Consider a couple that has one child but who, by dint of clinically diagnosed infertility, has been unable to bring forth another, and who arranges for IVF. For what reason, a Christian may ask, would God disapprove? The magisterium holds that every new human life is a product of divine-human collaboration. If human reason is also a divine gift, why would one not classify as a divine gift an embryo conceived by a husband and wife aided by a method devised by human reason? We apply our reason routinely in the practice of medicine to overcome what 'naturally' occurs. It is not clear why we should not do so concerning infertility.

One may also give a compelling response to the concern that the practice of assisted reproduction creates more embryos than are transferred. If this consequence renders assisted reproduction wrong, we should have to indict nature. Over their reproductive years, parents create more enabled embryos that die than implant. Creation *in vitro* of an embryo that later becomes a surplus embryo or epidosembryo does not harm the embryo. Creation cannot make the embryo worse off than if it had not been created, because in the nonsentient state in which a surplus embryo or epidosembryo exists, the embryo cannot experience discomfort, frustration, or any sense of a lost future so as to render existence worse than not having been created. Once an extracorporeal embryo exists, it would be rational to want for its sake that it develop into a mature human that enjoys a long and full life, but it is also rational to want and to be content for its sake that it not experience discomfort, frustration, or any sense of a lost future when, in the exercise of permissible discretion, the progenitors decline transfer of the embryo into the womb. This would seem to hold *a fortiori* if the embryo will thereafter be used in a humanitarian cause.

Donum Vitae specifically worries that condoning a privilege to designate an embryo as surplus and thereby doom it encourages that attitude about the role of human decisionmaking in reproduction that can foster eugenics. One may meet that concern without adopting Zygotic Personhood. One may distinguish fully voluntary use of germ line intervention from coercive practices in the name of eugenics. One may construct constraints on the practice of germ line intervention. One may impose a duty not to engage in reproduction by a means that the progenitors have reason to believe will likely produce an offspring burdened by a genetic defect that either would make life so miserable as not to be worth living, or would impose a severe deformity. In the next chapter, I assert this duty as to reprocloning. Other norms may evolve in discussion.

The foregoing are reasons that could lead a Catholic to the conclusion that assisted reproduction is not wrong. Let us now assume the contrary, that all assisted reproduction is wrong. I shall argue that donation of surplus embryos as epidosembryos is not wrong, and that donee use thereof in accordance with donative instructions does not effect complicity in the putatively wrongful creation of the embryos.

Once a fertility patient has authorized creation of extracorporeal embryos and embryos have been created, the putative wrong of their creation is a *fait accompli*. A decision against intrauterine transfer of one or more of them is an independent act – the right act, according to the church, since to gestate such an embryo would be to practice an illicit method of reproduction. The argument from nonenablement shows that, given a choice against intrauterine transfer of an embryo, donation as an epidosembryo is virtuous. Hence such a donation is not a wrong in which anyone can be complicit.

So we consider complicity in the creation of extracorporeal embryos. Receiving its fullest expression in Catholicism, complicity is said to obtain when a moral agent becomes blameworthy by dint of some nexus to a wrongdoer. Each of the following has been held to be a sufficient nexus: contributing to or inducing harm, cooperating with evil, tolerating wrong, making wrongful conduct more eligible in a perpetrator's mind, and effecting scandal. Not every nexus effects complicity. We do not regard parents as complicitous in all wrongdoing by their children. Benefit is not a sufficient nexus for complicity. We would condemn too much were we to condemn receipt of benefit consequent on wrongful conduct. For then we would condemn all organ transplants from victims of crime.

We do not test for complicity by asking, as would a court concerning an alleged tort or crime, whether there occurred proximate causation. Complicity falls short of causation.[88] Even the kindred but stronger notion of accomplice liability in crime does not require causation. We recall a game played by fathers with their young sons. The father takes hold of the boy's hands, strikes them against the boy's body, and asks, 'Why are you punching yourself?' In formal terms, the father causes the punches and the boy is coerced, or does not act at all. Analogously, if Brutus causes Felix to act wrongfully, Brutus is not an accomplice but a coperpetrator – or even sole perpetrator insofar as he coerces Felix. What distinguishes an accomplice from a perpetrator is what the accomplice does *not* cause. (In the language

---

[88] Here I draw on Guenin 2004.

of the law, the accomplice does not effect any act that is either necessary to produce the harm or that belongs to a set of nonredundant conditions that jointly suffice to produce the harm.) When at the urging of her lover Aegisthus, Clytemnestra kills Agamemnon, Clytemnestra causes the death, Aegisthus does not. An accomplice contributes to another's wrongful act, but does not cause it.

We inquire into the nexus between assisted reproduction and epidosembryo use. Women desiring babies and the physicians assisting them, including conscientious Catholics, had long been producing large numbers of surplus embryos before anyone knew how to obtain useful derivatives from human blastocysts. Research on epidosembryos does not constitute complicity in the putative wrongdoing of assisted reproduction when the investigators in no way induce creation of the embryos. Will surplus embryo use, consequent on assisted reproduction, express toleration of assisted reproduction, or make assisted reproduction more eligible in a perpetrator's mind? A prospect of helping research does not seem to influence people in choosing assisted reproduction, nor to affect how people view that practice. In the main, people do not think of assisted reproduction as availing research. They think of having a baby.

The objection to use of epidosembryos created by scientists from donated cells is not complicity in assisted reproduction. Scientists are the direct perpetrators, authorized by donors, in creating those embryos. Rather the teleological objection comes to bear, asserting that one may not use an oocyte for a nonprocreative purpose. I responded to this objection in Chapter 2, and shall provide a fuller response in Chapter 6.

(d) Escape from a dilemma

Suppose a Catholic who, against the argument from nonenablement, proposes that even as the magisterium condemns nonconjugal procreation in the general case, the magisterium should assert the Duty of Intrauterine Transfer secondarily. It should impose such duty on those agents who, albeit wrongfully, have created extracorporeal embryos. The proponent of this duty urges that the magisterium adopt this stance by parity of reasoning with its stance in respect of natural conception. The proponent refers to the stricture that anyone who has engaged in sexual conduct so as to risk conception must support the gestation of any conceptus that happens to result, even if the sexual conduct was wrong. But the magisterium usually errs on the side of caution. Mindful of how enormous is the number of its faithful, and how diverse are the cultures of the world, it tends to eschew any doctrinal concession that it thinks susceptible of stretching. It is keen to avoid slippery slopes. To preach a duty that every embryo in a laboratory should be transferred to some uterus would seem to condone, if not to encourage, a method of procreation that the church condemns. The magisterium declines the proponent's invitation. Instead it depicts a tragic dilemma. The horns are, first, that when a progenitor elects to freeze and store embryos produced artificially, this results in 'depriving them, at least temporarily, of maternal shelter and gestation,' not to mention the likelihood that they will perish as waste, and second, that when a progenitor arranges for transfer of such embryos into the womb, the progenitor practices an illicit method of procreation. The magisterium judges that it has no recourse but to assign blame for presenting this dilemma. It blames the practice and practitioners of IVF. They have visited on surplus embryos an 'absurd fate, with no possibility of survival which can be licitly pursued.'[89]

If the magisterium someday approves assisted reproduction, it could grasp the foregoing dilemma by the second of its horns. In such case there would follow the considerations adduced in §2.3(b) against asserting the Duty of Intrauterine Transfer, and in favor of recognizing progenitor discretion concerning intrauterine transfer. There would then follow by means of the argument from nonenablement the justification for humanitarian use of any embryos that become surplus, and by the same reasoning, of embryos created in research. The availability of an option to devote surplus embryos to the merciful work of medicine could assuage concern for their fate, a concern cited as one of the reasons for disapproving assisted reproduction. In the future, assisted reproduction could be seen as likely to confer benefit on human life no matter what happens. Another response to the dilemma also presents itself. That is to escape between its horns by recognizing epidosembryo use as a practice that in the case of surplus embryos follows upon, but in no case effects complicity in, assisted reproduction. Whereupon again the argument from nonenablement compels assent.

(e) Protecting a related stance

We have reviewed the considerations that, from the magisterium's point of view, have been or might be raised against epidosembryo use. None forestall the argument from nonenablement. The church recognizes the permissibility of – in fact presently insists upon – declining intrauterine transfer of an extracorporeal embryo. The argument from nonenablement

---

[89] *Donum Vitae* § I(5)–(6).

justifies the use of embryos that have been barred from intrauterine transfer. Their developmental potential is bounded such that they can never begin gestation. Their use in the merciful work of regenerative medicine would fulfill the church's fundamental commitments to love of neighbor and the law of charity.

I now want to dispel any concern that approval of epidosembryo use would undermine the church's stance against abortion. On the contrary, the present inquiry has brought to light a means by which, if the church wished, it could shore up that stance. I first comment briefly on attempts to assimilate epidosembryo use to abortion. Ejecting a conceptus from the womb interrupts a process that if not interrupted could result in a birth. Sacrifice of an epidosembryo barred from the womb and confined to the dish interrupts a process that if not interrupted will cease short of gastrulation. Anyone approving epidosembryo use may, if they wish, consistently condemn abortion. The notion that epidosembryo use is tantamount to abortion is an instance of the high price of conflation.

The magisterium's case against abortion has come to rest on Zygotic Personhood, a precept originated by inference from a papal decision about punishment. The magisterium's principal defense of that precept is ousted by a more fundamental belief that such defense contradicts. The other cryptic arguments for the precept fail. The appeal to Zygotic Personhood is further undermined when, echoing Boethius, the magisterium affirms that a person is a being constituted by a rational nature that is capable of self-consciousness and autonomy. Meanwhile the argument from nonenablement reveals that assertion of Zygotic Personhood is futile when a progenitor permissibly declines intrauterine transfer.

The description of a person as a being constituted by a rational nature that is capable of self-consciousness and autonomy is nearly a paraphrase of Kant. Herein lies an insight into how the church might extricate itself from its predicament, the predicament of lacking a compelling argument for its stance against abortion. The church could articulate and defend a duty that protects an embryo by assigning significance to an embryo's potential. In terms of the device that I have employed, the church could recognize in the general case a possible person corresponding to an embryo.[90] This correspondence, so the church without contradiction might add, *does* obtain regardless of time of ensoulment. Whereupon the church could assert the Duty of Noninterference. As defined in §2.1, this duty entails that in respect

---

[90] For a Catholic theologian's view that embryos should be protected as other than persons, see Donceel 1970.

of an embryo in a given circumstance, it is wrong to interfere with any current process of development of the sort that in such circumstance usually results in a person. Whereupon abortion may be declared wrong.

The Duty of Noninterference gives the church the resources, if it insists, for opposing abortion strictly. The church could continue to say that a conceptus is a gift of God bestowed by collaboration with humans and that its believers should not make bold to refuse a gift and expect another later. In the new idiom, it may say that to God belongs the privilege of deciding whether possible persons corresponding to enabled embryos shall become actual. As for exceptions, the church could insist that the Duty of Noninterference allows none. Or it could allow that God does not collaborate with a perpetrator of rape or incest. Or that He may not wish a woman to incur a serious risk of death in order to give birth. However strict the church chooses to be about it, the Duty of Noninterference will not collide with any bedrock belief, purport to answer a theological question declared intractable, or employ the assumption that personhood can only be attained instantaneously. The church does not need Zygotic Personhood to oppose abortion, and its case would be more cogent without the precept. Casting off the constringent mantle of Zygotic Personhood while asserting the Duty of Noninterference would buttress the church's stance against abortion while allowing it to endorse the charitable work of those who would relieve suffering by means of embryos to which no possible persons correspond.

5.6 RECOGNIZING COMMON GROUND

Even though the papacy exercises prescriptive authority – long a *cause celebre* in Catholicism's separation from Protestantism – and even though the church has branded some views heresy and excommunicated their proponents, clergy and laity have debated theological and moral ideas throughout the church's history. In the history of the magisterium with which I began, there appear more theologians than popes. If the Vatican seems to reason according to the rule 'if you give them an inch, they'll take a mile,' imagine that any of us knew that whenever we delivered ourselves of some view on a moral matter, more than a billion people would take what we say as doctrine. The century may be the unit in which the church measures change. But discussions have sometimes issued in doctrinal change. Many Catholics are thinking through the issue of embryo use, forming their own consciences. Various of them maintain their faith even as they reject the magisterium's condemnation of contraception, its exceptionless stance against abortion, or its declination to ordain women as priests.

I observed at the outset that if embryo use comes about, or is banned by, mere majoritarian rule, that may leave in its wake a conflict that society fails to resolve. Traveling along the wide path of public reason, the foregoing account offers an alternative to the unhappy outcome of moral discord. The argument from nonenablement does not invoke the tenets of any particular comprehensive moral or religious view, but it sounds in many. The argument states a basis on which, faithfully to Kantian morality and to Catholic teaching as a whole, one may conclude that epidosembryo use is permissible, virtuous, and a fulfillment of a collective duty.

As we recognize this conclusion for Kantianism and Catholicism, and as we take stock of the many less strict religious traditions within which the argument from nonenablement compels assent, we discern a salutary intersection of moral views. The argument from nonenablement occupies a place in an overlapping consensus. If I am correct about this, we are not relegated to asking if some value is overriding, or to balancing values, or to installing one moral or religious view over others, or to outvoting a principled minority while not satisfying their concerns.

CHAPTER 6

Clones

I have spoken of the generality of the argument from nonenablement, lately describing its force even within moral views often read to yield a contrary verdict. Earlier I noted that the argument's scope encompasses epidosembryos donated as such and epidosembryos formed from donated cells. In this chapter, I discuss issues peculiar to clones as epidosembryos of the latter sort.

To motivate the discussion, I shall first briefly describe the expectations for human nonreprocloning that have excited scientists and patients. As earlier defined, nonreprocloning consists in the creation of a clone embryo not transferred to a uterus. Apart from the objections to embryo use in general that I have thus far discussed, the principal direct objection to nonreprocloning is the teleological objection. I shall undertake to refute that objection. What I shall say will apply to the creation of embryos in research by other means as well. I shall then turn to the bogeyman introduced in almost any discussion of this topic, reprocloning. Fears of reprocloning, some well-considered and some exaggerated, demand attention in constructing a defense of nonreprocloning. There presently obtains a consensus that human reprocloning would be so unsafe as to be irresponsible in the attempt. I review the reasoning therefor. I then assume for the sake of argument that the day arrives when reprocloning is considered, in comparison with natural conception, relatively safe. I consider whether we should then prohibit reprocloning, or instead protect it as private. It has been proposed that we head off this issue by prohibiting all cloning now, this so that nonreprocloning will not propel us down a slippery slope to reprocloning. I consider and reject that proposal.

6.1 NONREPROCLONING

Investigators in regenerative medicine have imagined that use of nonreprocloning in experiments could augment fundamental knowledge and might serve as a means of delivering therapies. Among diseases and disabilities that investigators imagine combating are those many caused by undersupply of specialized cells of one kind or another.

Since reprogramming occurs in clones, a compelling reason arises for observing them. In reprogramming, the asexually-activated oocyte's cytoplasm turns off the gene expression program of the mature somatic cell from which came the source DNA, and turns on a gene expression program that directs early development. So it was discovered in the work that led to Dolly, which confirmed after a century of puzzlement that the hereditary material in a nucleus remains intact throughout development.[1] Discovery of cytoplasmic transcription factors that trigger reprogramming then enabled the generation of human induced pluripotent stem cells.

Nonreprocloning could enable the efficient modeling of heritable diseases. From a consenting patient affected by a disease, an investigator would obtain DNA with which to create a clone, then obtain from the clone an embryonic stem cell line. The investigator would then induce the embryonic stem cells to differentiate into the specialized cells whose insufficiency brings about the disease. Or the investigator might so direct the differentiation of induced pluripotent stem cells. The investigator would seek to observe how the disease develops in the derived cells, and how the cells come to differ from healthy specialized cells. Healthy cells serving as the control in the experiment could also be obtained by inducing differentiation of pluripotent stem cells. After designing a drug targeted at a disease, the investigator could test the drug on an exemplifying cell line. Availability of pluripotent stem cells could also accelerate drug development in general by allowing investigators to generate quantities of human cells of any desired type for use in drug testing. This could reduce the use of nonhuman animals in such tests. More generally, by the use of nonreprocloning, scientists might acquire a better understanding of cell growth and specialization. Such knowledge could enable progress against cancer. It may also avail for understanding aging.

One of the first imagined therapeutic strategies that would use embryonic stem cells would induce those cells to issue in transplantable specialized cells whose absence causes disease. But in the general case, a patient's immune system will reject entrants that it does not recognize as self. Some special cases arise that do not present this problem. Because of the blood-brain barrier, a transfer of nonself cells into the brain may occur without provoking an immune system response. Degenerative diseases of the central

---

[1] The history is recounted in McLaren 2000.

nervous system (e.g., Parkinson's) could yield to transplantation therapy using nonself cells. Scientists might also develop improved immunosuppressive drugs that produce less severe side effects. For the general case, in which rejection remains a roadblock to cell transplantation, biologists have devised an ingenious solution, *autologous transplantation*, envisioned to work as follows. A clinician first uses somatic cell DNA from a sick patient to form a clone of the patient. The clinician then derives embryonic stem cells from the clone blastocyst. An alternative technique is to generate induced pluripotent stem cells from somatic cells of the patient. If the patient's undersupply of specialized cells results from any genetic defect that might soon manifest, the clinician corrects the genetic defect, using the techniques of genetic engineering, in the cell line. The clinician then induces the stem cells to issue in the specialized cells needed by the patient. The clinician now transplants those cells to the patient, whose immune system recognizes them as self. Cells derived from a clone will not, in the general case, match the patient's mitochondrial genome, but this does not pose a major problem, since mitochondrial genes apparently do not code for anything on the cell surface, or if they do, the rejection problem is modest. The safety of transplanting cells that issue from induced pluripotent stem cells may be affected by any genetic and epigenetic alterations in the course of inducing pluripotency. In general, the theory is that a leap backward to the patient's earliest developmental stages might bring about the cure of a previously incurable malady.

Because many failures will occur for each success in producing patient-specific cells, it remains to be seen whether autologous transplantation will be practiced on a large scale. The outcome may turn on whether a procedure's consumption of time and resources is affordable. An economical alternative to the creation of cells peculiar to each patient would be to create banks of generic pluripotent stem cell lines. They would be generic in the sense that each line would be histocompatible with one of the alleles of the major histocompatibility complex. The major histocompatibility complex is a set of genes on chromosome 6 that code for antigens, the cell surface structures that signal that a cell is self. The number of alleles of the major histocompatibility complex genes is believed greater than the number of alleles for any other genes, but their distribution frequency may be such that a manageable number of cell line types might suffice to achieve close matches for a large majority of the population.

Lest it be thought that one could successfully pursue the foregoing avenues with surplus embryos from fertility practice, we may note the following. The insertion of a mature cell's nuclear DNA into an oocyte offers an unusual opportunity to observe full scale reprogramming of gene expression and regulatory mechanics back to an embryonic state. That opportunity does not arise with products of fertilization. Surplus embryos come from patients most of whom are young, affluent, caucasian, and infertile. These patients do not represent the generic diversity of the population. There is much to be gained from studying diversity. Surplus embryos will also not likely exhibit the genotypes of all the diseases that need to be studied. An investigator cannot use recombinant DNA technology to simulate a disease in the derivatives of surplus embryos unless the alleles implicated in the disease are known, which for most degenerative diseases is not the case. For many diseases, cloning or inducement of pluripotency in somatic cells may be the only means of procuring disease-specific pluripotent stem cells.

The foregoing illustrates how scientific ingenuity has set the stage for the use of nonreprocloning to make substantial contributions to the expansion of fundamental knowledge and the development of therapies.

6.2 THE TELEOLOGICAL OBJECTION

Nonreprocloning is the most prominent experimental method of embryo creation, and it is my main concern in this chapter. But what I shall say in this section will also apply to experimental creation of embryos by fertilization or parthenogenesis.

We recall Publius of §2.4. Publius contends that lack of intent to procreate casts a pall of wrongdoing over any scientist who induces an oocyte to begin dividing. Put differently, creation of embryos *ex vivo* is legitimate only if the cell donors intend to procreate. To this my reply was given earlier. Procreative intent plays no part in the argument from nonenablement. In the absence of procreative intent, the argument justifies creating epidosembryos in research. But Publius persists. He claims that the singular and divinely ordained purpose of human oocytes is reproduction. It is wrong to appropriate oocytes for any other purpose. Creating embryos in research is wrong intrinsically, wrong for its direct effects, and wrong for its symbolic effects.

Reprising an argument given earlier, we may maintain that activating an oocyte to create an epidosembryo for use in research does not harm the embryo. Creation cannot make the embryo worse off than if it had not been created, because in the nonsentient state in which an epidosembryo will remain, the embryo cannot experience discomfort, frustration, or any sense of a lost future so as to render existence worse than not having been created. While it is rational to want more for the embryo, it is also rational to be content for the embryo's sake that it be spared any unpleasant experience while serving as a research subject for benefit of other objects of rational care. But the teleological objection as stated by Publius would, if sound, survive this point about harm. In framing his objection, Publius seems to have put his finger on what appears the most plausible ground for the oft heard claim 'It is wrong to create an embryo in order to kill it.'

Aristotle held that 'nature creates nothing without a purpose, but always the best possible in each kind of living creature by reference to its essential constitution.'[2] Aristotle also imagined that 'every bodily member subserves some partial end, that is to say, some special action. . . .'[3] At various times in history, natural philosophers have thought that they knew *the* respective purposes of sundry human structures. From that supposition, it was a short step to the belief that the putative purposes were not accident, but divine design. If, by the end of the eighteenth century, Aristotelian teleology no longer held sway, then after Darwin, such view has lost its grip on our thought. Granted, when we take a static view, when we observe an organism at a moment in evolutionary history, we think that we discern purposes for its sundry components. We say that a bird's wings subserve the purpose of flight. We may also fail to discern some functions that components perform. We shall surely fail to anticipate all functions over the course of evolutionary history. We have learned how to account for structures and functions as outcomes of evolution. The theory of natural selection sends by the board the notion that for an organism or parts thereof, there is any target toward which evolution progresses. Life forms do not evolve toward targets.[4] Evolution, it has been said, is merely chaos with feedback. We would narrow our vision improvidently were we to ascribe a fixed purpose to any structure or cell type. Philosophers of biology nowadays debate whether a function of a feature is a causal role, or instead an effect for which the feature is an evolutionary adaptation. That is a post-Darwinian conversation. The single-purpose teleological view to which I am responding is pre-Darwinian.

Some who reject the theory of evolution, and even some who believe something of it but do not want to acknowledge that there occurs no purposive process, may continue to maintain that gametes bear ordained singular purposes. For them, laboratory manipulations of gametes defy

---

[2] *Progression of Animals* 704b14–16. [3] *Parts of Animals* 645b14–15.
[4] A point made in Kuhn 1970, pp. 171–172.

nature or divine will. We may not permissibly direct an oocyte to serve something other than its 'natural end.' Adherents of one modern incantation of teleology, the intelligent design version of creationism, are apt to say that each thing exists for a purpose and that bad consequences flow from not honoring a thing's purpose.

Yet all of us recognize man's folly about what man knows. Our forbears thought that the purpose of our bones is to hold us up. Now we also look upon the marrow as a blood cell factory. Not merely as a *façon de parler*, our forbears referred to blood as person- or family-identifying. Our speech retains some of their idioms (e.g., 'flesh and blood' and 'the blood line,' the latter assigned significance emotively and in the law of inheritance). We now know that blood of one human will function in the body of any other human whose blood is of the same generic type. The healer's art has revealed that human bodily components exhibit remarkable adaptability. Surgeons have shown that skin from one part of the body can engraft at another. Arteries of the leg can function when relocated to the vicinity of the heart. An entire organ can operate in a body other than that in which it originated. We are learning how to redirect proteins and cellular processes, and how to induce them to serve ends that we choose, including therapies and repulsion of pathogens. We call this 'conventional drug therapy.' Recent observations about biological adaptability have stood on their heads many earlier suppositions about biological function.

Even if cells of a given type ordinarily performed only one function, and even were we to know that function, it would not follow that it is immoral to deploy a cell of that type for another function. To borrow a trope from Daniel Dennett, a human body consists of a team of a few trillion cells. If it can help the team, it seems reasonable to deploy as a defensive back a quarterback who would otherwise languish on the bench. We might deploy a surfeit of oocytes in service of ends other than procreation. One who holds this wrong on teleological grounds will have to explain what purpose is served by the endowment of immature oocytes of the order 10^5 that every human female possesses from birth. A woman will ovulate only a few hundred of these over the course of her reproductive years, and that number will vastly exceed her feasible number of children.

Possession of an abundance of immature oocytes might be explained as an evolved characteristic enhancing reproductive success. Salmon lay vast numbers of eggs. Human males produce vast numbers of sperm. Still it is the case that most human oocytes are never ovulated. Physicians can stimulate oocyte development by drugs, and scientists can nurture oocytes in the laboratory. If one is imputing purposes, how can one ignore that unovulated oocytes could serve the purpose of relieving suffering? Unless we think it advisable that every woman bear vastly more children than she wishes, it would seem that procreation cannot be the sole purpose to which oocytes may rightfully be put.

According to a teleological view, some purpose must be served by human reason. Aristotle elevated reason to 'what is peculiar to man,' declaring that the function of a human as a whole consists in the active exercise of rationality.[5] Our selves are among the subjects about which we reason. The function of the faculty of reason includes, *inter alia*, the choosing of one's ends. In implementing our choices of ends, we effectively devote our bodies to our chosen purposes. A teleological account seems compelled to acknowledge that the respective purposes of our bodily parts include the service of ends that we rationally choose. Ends that we might rationally choose include humanitarian aid to others. One means that we might choose consists in donating parts of ourselves, including oocytes.

If we consider teleology from a religious point of view, suppose it is thought that we must use our reason only insofar as we respect divinely chosen purposes. Who can know the mind of God about purposes? Imagine again that we could have a conversation with God. We report that in 1998 we humans discovered how to maintain a culture of embryonic stem cells. He might first observe, 'It took you long enough.' But suppose that we explain how we think that research may lead to the relief of suffering. Would He respond that His purpose in endowing human females with oocytes was exclusively procreation? For the reasons indicated, such a restriction would seem odd for an endowment of the order 10^5. If God allowed such abundance to evolve (or designed it), it seems doubtful that He expected and preferred that every oocyte would take an active part in reproduction. It seems implausible that an omniscient, all-loving, and all-merciful God would wish that we not use our reason or any of this vast corpus of oocytes to help our neighbors in distress. It is plausible that God would commend epidosembryo donors, that He would encourage our humble progress thus far with nonreprocloning, that He would regard our efforts as expressing esteem for human life.

6.3 REPROCLONING

Even when nonreprocloning and reprocloning are sharply distinguished, fears arise that the former will lead to the latter. I shall respond to this by

[5] *Nicomachean Ethics* 1098a13.

arguing that reprocloning is presently unsafe and rightly condemned, that if reprocloning becomes safe, it will not be a foregone conclusion that the procedure is wrong, and that the possibility or likelihood that reprocloning eventually will be safe but wrong does not constitute a sufficient reason to forbear from clone epidosembryo use.

(a) Hazards

The consensus present objection to reprocloning is that at the present state of technology, the risk of producing a deformed offspring and the risk of harm to the mother would be so high that reprocloning would be irresponsible in the attempt. The embryo that developed into Dolly, the first mammalian clone born alive from an adult somatic cell, was the only one of 277 experimentally-created clone embryos that attained birth and developed normally. If human reprocloning were practiced, we should have to expect that most clones would die before implanting, or by miscarriage. Of those clones that reached the fetal stage, it is probable that a high proportion would be afflicted by severe genetic abnormalities and hampered by placental defects. For any that survived to birth, there would obtain an abnormally high chance of severe defects. It is a grim picture.

We do not have to look far for an explanation. Clones suffer from abnormal expression of genes in consequence of abnormalities in imprinting and in other processes that restrict expression.[6] Imprinting is a process that occurs in mammals with placentae (but not in egg-laying animals). It is a process that epigenetically modifies a small number of alleles so as (in most cases) to suppress expression of the allele. The process does not alter the nucleotide sequences of chromosomes, but instead attaches methyl groups. These are the imprints. The imprints prevent transcription of the alleles to which they are attached. In a zygote formed by natural conception, the maternal and paternal chromosomes have recently emerged from gametogenesis, in the course of which all imprints were erased and new imprints were attached. The imprints attached to the maternal chromosomes will subdue growth-promoting genes, while the imprints attached to the paternal chromosomes will silence growth-reducing genes.[7] As a result of imprinting, paternal alleles play a lesser role in embryonic structures than do maternal alleles, while paternal alleles play a greater role in extraembryonic structures such as the placenta. In a clone, the source DNA bears the

---

[6] I thank William Lensch for conversation concerning this.
[7] For which point I am indebted to Shirley Tilghman.

cumulative results of imprinting throughout the process of differentiation that formed the mature specialized cells of its type. This mature DNA possesses a significantly different combination of imprints than those of a zygote genome, and also embodies the effects of aging and mutation. As the clone cytoplasm operates on the source DNA, it strips some imprints that should not be stripped. It adds others that should not be added. So rapidly does the cytoplasm reprogram the source DNA that errors seem inevitable. All sorts of things then go wrong. Expression of abnormally imprinted genes and other genes is so aberrant as to cripple development. It also appears that in primate cloning, the process of removing the oocyte nucleus removes proteins lying in the vicinity, and that as a result the ensuing process of cell division produces cells possessing a nonstandard number of chromosomes.[8]

Failure in cloning does not seem surprising for animals that ordinarily do not reproduce asexually. In the words of the scientist who cloned Dolly, reprocloning 'is a lottery, a stochastic process. Several coins are thrown and must all come up as heads if normal life is to result.'[9] The developmental biologist Rudolf Jaenisch has often said, 'There are no normal clones.' Clones suffer from defects in vital organs, respiratory distress, immune system deficiencies, and serious problems in later life. Dolly became obese, arthritic, and may have aged prematurely. Distinctive features of human biology suggest that human reprocloning would be at least as, if not more, difficult and risky as reprocloning of other mammals.

The poor developmental prospects of a clone if transferred to a uterus have sometimes been invoked as if they alone would justify nonreprocloning. I do not offer that defense. The burden upon anyone who predicates the morality of using a product of activation on its putative birth probability would be to define a function assigning probabilities to products of activation undergoing organismic development, then to specify some probability p such that any product whose birth probability is lower than p is eligible for use. Whatever p they specify, fertilization will doubtless produce some embryos so defective as to fall below p while improved cloning techniques may produce some clones above p. With the benefit of recombinant DNA techniques employed in forming a clone, it would be nomologically possible for a clone to develop without substantial change into a person. That will become manifest as and when, by means of genetic engineering, someone effects a live birth of a human clone. Whereupon the Duty of Noninterference will be asserted as to a corresponding possible

[8] Simerly *et al.* 2003.   [9] Wilmut 2002.

person. So will the duty not to kill predicated upon Zygotic Personhood. These assertions will not be met by citing a nonzero birth probability, even if said to be vanishingly small, since the reply will be that birth is nomologically possible upon transfer to a uterus. Those asserting such duties will argue by analogy that we do not condition the personhood of an adult on actuarial tables. Going out on a limb to predict which products of activation would, if transferred to a uterus, develop into healthy fetuses, and which would not, will yield only an insecure moral defense for any treatment of them. The ground of my defense of nonreprocloning lies elsewhere. It consists in a permissible exercise of discretion such that transfer to a uterus will never occur.

So we return to reprocloning. It may be argued that we have a duty not to engage in reproduction by a means that we have reason to believe will likely bring forth an offspring burdened by a genetic defect that either would make life so miserable as not to be worth living, or would impose a severe deformity. As to the latter possibility, that duty may rest on a non-person-affecting principle, one that binds even when, because an offspring's life burdened by a severe deformity is not worse than nonexistence, birth could not be said to harm the offspring. The duty is not owed to anyone in particular but is a duty nonetheless. It may be said to forbid use of a relatively unsafe method of reproduction when there is available an alternative (e.g., natural conception) presenting a high probability of a healthy baby. Thus suppose that a couple, after being apprised of the risks, brings forth a clone, which as it happens is mentally retarded, yet happy. For the parents to have refrained from reprocloning would have been worse for the child than the child's retardation: refraining would have assured that the child would not exist. Still the parents have arguably acted wrongly. They have breached the above described duty.

By the foregoing line of reasoning, we may be said to have a duty not to reproduce by reprocloning. Already in polities that give a wide berth to personal liberties, anticonsanguinity laws prohibit marriage between blood relatives within a specified range. The reasonableness of these laws rests on the significant probability that mating of blood relatives will produce offspring affected by recessive diseases. A physician also has a duty not to perform an intrauterine transfer of a conceptus that will subject the fertility patient to unreasonable risk. Were a physician to practice on humans any other medical procedure that had produced as high a rate of disastrous consequences in nonhuman animal tests as has reprocloning, few would hesitate to pronounce the physician reckless.

As a person may have a moral duty relating to future persons, the state may be given responsibility to protect future persons. Scientific consensus on the dangers of reprocloning warrants state action prohibiting the practice so long as unsafe. When reprocloning has been interdicted,[10] it will be a rare physician who risks prosecution and probable loss of career to attempt it.

It is not clear how anyone could change this situation by improving reprocloning in a morally permissible manner. If human reprocloning is not rendered safer than it now is, it will be impermissible to attempt it. If no one attempts it, it may never become safe enough to be permissible. Biologists' usual way of escaping through the horns of such a dilemma is to experiment extensively on nonhuman animals. Often they find an animal model that appears so close to the human in its pertinent characteristics that, after they have attained success, a leap to human trials seems warranted. But it is unclear what may ever warrant a leap to human reprocloning trials.

(b) Nonsafety objections

So that we may better understand the morality of human reprocloning, let us assume that the daunting technical challenges have somehow been met. Human reprocloning has been improved even to the point that safety and deformity rates are not markedly less favorable for reprocloning than for natural reproduction. Reprocloning has become a relatively safe way to have a baby. Providing an account of what is 'relatively safe' is a task that I do not undertake here. For my analytical purposes here, it suffices to assume that we would not countenance a claim of relative safety until there obtains a scientific consensus that the practice is safe. Before any decision were taken predicated on extent of safety, we would insist on a rigorous understanding of the concept applied to pertinent evidence.

Against reprocloning when relatively safe, there will come to bear another set of objections. Some people will assert that reprocloning is a bad idea whose time should not come. If we allow the practice, we shall pave the way to abuses so awful that we shall later regret that anyone ever began it. Already such forebodings have become a mantra for some advocates. They importune legislatures to prohibit reprocloning under all circumstances. I shall first relate the objections. I shall then explore what might motivate reprocloning, this with a view to imagining its likely incidence as we assess

[10] For example, the Food and Drug Administration has effectively interdicted reprocloning in the US, rendering its likely incidence nil. In Guenin 2005a, I present and defend the rationale and authority for this action.

objections. Hereafter I shall refer to the person who contributes source DNA for producing a clone as the *source* or, where the context is not clear, the *cloning source*.

A leading objection is the speculation that a clone will experience an identity crisis. The concern seems to be that when a clone discovers that the clone's nuclear genome is the same as the source's, the clone may not fully see itself as a distinct or unique person. Imagine the source saying to the clone, 'When I was your age, ...' At the outset, this speculation seems to betray, as does much cant about reprocloning, an exaggeration of the extent to which a clone and source will resemble each other. One who plants a twig may produce a plant identical in genome to that of the plant from which the twig comes, but a clone formed by nuclear transfer will not be genetically identical to the source. The mitochondrial genomes will differ (save only in the case in which a woman has cloned herself or a maternal ancestor and no relevant mitochondrial mutations have occurred). While known for its role in the etiology of diseases, mitochondrial DNA also encodes nondisease traits that would likely be noticeable in gross even if a clone and source were the same age.

If we look to nature, to a case of even greater genetic homology, we see no cause for concern. Monozygotic twins are commonly said to be identical, by which presumably is meant that their genomes are exactly similar, but as Leibniz wrote,

There is no such thing as two individuals indiscernible from each other. An ingenious gentleman of my acquaintance, discoursing with me, in the presence of her Electoral Highness the Princess Sophia, in the garden of Herrenhausen, thought he could find two leaves perfectly alike. The Princess defied him to do it, and he ran all over the garden a long time to look for some; but it was to no purpose. Two drops of water, or milk, viewed with a microscope, will appear distinguishable from each other.[11]

Leibniz also spoke presciently of eggs:

I have said that it is not possible for there to be two particulars that are similar in all respects – for example two eggs – for it is necessary that some things can be said about one of them that cannot be said about the other, else they could be substituted for one another and there would be no reason why they were not called one and the same.[12]

[11] Alexander 1956, *The Leibniz–Clarke Correspondence*, p. 36. In respect of the supposition that monozygotes are exactly similar, I mention these remarks by way of empirical caution, apart from the identity of indiscernildes.
[12] *Fragmente zur Logik*, pp. 476–477.

We earlier noted that sometimes one monozygotic twin inherits a genetic disposition to a disease while the other twin does not, and that on rare occasions, monozygotic twins even differ in sex. Sometimes a genetically-linked abnormality will beset one monozygotic twin but, by virtue of the phenomenon of incomplete gene penetrance or variable expressivity in which an allele is present but does not manifest in the disease phenotype, the other twin will not exhibit the abnormality.[13] Monozygotes may also differ in number of mitochondria. Mutation begins immediately in each twin, and the results will differ between them. Even so, monozygotic twins will usually be so similar that we can barely tell them apart. So if homology is a social or psychological problem, we have far more reason to worry about monozygotic twins than about a clone and its source. By and large, we do not worry about monozygotic twins. The ostensible reason is that we do not believe in genetic determinism. Identity in genotype does not entail identity in phenotype. Both an individual's epigenetic systems and the external environment influence phenotype. We know from everyday observations how monozygotic twins encounter different experiences, make different choices, and thus distinguish themselves. In monozygotes, as Stephen Jay Gould has said, we effectively 'have known human clones from the dawn of our consciousness.' Much cant about cloning neglects the influence of environment on phenotype. Monozygotes 'provide sturdy proof that inevitable differences of nurture guarantee the individuality and personhood of each human clone.'[14] A clone will be a sort of delayed twin – most commonly, we may assume, delayed by about a generation. The environment in which the clone matures will differ from the environment in which the source matured. The clone will have ample reason to see itself as possessed of its own identity.

Concern about clones is sometimes expressed by imagining that they will be deprived of what Feinberg has called an 'open-ended future.' It has been suggested that it is optimal to be ignorant of how genome will shape one's future and that one will be denied that blissful ignorance if someone possessed of the same nuclear genome precedes one and resides in one's home. It is imagined that a clone must deal with the expectation that anything less than the source's accomplishments will constitute the clone's failure 'to be what he or she can be.' This objection too seems mistakenly to assume genetic determinism. One's genome does not determine one's future. *Any* child may encounter difficulty in trying to live up to expectations of those to whom the child bears a family resemblance. Will

---

[13] Machin 1996. I thank Jonathan Beckwith for discussion of this and other topics hereafter.
[14] Gould 1998, p. 48.

a perception of nuclear genetic identity with a forbear affect a clone *more than* being the spitting image of a parent or the monozygotic twin of a sibling affects a nonclone? We lack empirical observations to answer this. It could boost a clone's confidence to know that the nuclear genome of an esteemed forbear lies within. The clone could even surpass the forbear. Richard Dawkins, imagining an Einstein clone, observes wryly that 'Old Einstein, however outstanding his genes, had an ordinary education and had to waste his time earning a living in the patent office. Young Einstein could be given an education to match his genes.'[15] The mere occurrence of discussion about a clone's self-image might go a long way toward solving the problem. Alerted by a spate of publicity on the topic, parents of clones might take pains to reinforce in each child a sense of self, urging each to follow his or her own star. By the way, asks the biologist Lee Silver, mindful of antipathy to social welfare programs, why is it that so many politicians seem to care so much about cloning, but so little about the welfare of children in general?[16]

A clone could feel disappointment at what may appear as elective genetic constraints. 'Why did you make me a clone of Uncle Percival?' says Tom to his mother. 'I have long skinny fingers. I do not want to be a pianist. I want to play linebacker for the Michigan Wolverines.' Tom will also know that if his parents had not chosen to clone Percival, Tom would not be here. His parents might have had another baby, but it would not have been Tom. Supposing that instead they bring forth a child Ann who suffers from a serious inherited disease, Ann's question may be, 'Why did you pick an unhealthy source?' Should it happen that Ann gets a look at the medical files revealing details about her parents' reprocloning decision, there may be some explaining to do. But if genetic determinism is assumed, any reproductive decision may be construed as imposing elective genetic constraints.

Some people have decried reprocloning as narcissism. This charge of course could gain traction only as to parents who clone themselves. Another objection lodges by subsuming reprocloning within the practice of designing children. That practice, we may hear, constitutes eugenics. Reprocloning would be an instance of 'playing God' in which parents fail to show reverence for life as a gift. Another complaint is the mere fact that reprocloning is asexual. Of course monozygotic twinning is asexual, but that does not rouse moral compunctions because such twinning is seen as a 'natural' phenomenon and is immediately consequent on sexual reproduction.

---

[15] Dawkins 1998, p. 56.   [16] Silver 1997, p. 143.

What is wrong with asexual reproduction? According to the Catholic magisterium's account, children originating by nonconjugal methods (IVF, reprocloning, or other) are shortchanged in parental bonding. As earlier remarked, this seems implausible, since pregnancy and childbirth run the same course regardless how conception occurs. Parents might even bond more to a child to whose conception they have devoted unusual effort. More telling is the magisterium's admonition that children should be born and raised 'within marriage and from marriage.' A woman who selects a female DNA source could bear a clone without recruiting a man for the project. The dramatic way of presenting this prospect is to say that if cloning without men becomes prevalent, men will be threatened with reproductive obsolescence. This fires the imaginations of futurists who now begin to speak of societies in which fathers play only a minor role.

Lastly, genetic diversity avails a species as a means of surviving disease and other assaults. Sexual reproduction's genetic lottery increases genetic variety. Sexual reproduction has evolved in many species by virtue of that advantage. It has been suggested that by asexually bringing into being humans who are 'copies' of each other, reprocloning would diminish human genetic diversity.

(c) Considering probable incidence

Before we explore the objections, or rush to embrace the conclusion that any of the envisioned ill effects would be visited upon us, we ought to inquire into reprocloning's probable incidence. We can get a handle on this by exploring incentives and disincentives for reprocloning at such time as it may be considered relatively safe.

Nowadays in developed countries, the preponderance of children conceived naturally are born healthy. We attribute this salutary result to the general state of public health, advances in prenatal care, and other circumstances. Consider couples of which the following is true. (Here I use the term 'couple' for a pair of prospective parents.) If they give reprocloning a thought, it holds little appeal for them. They face no special situation that evokes a desire to bring forth a genetic replica. They imagine bringing forth *new* people. So they conceive the old-fashioned way. They assume the risks of natural conception. Though they may not investigate the biological details, they understand generally that reproduction is a kind of genetic lottery. They understand that in selecting each other as mates, they have confined the genetic sources to two. Even so, the combinatorics are such that the range of different genomes that they as a couple can create is astronomical in number. They also understand that things can go wrong. The genome of their offspring could contain alleles implicated in disease or exhibit aneuploidy (an abnormal number of chromosomes).

For some of these prospective parents, acceptance of the natural lottery is provisional. They contemplate that during a pregnancy, they will procure genetic testing of the fetus via chorionic villus sampling in the first trimester or amniocentesis at a later stage (or, when the technology arrives, by testing of fetal cells circulating in the maternal bloodstream), and, if the tests reveal a serious defect in the conceptus, they will consider terminating the pregnancy. Others reject any thought of abortion and plan to welcome any child that they conceive. They will also accept infertility should that be their fate. Still others proceed contentedly in the belief that because they and their forbears have been healthy, the risk of transmitting a significant genetic defect is low. If any of these prospective parents give reprocloning a thought, they see little in it that appeals to them. They find much cause for concern over its burdens and risks. In poor countries, the question will seldom arise, as the cost of assisted reproduction will be prohibitive. It seems probable that, for one or another of the foregoing reasons, the preponderance of couples will lack an incentive for reprocloning, and hence will reproduce by natural conception.

A couple that might consider reprocloning would seem to fall within one of the following categories: (1) fertile couples for whom reprocloning is an alternative to natural conception, (2) infertile couples for whom reprocloning is an alternative to assisted sexual reproduction, (3) prospective parents affected by or carriers of a hereditary disease, and (4) single women and female couples. In the following, I consider the incentives for people in each category, this so that we might surmise how frequent might be the practice.

(1) The stereotypical case that opponents of reprocloning seem to have in their sights is that of a couple capable of conceiving a child naturally who prefers reprocloning for no reason other than a desire to create what they understand to be a replica of an esteemed person.

If any fertile couple considers reprocloning, in their path lie the following burdens and risks. Reprocloning demands a great deal of the prospective mother. She must undergo the same regimen of ovarian stimulation, oocyte retrieval, and intrauterine transfer, with attendant risks, discomfort, and expense, as a fertility patient. To avoid this, the prospective mother could accept and use a donor's oocyte, but the fact that a child derives its mitochondrial DNA from the oocyte provides a compelling reason to recover and activate her own.

If the thought of this inconvenience does not quell enthusiasm for reprocloning, an appraisal of the risks may. We are assuming for the sake of argument that reprocloning is 'relatively safe,' but anyone attempting reprocloning will always be running uphill. They will be dependent on an elaborate suite of laboratory gymnastics so as to overcome problems inherent in trying to perform asexually what the evolved organism accomplishes sexually. At stake is the offspring's health, not to mention the mother's. It will give pause to any prospective parent to hear, 'There are no normal clones.' To proceed, a fertile couple will have to take on risks that, so they know, would not arise if they conceived naturally.

Prospective parents would also need a heavy dose of genetic determinism to sustain any belief that a clone will mimic the source. Heritability of a trait (the ratio of genetic variance to phenotypic variance) is routinely less than unity, and for some traits, is less than 50%. Some people with an allelic pairing linked to a disease never contract the disease. Heritability is defined relative to an environment. Environment and the gene-environment interaction profoundly influence traits. The phenotype of a clone will reflect the variable penetrance of the many genes associated with most traits of interest.

Prospective cloners cannot even be sure what lurks within a cloning source by way of genetic predispositions to disease. They might think that because source DNA passes a screening test for alleles then known to correlate with diseases, the source DNA does not possess any genetic predispositions to disease. That expectation could crumble sometime after birth of a clone when the source first manifests an inherited disorder, a disorder that the screening missed because no one then knew the associated alleles. Prospective parents will also know that many people condemn reprocloning. Social attitudes could menace a clone and its parents if anyone learns how the child was conceived. All these considerations may persuade someone who at first contemplates reprocloning that it is not worth the trouble.

Such is the situation before considering alternatives. The first alternative would consist in conceiving by IVF (where from here on I use 'IVF' to encompass all sexual methods of forming an extracorporeal embryo) and then procuring preimplantation genetic diagnosis ('PGD'). In PGD, a fertility technician removes a blastomere from a candidate embryo at or before the eight-cell stage. It is remarkable that from a microscopic conceptus anything could be removed by pipette without destroying the conceptus. But in many though not all cases, embryos survive removal of a blastomere with no diminution in likelihood of normal preimplantation development. Physicians perform PGD on this supposition.[17] After removing a blastomere, a fertility technician will screen its DNA for sequences of interest. Depending on the test results, the parents may reject the tested embryo for transfer, elect to transfer the embryo to the uterus, or elect a genetic intervention followed by transfer. Although PGD is not a method of DNA assembly, and although PGD was originally employed to screen for disease-linked alleles, PGD may be used to select for any allele. As scientists mine the sequence data yielded by the Human Genome Project, knowledge of links between alleles and traits seems likely to burgeon. That will give physicians an ever growing list of alleles for which to screen. Of course the more alleles for which a couple elects to screen, the less the chance of finding an embryo that possesses every allele desired. But IVF–PGD offers advantages over reprocloning. Many people, if they had their druthers, would bring forth children for whom they might select some alleles but which they would still see as 'new' people. Others may oppose reprocloning. PGD not only follows upon sexual reproduction, but reduces the risks associated with it.

Someone might interject that cloners, in comparison with those who opt for IVF–PGD, get the opportunity to select for more alleles. Only in a weak sense of 'select' is that true. Cloners must make an all-or-nothing choice, imparting to their children vastly many alleles that the cloners do not discern. In a more familiar sense of selection, one who selects an allele chooses an embryo in which one detects the allele or into which one inserts the allele.

Could cloning increase the odds of finding a desired set of alleles when screening embryos? Suppose that as of the relevant time, scientists have linked N alleles to phenotypes. We imagine a couple that has designated $n < N$ disease-linked alleles for which, were they to procure PGD, they would test. The prospective parents compare options. They could arrange for genetic testing on a cloning source's nuclear DNA and on the prospective mother's mitochondria, and if the results are satisfactory, form a clone of the source, or they could form a clone and then perform PGD on the embryo. Or they could proceed with IVF–PGD. Is cloning more likely to produce an embryo that passes n tests than is IVF–PGD? A given cloning source has no greater chance of passing n tests than does an embryo formed by IVF. It might sometimes occur that after designating n alleles, a couple hits upon a prospective cloning source that passes all n tests and that meanwhile no embryo that they have formed by IVF has passed all n tests.

---

[17] Handyside *et al.* 1992; Hardy *et al.* 1990.

But rarely, so it would seem, would this be the end of the story. While the set of prospective cloning sources available to any given couple may be as small as their family and intimates, the set of different embryos that they could produce from their own gametes is enormous. By repetitious IVF cycles, or by fertilizing a large quantity of immature oocytes harvested in a single procedure and matured in a laboratory, the couple may create many embryos for screening. Risks of asexual reproduction inherent in cloning would seem ample motivation for the IVF–PGD alternative. It would not be fatuous for a couple to think that eventually they will obtain an embryo that, so far as PGD can reveal, lacks any of the then characterized genetic predispositions to disease. The chances of attaining or approaching this salutary result will increase as methods emerge for maturing immature oocytes in the laboratory.

The second alternative is *germ line intervention*. Genetic intervention consists in the use of recombinant techniques to alter nucleotide sequences in a genome. Somatic cell genetic intervention affects only targeted nongametic cells. Genetic intervention that occurs at such an early stage of embryogenesis that the change takes effect in all cells of the body is classified as germ line intervention. In germ line intervention, one might insert into an embryo an allele thought to be associated with a trait. Critics have imagined the use of germ line intervention to produce, in a popular sobriquet, 'designer children.' As soon as germ line intervention comes along, it will offer a flexibility that neither PGD nor reprocloning can achieve. But genetic intervention poses its own complement of safety problems, including the risk of inserting sequences at the wrong loci and of inserting an abnormal number of copies. It has been said that early somatic cell gene therapy enthusiasts promised much and delivered little. Germ line intervention involves risk not just to one offspring, but to a lineage. From the first mention of germ line intervention, scientists have approached the prospect gingerly.

One proffered technique consists in constructing and introducing auxiliary chromosomes.[18] Into an embryo formed by IVF, there would be inserted a forty-seventh chromosome or twenty-fourth chromosome pair. An auxiliary chromosome would be an artificial chromosome constructed either from scratch or by truncating a human chromosome. To an artificial chromosome, a clinician would add alleles and regulatory sequences associated with traits chosen by the prospective parents. The technique could avoid the mischief of sequences inserting in native chromosomes in

[18] This strategy is explained in Stock 2002.

the wrong places or in too many copies. It is also thought that a clinician may put larger sequences into an artificial than into a native chromosome. At first one might reliably add to an auxiliary chromosome only a small number of alleles and regulatory sequences, presumably ones already found in living humans and plausibly correlated with traits. As knowledge of links between alleles and traits increases, parents could be given a larger universe of alleles from which to select, including alleles not copied from existing genomes. Upon including in an auxiliary chromosome an allele of a given gene, it may be necessary to block expression of other alleles of that gene. An auxiliary chromosome could include antisense sequences designed for that task.

The use of auxiliary chromosomes poses technical challenges – how to insert into blastomeres the large molecules that auxiliary chromosomes would constitute, how to insure that auxiliary chromosomes replicate but do not insert into native chromosomes or interfere with replication or expression of the latter, except as the intervening clinician designs, and doubtless many further problems.[19] Failure could produce havoc. We know what can occur in consequence of extra copies of chromosomes (e.g., Down syndrome). But in theory, a person born with an auxiliary chromosome could control expression of its genes by taking drugs designed for that purpose. The person might choose to activate, only late in life, genes that work against eventualities only then occurring. An advantageous move would provide the option of deleting an auxiliary chromosome from gametes. Deleting could minimize the risk that after something goes wrong, the auxiliary chromosome burdens a lineage. Suppose an embryo formed by IVF. After the embryo forms, clinicians insert an auxiliary chromosome containing two marker sequences, one at each end of its centromere, which mark the centromere for deletion. The auxiliary chromosome also includes a gene for an enzyme that cleaves at those markers, a gene that can be activated only in gametes. The embryo develops into an infant named Jane. When as an adult, Jane contemplates having a child, she will have the option, exercised by taking a drug that activates that enzyme gene, to omit the auxiliary chromosome from her oocytes. That will insure that Jane's child will not inherit the auxiliary chromosome (although the child might not inherit it anyway if the father does not have a homologous auxiliary chromosome).

Thus compelling reasons obtain for a couple to choose either IVF–PGD or germ line intervention, not reprocloning, as a method of selecting

<hr>

[19] Willard 2000 and Choo 2001.

alleles. IVF–PGD is already available, is safer than reprocloning in virtue of employing but not interfering with sexual reproduction in which both parents contribute, offers the ability to select against well-characterized genetic predispositions to disease or abnormality, and offers the ability to select for sex and for an ever growing list of alleles associated with phenotypes. Germ line intervention when perfected will afford more flexibility, allowing parents to insert alleles so as to generate combinations that even the astronomically large set of their possible embryos does not contain.

To take a situation sometimes posed as an incentive for reprocloning, consider fertile parents bereaved by the death of their daughter Marie at a young age. If Marie had suffered from a disease or abnormality, that would militate against replicating her genome. If Marie had been healthy, then although the parents may dream of replicating her, will they risk an unhealthy replica when they might conceive naturally? To take another case, suppose parents think of conceiving a child who could be available as a histocompatible organ or tissue donor to a sick child. It has already happened that parents have conceived naturally and brought forth children hoping for histocompatiblity with earlier children. Other parents, after using PGD to select a histocompatible embryo, have stored umbilical cord blood obtained during the birth of a new baby. Some people have questioned the motives of these parents. We might instead allow the possibility that those who bring forth a child thinking that the child may under some exigency become a histocompatible donor to a sibling may also fully treasure the newborn as a person. The parents may discipline any thought of a cell or organ donation by the same reasoning, taking into account the welfare of each child, that they would apply if, *after* the births of two or more children, an illness of one moved them to consider a living sibling's ability to help. In any case, the likely number of parents seeking to replace a deceased child or to bring forth a child who could donate to a sibling would not seem large enough to exert a significant effect on a population. For the reasons given, it also seems dubious that reprocloning by fertile couples in general will have a significant effect on a population.

(2) We may now consider couples experiencing infertility. To them, reprocloning will present the same congeries of burdens and risks as in (1). If such couples elect IVF, or at some future time, genetic engineering, they may select some particular alleles, but will still see themselves as bringing forth new people. To these couples, there applies the same analysis as in (1).

There is one special case. Some women do not produce oocytes that are sufficiently developed or of good quality. There also exists a small but nonempty set of men who do not produce sperm. (These are to be distinguished from men who produce sperm of insufficient motility, for whom fertility physicians can achieve fertilization by intracytoplasmic sperm injection.) Suppose a couple encountering both problems. They could avail themselves of both donated sperm and oocytes. But if they want to insist that at least one of them make some genetic contribution to the offspring, they might consider reprocloning of one of them using a donated oocyte. The number of couples for which both such problems obtain is very small, and seems likely to dwindle as current research pursues the procurement of patient-specific pluripotent stem cells that may be induced to issue in sperm and oocytes (provided that conception by means of such gametes would be safe[20]). If only one of the prospective parents does not produce usable gametes and wishes to become a biological parent, reprocloning of that prospective parent might be chosen so that such parent could make a genetic contribution. But IVF using donated gametes will be safer and will avoid the problems associated with reprocloning.

(3) Prospective parents who are affected by or carriers of hereditary diseases might consider reprocloning as a means of copying a putatively healthy nuclear genome in lieu of risking the creation by them of a new genome. Should it happen that a disease in point is a mitochondrial one that afflicts the prospective mother, that would render her oocytes unsuitable for reprocloning. In that case the couple might consider use of a donor's oocytes. I shall concentrate on nonmitochondrial diseases. We may define four pertinent situations. (i) If either but not both of the spouses possesses the allele for a dominant disease (e.g., Huntington's or muscular dystrophy), then instead of taking the at least .5 chance that a baby conceived by them will inherit at least one copy of the disease-linked allele, the couple might choose to clone the spouse not possessing that allele, or to clone anyone else other than the spouse possessed of the disease-linked allele. (ii) If both spouses possess the allele for a dominant disease, then in lieu of the at least .75 chance that a baby conceived by them will inherit that allele, they might clone someone other than themselves. (iii) If both spouses are carriers of a recessive disease, i.e., they are heterozygous for an allele linked to that recessive disease, then rather than take the .25 chance that a baby conceived by them will be homozygous for the recessive allele, they might clone either of themselves. (iv) If both spouses are homozygous in respect of the allele for a recessive disease, then rather than conceive a child who is also a homozygote for the recessive allele, they might clone someone other than themselves.

---

[20] As discussed in Testa and Harris 2004.

Possession of a pair of alleles characterized as conferring a genetic predisposition to disease does not guarantee disease. By virtue of a variety of phenomena and mechanisms – biologists know them as lack of dominance, partial dominance, codominance, variable expressivity and incomplete penetrance, epistasis, and epigenetics – the probabilities that a child will be affected by a hereditary disease are less than those yielded by the simple Mendelian analysis assumed in the previous paragraph. But whatever the odds, two noncloning strategies present themselves. Each seems superior to reprocloning. The first strategy is less risky than reprocloning. Prospective parents could conceive by IVF and immediately thereafter procure PGD. Using PGD, physicians may select for intrauterine transfer only embryos that have not inherited a pairing of alleles known to predispose to disease. In the second strategy, if the prospective parents' views concerning abortion allow for this, they may conceive naturally on the understanding that if genetic tests during pregnancy reveal a predisposition to disease or any other defect, they may elect to terminate the pregnancy. Either the first or second strategy will work for all diseases with which scientists have correlated predisposing alleles – of which ever more will be known as genomics operates on the fruits of the Human Genome Project. Both strategies will issue in children to which each parent has made a genetic contribution. Both strategies will avert the risks inherent in asexual procreation. For people affected by or carriers of hereditary diseases who come to know of these strategies, reprocloning may have little to commend it.

In the relatively rare case of (iv), two persons who are homozygous for a recessive disease allele have married, they wish to have a child, and the woman is healthy enough to bear one. Neither of the foregoing two noncloning strategies will work. In the short run, this presents an incentive for reprocloning. In the long run, a couple in this situation is likely to prefer germ line intervention. By the time reprocloning has become safe, germ line intervention will likely have become reliable in some domains. Germ line alterations of an embryo formed by IVF could eliminate or prevent expression of the recessive allele. Thereby the prospective parents could bring forth a child not genetically predisposed to the disease and to which each parent has contributed genetically. But even before the availability of germ line intervention diminishes their number, the instances of (iv) will probably be too few to result in a significant effect on a population.

(4) Some single women, and female couples, may wish to bear and raise clones. If this practice became prevalent, would it undermine the role of the family? Reprocloning seems unlikely to effect a significant increase in the number of children reared outside a marriage of man and woman.

Here again, in view of reprocloning's burdens and risks, presently available technology seems preferable in both convenience and extent of risk. Single women and female couples can achieve pregnancy by means of artificial insemination using sperm available from sperm banks. Thereby they can spare themselves ovarian stimulation, oocyte retrieval, and intrauterine transfer, as demanded in IVF or reprocloning, and spare their offspring and themselves the risks of asexual reproduction. Even when a single woman or female couple would prefer a clone to a product of fertilization by a stranger's sperm, they would confront the same considerations that come to bear for anyone else thinking of reprocloning. When prospective parents think about the risks posed in reprocloning to the offspring, they will recognize a compelling case for sexual reproduction.

In the foregoing, I have tried to offer a dispassionate analysis of the incentives for reprocloning so as to enable us to infer something about its probable incidence. I may have erred in imagining incentives, or in assessing their relative strengths. Even so, I hope to have illustrated the sort of analysis on which we should insist before anyone rushes to embrace any of the speculations that can be heard about reprocloning's effects. To summarize, it seems that the preponderance of couples would be unlikely to bear clones even if reprocloning were free of burden and risk. Given incentives ranging from pleasure to principle to avoiding unnecessary expense, they would just as lief bring forth children the old-fashioned way. Reprocloning also seems an inferior strategy for those affected by or carriers of hereditary diseases, except in rare cases of spouses both homozygous for a recessive allele. For a fertile couple, reprocloning seems extremely burdensome in comparison with natural conception. There may be couples who might like to replicate the nuclear genome of someone they admire. There may be single women who prefer to bear someone's clone rather than a sexually-created conceptus. But anyone who would substitute artificial for natural conception so as to engage in genetic selection would take on greater risks by choosing reprocloning than if they chose assisted sexual reproduction followed by screening for genetic defects. Another consideration is that the all-or-nothing choice of relatively safe reprocloning will offer less selectivity than will genetic engineering when it is relatively safe. For the same reasons, infertile couples will likely prefer assisted sexual reproduction to reprocloning, the latter being only a last resort. Considering that only in unusual circumstances does reprocloning appear preferable to alternative reproductive methods, we may surmise that the incidence of reprocloning, as and when relatively safe, will be low.

(d) Assessing the objections

Having heard the objections to reprocloning, and surmising but not knowing that the incidence of reprocloning may be low, what shall we say to urgings that we condemn reprocloning in all events? Should the state prohibit it?

By way of objections, we have heard speculations about how the lives of clones might go. The closer one looks at the speculations, the more contrived they seem. Most seem to betray an overdose of genetic determinism. None of us have ever met a clone. We have known happy monozygotic twins. Even though we often have trouble telling such twins apart, no amount of speculation about identity crises would lead us to question whether monozygotic twins should have been born. There is arguably less cause for concern about clones, since a clone's age may differ by decades from that of the source, and the mores and places in which they are respectively reared will differ. I do not imply that we should ever neglect any psychological or social difficulties that ensue if clones someday come forth. I do think it appropriate to train a sceptical eye on the claim that, by virtue of its effects, reprocloning will always be wrong. In canvassing those unusual circumstances in which reprocloning might be preferable to reproductive alternatives, we have found little that seems worthy of condemnation – not the desire of spouses homozygous for a recessive disease to spare their child from the disease, not the desire of prospective parents to make a genetic contribution to a child, not the cloning of a deceased child. Each of the objections that predicts an effect on a population or society collapses if the incidence of reprocloning is low. Reprocloning does not seem a threat to undermine marriage and sexual union as the predominant method of reproduction. If clones will not constitute a significant portion of the population, they will not significantly diminish the genetic diversity of the population. We might even surmise that in a crisis, reprocloning could serve as a means of distributing alleles for which the gene pool is understocked. AIDS has reminded us that, despite our knowledge of microbiology and success in devising vaccines, a virus can appear that we do not immediately know how to defeat. If, as bubonic plague once did, a highly infectious and virulent virus began to devastate the human race, and if some humans were resistant to the virus but the then state of science did not explain how, the ability to clone people who were resistant might be a mercy. As for suspicions of narcissism, for others to pass judgment on someone's motive for having a child is a dubious limb out on which to go. To object to narcissism may be to impugn many instances of natural conception.

Turning to a religious point of view, we observe that according to Christian belief, Christ was born by parthenogenesis. The word 'parthenogenesis,' in the Greek, reads 'virgin birth.' People may think about this in different ways. Human parthenogenesis could be understood as a process reserved for Christ. (His birth would differ from parthenogenesis as we understand it, which, because an oocyte lacks a Y chromosome, can produce only females.) Or the method of Christ's birth could be taken to refute the claim that human asexual procreation has never occurred and should not occur. In any case, if we could discuss reprocloning with God, we would be talking about a method of conception that He had allowed us to discover. Would He say that He prefers that we not use the method? We, none of us, can confidently claim to know that, when pregnancy and maternal bonding would ensue in any case, He would wish us to shun any particular method of conception.

A more general objection is that we should condemn germ line intervention and therefore reprocloning as its global version. Or it may be contended that parents should not avail themselves of germ line intervention for enhancement insofar as enhancement may be distinguished from therapy. To attempt enhancement would betray hubris challenging the genetic choices of God. When it comes to tampering with reproduction, less is more. For those who take this view, it is cold comfort that selective genetic engineering is preferred over reprocloning. They fear that contributions to knowledge gained by studying germ line intervention will foster reprocloning, and vice versa. But any prediction that reprocloning will pave the way to designing children would betray a misapprehension. The pressures exerted by diseases have long propelled efforts to accomplish germ line intervention. We shall not reach germ line intervention via a slippery slope that descends from reprocloning. We are already headed there directly. Genomics is likely to yield the sequences and loci of predisposing alleles for an ever longer list of diseases. The day could arrive at which germ line intervention reliably corrects or blocks expression of those alleles. It allows parents to bring forth children of their own making while incurring a much lower risk of defects than they would incur in natural conception. For couples who conceive by IVF, it would seem dubious to bar their physicians from intervening genetically to avert disease if the odds of the intervention's success exceed the odds of any treatment after birth. It may further be argued that prospective parents to whom germ line intervention is available bear moral responsibility for their children's genetic endowments to the extent that they choose or do not choose such intervention. Whereupon it becomes virtuous for prospective parents to conceive by IVF and to arrange for genetic testing followed by germ line intervention to fix any detected defect.

A rational creature, so it would seem, would not accept the chance results of a genetic lottery if by exercise of its faculties it had found a more efficient way to endow its offspring with advantageous genes. That is to say that rational creatures would effectively direct evolution to the extent that they can. Those who would act to avoid transmitting maladies, to ward off threats, and to give their offspring other genetic advantages would fulfill their nature as rational beings. To restrain them from doing so could not plausibly be defended on grounds of insisting on the natural. Rawls remarks that the pursuit of reasonable policies to insure 'the best genetic endowment' is something that earlier generations owe to later.[21] From a religious point of view, it is not obvious that selecting alleles encroaches on a divine prerogative. Even in traditions that foster arranged marriages, the belief prevails that God allows humans to decide who marries whom. By selecting mates, humans greatly affect the genomes of human offspring. By what token would one know that God disapproves of further selectivity? One common religious view of reproduction is that it is a divine-human collaboration. The notion of collaboration implies more than passivity by each collaborator. One might even argue that responsible human collaboration demands that we heed what we know. We ought to take action to prevent maladies that we know how to prevent, if not to enhance our children as best we know how.

To this we may hear the objection that enhancements will foster invidious discrimination against those not enhanced. But genetic engineering will not invent discrimination, a practice already thriving as to traits in general. The temptation to be invidious should remind us, as do Kant and many religions, to recognize the dignity of each person.

The conventional explanation of why sex evolves in species is that sexual reproduction allows an enormous number of combinatorial possibilities, producing such variety in individual genomes that the species as a whole thrives and survives new threats. Germ line intervention following IVF would not sacrifice this advantage. Following upon creation of a new genome by syngamy, germ line intervention would only effect a modicum of allelic changes. Knowing how easily things can go wrong, the incentive would obtain to perform only those modifications that could reliably be done with predictable effects. The results might confer important competitive advantages. We could imagine, for instance, that designed

---

[21] Rawls 1971a, p. 108.

modifications endow humans with the ability to withstand threats resulting from global warming. We can also imagine that as rational creatures design, they will make mistakes. They will pick alleles that produce disadvantages.

If prospective parents have a duty not to use a method of reproduction that risks bringing forth a severely abnormal child, it may even be argued that germ line intervention is obligatory if and when artificial conception has been perfected to the point that it poses less risk for offspring than does natural conception. But germ line intervention requires that conception occur artificially. Although one could alter some gamete nucleotide sequences,[22] in natural conception one cannot control or predict which of the at least 4^{23} different spermatozoa that a man is capable of producing will fertilize which of the at least 4^{23} different oocytes that a woman is capable of ovulating. Hence one cannot know which of 4^{46} possible zygotes will form. To arrange reliably that an offspring will bear a substantial number of engineered sequences in all its cells appears infeasible unless an opportunity arises for genetic engineering immediately after conception. To perform that, the conceptus must be accessible. Absent a feasible way to perform genetic engineering *in utero* – presently one cannot even detect natural conception until after implantation – one must arrange for conception to occur outside the body. Of course the notion that artificial conception is obligatory and natural conception reckless would threaten the emotive value that we attach to conjugal reproduction. For present purposes it suffices to observe that the chance that a plausible claim might someday be stated merely that germ line intervention is less risky for the offspring than natural conception should give considerable pause to anyone who would condemn germ line intervention in all circumstances.

The circumstances that germ line intervention can only be accomplished when conception is achieved artificially, that humans prefer natural conception, and that many could not afford anything else will constrain the population-wide effect of germ line intervention. Though I cannot pursue further the morality of germ line intervention, it seems to me that there obtains a plausible moral defense of germ line intervention such that reprocloning should not be condemned because it is a version of that practice. Whether germ line intervention in general and reprocloning in particular are moral depends on empirical information – about safety, individual consequences, and societal consequences. We do not know all the pertinent facts. The morality of reprocloning when relatively safe will be an issue for

---

[22] In one technique demonstrated in mice, testes can be made to produce only genetically engineered spermatozoa (Brinster and Avarbock 1994).

another era. The case has not been made that reprocloning will always be wrong.

(e) Prohibition and privacy

'A frontier must be drawn,' wrote Isaiah Berlin, 'between the area of private life and that of public authority. Where it is to be drawn is a matter of argument, indeed of haggling.'[23] At least two senses of privacy appertain here. One is secrecy of information, the other is an inviolable domain of liberty. A prohibition of reprocloning would infringe privacy in the latter sense. Compelled disclosure that a child is a clone would thwart an expectation of privacy in the sense of secrecy, and may exert a chilling effect on privacy in the sense of an inviolable domain of liberty.

I assume that any tenable theory of justice provides for allowing each person some range of action consistent with allowing a range of action for others and as to which it bounds the extent of interference by others or the state.[24] Recognizing reproduction as a personal liberty follows from a plausible line of reasoning for a Kantian who holds oneself obligated to respect the autonomy of rational beings pursuing self-chosen ends, for an intuitionist who recognizes prima facie moral principles, for a contractarian who respects the equal liberties of persons each capable of forming and revising a conception of the good, for a utilitarian who adopts those policies about liberty that maximize aggregate preference satisfaction, and for a proponent of virtue ethics who respects individual liberties in order to promote human flourishing.

At such time as reprocloning is safe, protecting the physical welfare of offspring and the public health will collapse as a rationale for banning reprocloning. In respect of legislating against the immoral, even if that were established as proper, our review of the objections to reprocloning has not detected, within an overlapping political consensus, a compelling case against reprocloning. Rawls holds that it lies within public reason to assert that government should protect 'the orderly reproduction of society over time,' of which the family is the basis, but he adds that it would step outside public reason to condemn, for instance, same-sex marriage.[25] According to common sense morality, few things are as private – in the sense both of conduct appropriately shielded from probing eyes and of conduct that we should respect as the exercise of liberty – as procreation.

[23] 'Two Concepts of Liberty' in Berlin 1969, p. 124.
[24] As Rawls observes, a domain of privacy is not a prejustitial given (2001, p. 166).
[25] Rawls 1999, pp. 587, 595–596.

Here we are not concerned with government restraints with respect to a conceptus already in gestation, i.e., the issue of abortion. Rather we are concerned with decisions concerning whether and how to conceive. For a given couple, such a choice is theirs. No one else may dictate to them. Decisions by people about natural conception – about whom to marry and whether and how to conceive – produce profound population-wide effects, but insofar as we respect privacy, we do not collectively dictate those decisions. If we would object to a restraint on natural conception because it restrains liberty, then by parity of reasoning we ought to object to a prohibition of reprocloning when relatively safe.

'If the right of privacy means anything,' the Supreme Court of the United States has said, 'it is the right of the individual . . . to be free from unwarranted governmental intrusion into matters so fundamentally affecting a person as the decision whether to bear or beget a child.'[26] The Court originally declared a right of privacy when it held unconstitutional a statute prohibiting contraception.[27] The Court located such right within, as it put it, the 'penumbra' of the Bill of Rights of the U.S. Constitution, most especially the Fourteenth Amendment's provision that no state 'shall deprive any person of life, liberty, or property, without due process of law.' To beget a child would seem to be a quintessential liberty warranting protection from governmental intrusion. Courts have also held that where a physician's assistance is ordinarily needed to take some action protected by this inferred right of privacy, the zone of privacy includes a physician's assistance. At any given moment in history, a court may or may not extend this line of reasoning, which has unfolded in cases concerning contraception and abortion,[28] to asexual reproduction. One can envision the contention that judges of yesteryear imagined only sexual reproduction and that their successors ought not extend to asexual reproduction protections fashioned on the supposition that all reproduction is sexual. We may anticipate that in many quarters, including courts, a dim view will be taken of asexuality.

Precedents do obtain for legal restraints on conception – among them laws that bound how many children a woman can bear, that compel sterilization of those thought to breed undesirable characteristics, and that implement other eugenics programs. But it may be rejoined that except for laws such as anticonsanguinity statutes that protect the public health, legal restraints on whether and how to conceive have no place in a free society. Overweening laws about conception are among the hallmarks of

---

[26] *Eisenstadt v. Baird*, 405 U. S. 438 (1972).   [27] *Griswold v. Connecticut*, 381 U. S. 479 (1965).

[28] E.g., *Planned Parenthood of Southern Pennsylvania v. Casey*, 505 U. S. 833 (1992). Concerning this I have benefited from discussions with Laurence Tribe and John Mansfield.

totalitarian regimes. As Mary Warnock once said of laws against artificial insemination, enforcement of a law against reprocloning would install 'a band of snoopers or people ready to pry into the private lives of others, which might well itself constitute a moral wrong.'[29] Transgression of such a ban would put physicians and parents in jeopardy of fine and imprisonment for using what, so we are assuming, has become a relatively safe method of conception.

If what I have conjectured about the extent to which couples would prefer reprocloning over alternatives were to be approximately correct, then the following case would be analogous. Suppose that someone in an industrialized democracy proposes a law that no couple may produce more than a dozen children. It may fairly be asked what need obtains for the restraint. As a result of numerous disincentives against large families, relatively few couples wish to bring forth more than a few children. Hence there is no substantial problem of supernumerary families about which to worry. In such case, why bar the unusual couple that has brought forth a dozen children from having another?

To endorse a ban on reprocloning when relatively safe is impliedly to hold that even if other instances of procreation are private in the sense of inviolable, cloning is not. The burden on a proponent of such a ban is to adduce convincing nonsafety grounds that warrant this view of privacy. The common sense view says that assisted asexual reproduction is just as private as assisted sexual reproduction.

6.4 STRATEGIC PROHIBITION OF NONREPROCLONING

What we have just reviewed will illuminate a pragmatic argument to which I now turn. The argument has been advanced for the proposition that even if nonreprocloning is moral, the procedure should be prohibited anyway. The argument begins with the prediction that use of nonreprocloning in research and therapy will boost scientific knowledge about reprocloning. This knowledge will hasten the day when reprocloning becomes so reliable as to tempt our mercurial descendants to remove all legal obstacles, embark on the practice of reprocloning, and visit on humankind its putative deleterious consequences. A slippery slope descends from nonreprocloning in regenerative medicine to reprocloning. A sovereignty could nip the development of reprocloning in the bud by prohibiting nonreprocloning. It is

---

[29] Warnock 1985, p. xii.

therefore concluded that all use of cloning by nuclear transfer should be prohibited by national laws, and by treaty among nations.[30]

Support for this argument's opening premise may arise if investigators using nonreprocloning to learn the secrets of reprogramming generate knowledge that bears upon reprocloning techniques. Let us grant the premise that the practice of nonreprocloning could yield some knowledge facilitating improved techniques of reprocloning. Not every decisionmaking surface is slippery. As Hare once noted, when the US adopted the rule that automobiles may turn right after stopping at red traffic lights, there did not ensue significantly more accidents involving right-turning vehicles. The slippery slope is an overworked metaphor. The public, so politicians are quick to point out, easily summons the collective will to prohibit reprocloning. Making reprocloning relatively safe will be a tough row to hoe. Attempts would likely produce miscarriages at best and badly deformed babies at worst. Public condemnation of that could stop reprocloning in its tracks. If somehow the day arrives when reprocloning has become relatively safe, a collective resolve against it could hold firm on nonsafety grounds. It is not a foregone conclusion that if reprocloning becomes safe, a majority will condone it.

But the salient defect of the slippery slope argument is not its prediction that reprocloning will prove irresistible. Rather the argument founders on the premise that governments can nip reprocloning in the bud if they forbid nonreprocloning. On the contrary, knowledge useful for human reprocloning may accumulate inexorably. Cloning of nonhuman mammals has been pursued in animal husbandry for decades, and is now a subject of keen scientific interest. Research on reprocloning of other animals, particularly as it progresses with primates, may constitute a direct source of knowledge bearing upon how reprocloning could be accomplished in humans. Only in the improbable event that prohibitions of nonreprocloning are imposed worldwide and everywhere enforced would there not occur knowledge dividends that could be cashed by reprocloning aspirants. Wherever originated, new scientific knowledge will travel rapidly through the pages of journals.

We should appreciate that it may be infeasible to prevent the practice of reprocloning if ever it becomes relatively safe and widely sought. For the reasons that I have indicated, other methods of germ line intervention may be preferable to reprocloning, and if reprocloning is not widely sought, we need not be concerned about its effects. But suppose for the sake of argument that reprocloning does become popular and achieves some advantage.

[30] The following response to this argument is discussed more fully in Guenin 2001b.

Consider a reprocloning prohibition of the widest sweep, an international treaty in which the signatories covenant to enact legislation that forbids reprocloning. If merely a few sovereignties were to decline to enter into this treaty, or if any signatories were not to install effective anticloning law enforcement mechanisms, reprocloning could be pursued. Suppose then that someone, whether an individual or group or nation, manages by reprocloning to produce offspring perceived to possess some advantage as viewed by rivals. Rivals acting rationally would then seek to practice reprocloning. Prospective parents who happen to desire reprocloning in jurisdictions where it is prohibited would travel or emigrate to jurisdictions where no prohibition obtains. Sovereignties would behave similarly, rushing to follow the first entrant. If by any technique, a country succeeds in producing genetically enhanced citizens, their competitors, military or economic, would not want to risk falling behind. So strong are the incentives for rational agents to follow suit under threat of genetic inferiority that in the long run, national laws against any popular technique of reproduction may be unenforceable.

Even if it could be shown that some ban on nonreprocloning would impede progress toward reprocloning, the slippery slope argument does not justify such a ban. The argument relies upon the assumption that reprocloning is always wrong. As and when reprocloning becomes relatively safe, one could plausibly maintain on behalf of at least some prospective parents that reprocloning is permissible. In default of any showing that the targeted reprocloning conduct is wrong, the slippery slope argument provides no warrant for a ban that sweeps nonreprocloning within its maw at the cost of foregone humanitarian benefits. Viewed from the perspective of years hence, the measure of damage wrought by a jurisdiction's forbearance from nonreprocloning in research could be the amount of suffering that would have been relieved had its research enterprise joined a worldwide effort.

CHAPTER 7

Analyzing alternatives

I now wish to discuss some proposed courses of action that, by their propo-nents' lights, would allow the polity to reap benefits such as what publicly-supported embryo use might provide, but which would not require us to resolve collectively whether embryo use is moral. The rationale for one such course of action speaks of noncomplicity of experimenters downstream from embryo use. Other imagined alternatives to embryo use purportedly would issue in functional equivalents of embryonic derivatives. I shall be concerned in particular with the proposition that one or more of the pro-posed courses of action would be morally superior to embryo use. We shall see that this proposition has been floated but not sustained, and that the justification of epidosembryo use still commands our attention.

7.1 PUTATIVE NONCOMPLICITY

Let us first consider the following proposed intermediation scheme. As a standard practice, when progenitors choose to donate epidosembryos to medicine, their attending physicians transfer the embryos, or cells donated for creation of embryos, to intermediaries. Two attributes qualify an agent as an intermediary for this purpose. The first is that the agent knows how to obtain derivatives (e.g., stem cells) from embryos. The second is that the agent is not, qua intermediary, a public scientist. For this purpose, a public scientist is a scientist for whose research in regard to embryos the state directly or indirectly provides funds. Upon receiving donations, intermediaries obtain derivatives from the embryos donated as such. With the donated cells, the intermediaries create embryos, then obtain derivatives from them. The intermediaries conform their procedures to what they believe will generate derivatives desirable for investigators to study. The intermediaries supply what they derive to public scientists.

This intermediation scheme, it is thought, will accommodate the con-cerns of citizens who hold that embryo use is wrong. It is claimed that this scheme saves from complicity in destruction of embryos the participating public scientists, the government that funds their work, and the taxpayers that fund the government. It is as if there stands a culpability firewall between the intermediaries and downstream experimenters. This scheme was not born of moral analysis. It was introduced to ground a Pickwickian claim that a policy providing funds for studies of embryonic derivatives would comply with a law prohibiting funding of 'research in which a human embryo or embryos are destroyed.'[1]

Stated in regard to the embryo rather than the investigators, a distinction between obtaining embryonic derivatives and using such derivatives is a distinction between sacrificing embryos and using the remains. The sacrifice of epidosembryos is either wrong or not wrong. If, as I maintain, epidosembryo sacrifice is not wrong, then the imagined firewall is superfluous, the intermediation scheme pointless. Suppose, contrary to what I have argued, that epidosembryo use is wrong. As we earlier saw, complicity arises in virtue of a nexus between a wrongdoer and an accomplice. If s_i, who derives and studies embryonic stem cells without use of public money, sacrifices an embryo in order to meet a request for embryonic stem cells from some public scientist t_i, s_i and t_i are effectively collaborators (and will probably call themselves such). Another s_j's sacrifice of an embryo may not correspond to any particular public scientist's request. It may be that s_j sacrifices embryos so as to develop cell lines for s_j's own work, and, in fulfilling requests from other scientists, s_j may split off and ship cells from already created, indefinitely propagating lines. Still another s_k might be a nonprofit institution that regularly sacrifices embryos as s_k develops and stockpiles embryonic stem cell lines in anticipation of demand from public stem cell scientists. Public scientists who receive cells form s_i, s_j, or s_k must provide assurances to their institutional review boards concerning their sources of embryonic derivatives. Hence in their research protocols, public scientists will identify these intermediaries as their sources.

In each of the foregoing cases, public scientists have induced supply. Demand for embryonic derivatives induces supply not only directly, but as an invisible hand effect of the independent actions of prospective

---

[1] This prohibition was imposed in the US in Pub. L. 104–99, §128, 110. Stat. 26, 34 (1996), and verbatim perennial successors, becoming the rate-limiting step of federally-funded embryonic stem cell research. I have elsewhere noted that an evident legislative intent to avoid government or taxpayer complicity in embryo sacrifice would importune construing 'research in which' to capture any research project of which embryo destruction is a direct, collaborative, or induced stage (Guenin 2001a and 2005c). The referenced policy is set forth in 'NIH Guidelines for Research Using Human Pluripotent Stem Cells,' 65 Fed. Reg. 51976 (2000), as reprised in legislation (e.g., S. 5, 110th Cong., 1st Sess. [2007]).

investigators. In respect of a given investigator t_i, it might be thought that embryo sacrifice would doubtless occur even if t_i did not seek embryonic derivatives. But there is no denying the invisible hand effect of the set $\{t_1, t_2, \ldots, t_i, \ldots, t_n\}$. We have seen this illustrated in another controversy in which complicity is pivotal. A furrier acquires coats from wholesalers at the end of a distribution chain composed of multiple intermediaries. The furrier never lays a hand on an animal, but the furrier's demand for coats, and that of other retailers acting independently, produces a retail demand function for coats. This supply-inducing effect renders the retailers complicit in animal killing. Antivivisectionists would add that consumers who buy fur coats are also complicitous in animal killing, this by an invisible hand effect creating the consumer demand that engenders retail demand.

Complicity transmits through the channels of inducement. When a chain of induced supply runs from investigators who sacrifice embryos to investigators who experiment with the sacrificed embryo's derivatives, the downstream investigators are complicit in embryo sacrifice. From a moral point of view, the source and the recipient ride in the same boat. A proponent of the intermediation scheme might rejoin that what renders furriers culpable is complicity in inducing the deaths of animals whose demise is not otherwise imminent. We should exonerate downstream investigators who induce the sacrifice of surplus embryos that would otherwise soon die. This rejoinder does not buttress a claim of noncomplicity. Rather it offers imminent death as a justification for embryo sacrifice. Imminent death, as we saw in §2.4, is not alone a justification for killing.

Because scientists working on embryonic derivatives collectively induce the sacrifice of embryos, the intermediation scheme's firewall is only an illusion of moral shelter. If using an embryo in research is not permissible, then whether a scientist sacrifices embryos, or instead induces someone else to do so, will make no moral difference. If embryo sacrifice is not permissible, then the intermediation scheme leaves downstream investigators, and any government that supports their research, complicitous in wrongdoing. Notwithstanding whatever attempts might be made to imagine other noncomplicity schemes,[2] it appears that the circumstances of research are such that there is no practical scheme for supplying embryonic derivatives to funded projects that will immunize the projects' investigators or funding grantors from complicity in embryo sacrifice. Embryo-based research without complicity in embryo use is infeasible.

---

[2] Another scheme takes the form of a policy to provide funding for studies of only those derivatives obtained before announcement of the policy. In Guenin 2004 and Guenin 2005c, I analyze this as another venture toward noncomplicity that fails to achieve it.

Notwithstanding that a putative noncomplicity scheme may be struck in the foundry of political compromise, it provides embryo-based research an insecure rationale. Such a scheme reinforces the belief that using embryos in experiment is wrong. That the scheme then brings complicity in its train renders the scheme futile. That it exacts a cost in progress of research at no moral gain renders it worse. It will likely impose arrangements as artificial and constringent for the working scientist as they are unavailing from a moral point of view. We would not commission a team of particle physicists to collect data from a detector but suggest that they not build it. In stem cell research, a challenge looms to discover what is the optimal composition of a culture medium and to learn what biochemical pathways need to be stimulated or enhanced.[3] The artificial division of labor effected by the intermediation scheme thwarts the acquisition of knowledge that public scientists would acquire were they themselves to derive the cell lines that they study. The intermediation scheme bars public scientists possessed of expertise in diseases from themselves developing cell lines that model the diseases. The scheme constrains the number, robustness, and genetic diversity of available cell lines.

Failure of the noncomplicity gambit reminds us that an effective defense of embryo-based research must be direct. Some people might be taken in for the moment by the illusion of a complicity firewall, but in the long run, one cannot construct a stable consensus on an illusion. If one is going to perform research using embryonic derivatives, one must justify embryo sacrifice. We may justify studies of embryonic derivatives, but it is no part of that defense to deny complicity in embryo sacrifice. According to my defense thereof, epidosembryo-based research is moral not because obtaining derivatives and studying them are separable, but because both are permissible.

7.2 STUDYING THE DEVELOPED HUMAN

I turn to an objection to embryo use that, in the public arena, has gotten as much attention as the fundamental question of permissibility. That is the objection that the question of permissibility is moot because one does not need to use embryos to achieve what has been sought from them. The objection has first arisen for the case of stem cell research, presently the vanguard of embryo use.

---

[3] I am indebted for this insight to George Daley.

Cato, a propounder of this objection, opposes embryo use in principle. To enhance his case against embryo use, he also stakes the claim that regenerative medicine may succeed by studying stem cells that he designates by the term 'adult.' On this ground, he advocates that stem cell research confine itself to the study of these cells, and urges that embryo use be barred. Cato's use of 'adult' here disserves clarity, because the stem cells of adults are, in plasticity, alike those of other developed humans, including fetuses, children, and adolescents – they are multipotent or unipotent. I shall instead draw a distinction between cells obtained from developed humans and cells obtained from embryos. Cato goes on to assert the general precept that when we are given a choice between functionally equivalent alternatives, we ought to choose the least morally problematic alternative.

It cannot be gainsaid that embryo use gives pause. But in consequence of my earlier arguments, epidosembryo use occupies moral high ground such that, as the suffering of others places moral demands upon us, there would obtain comparable cause for worry about neglecting epidosembryo use as about implementing it. Since I have already developed that ground, I consider here only the following premise by reason of which Cato thinks his precept applicable. Cato contends that there exist stem cells in the developed human that are functionally equivalent to embryonic stem cells. I refer to this premise as 'functional equivalence.'

We ought to resist the temptation to say flatly that the weight of scientific evidence gives the lie to functional equivalence. What scientists now think that they know could hereafter seem ephemeral, a collection of preliminary results later eclipsed. Yet the claim of functional equivalence is implausible on its face. Although stem cells in the developed human may be capable of differentiating into one or more cell types, multipotency is a far cry from pluripotency. Pluripotent stem cells are the natural athletes of cellular generation. They can play any sport. Multipotent stem cells are lineage-restricted. They can play only a couple sports, and are bounded in their ability to self-renew. Stem cells in the developed organism also embody the effects of aging. Mutations accumulate. The biologist George Daley has observed that

On the basis of the data, no credible biologist would accept the idea that embryonic and adult stem cells have the same intrinsic or native developmental potency. It is incontrovertible that embryonic stem cells can generate all tissues, whereas it has never been shown that any form of unmanipulated adult stem cell has the same unbridled potential.[4]

[4] Daley 2003.

Even pluripotent embryonic germ cells appear less versatile than derivatives of blastocysts, this because the former originate from a later embryonic stage. Stem cells taken from amniotic fluid during amniocentesis have been characterized by their discoverers as 'an intermediate stage between pluripotent ES [embryonic stem] cells and lineage-restricted adult stem cells.'[5] These amniotic fluid cells do not form teratomas, which on the one hand is desirable, but which shows to their disadvantage insofar as forming teratomas is a telltale indicator of the robust plasticity of embryonic stem cells. Cato also suggests use of cells from spontaneously aborted fetuses, stillborn fetuses, and umbilical cord blood. Those cells arise yet later in development, not to mention that the genomes in the first two cases are doubtless defective, or so pregnancy's early end seems to indicate. To illustrate the point being made here, suppose that a fantastic new technology allowed each of us to replace some of our skin, in a procedure that does not produce any discomfort whatsoever, with skin proliferated in the laboratory from cells procured from a donor through a procedure that also does not produce the slightest bit of discomfort. Whose skin would each of us rather receive, that of our grandmother, or that of our infant niece? As it is for skin, so it seems for stem cells. The earlier, the better.

For some critically important cell types, among them cardiomyocytes and pancreatic β cells, no stem cells have yet been found in developed humans. For other types of specialized cells, the quantities of corresponding stem cells in our bodies are small, the populations difficult to find, and the means of retrieval intrusive. Even after retrieval, it may be very difficult to grow a large quantity of cells in the laboratory. Multipotent stem cells evidently do not propagate as well in the laboratory as do embryonic. Stem cells also vary in the extent to which scientists can direct their differentiation. Merely because a population of stem cells *can* differentiate toward a given fate does not guarantee that the cells *will* so differentiate, as and when a clinician wishes. Embryonic stem cells may prove easier to direct and control.

In the competitive marketplace of ideas, if embryo research did not hold special advantages, it would wane. If functional equivalence seemed likely, we would expect to see investigators rushing from controversial embryo use to the putative equivalents. The inexorable conclusion is that it is wishful thinking to suppose that the scattered stem cells of the developed human are functionally equivalent to the pluripotent embryonic. 'Wishful thinking,'

---

[5] De Coppi 2007.

as Israel Scheffler has written, 'is not a sound method; it must be tempered by collision with the stubbornness of facts.'[6]

Still clinging to the notion that embryos offer no scientific advantage, Cato is wont to trumpet any report appearing in the scientific literature that suggests plasticity of stem cells other than embryonic. He also accentuates any report of failure in embryonic stem cell research. He seeks to let the air out of the tires of those who urge his government to support such research. He exaggerates the words of embryonic stem cell investigators who circumspectly qualify their published findings and advert in public comments to how little they know. These remarks Cato portrays as admissions that their line of inquiry is futile. We have learned from encounters with such ventures as 'creation science' that we must be sceptical when advocates offer purported analyses of scientific information to reinforce conclusions that they have already reached on nonscientific grounds. In respect of candor in science, I have elsewhere presented an account of a duty of nondeceptiveness in one's assertions, arguments, and Gricean implicatures.[7] An objection to embryo research on moral grounds is quintessentially pertinent here. But insofar as one thinks that the moral permissibility of an action may depend on that action's probable success in achieving a scientific result, one should take counsel about that probability. The voice of science's mainstream has been resounding. It has described a significant probability of scientific and therapeutic rewards from the use of embryos. We could fail to apprehend the mainstream consensus on the singular promise of embryo use only by putting our heads in the sand.

It therefore seems plain that, to understate the point, embryo use meets the minimal condition of presenting such reasonable prospect of success as to warrant pursuing it alongside other avenues considered to meet that standard. We need not decide that some avenue is best or greatest. Contrary to a popular tendency to think that every set of desirable things has a best member, there is no 'better than' ordering of books in the library, and there may be no 'better than' ordering of stem cells. Biomedical research could reveal advantages for many types of stem cells – one type for one disease, another type for another disease, and so forth. We may take instruction from the history of science. It is usually not known, in advance of exploration, which avenues of inquiry are the most fruitful. Scientists have independently followed whatever paths they respectively have thought promising. Sometimes cross-fertilization produces results. Several new subfields of

---

[6] Scheffler 2001.
[7] Guenin 2005b. For an argument that Kantian duties are violated by many claims offered in support of Cato's view, see Wood 2005, pp. 323–324.

mathematics contributed to the progression of thought in which Andrew Wiles proved Fermat's Last Theorem. Sometimes great advances occur serendipitously. Roentgen discovered x-rays without looking for them. Cellular regeneration is a door for which we do not yet have the key. When delay is measured in death and suffering, we ought to seek progress on all fronts simultaneously.

Cato rejoins that embryo use has not yet cured anything. He argues that even if moral views contain remarkably similar versions of a duty of mutual aid, and even if it would fulfill that duty to aid others by using entities to which no possible persons correspond, embryo research could be a bubble. To this investigators will reply that the present agenda in embryo studies is basic research. Research on embryonic stem cells was stymied by US law from the moment at which the line of inquiry became feasible. First came the aforementioned prohibition of the use of public funds for research in which embryos are destroyed. Prohibitions of cloning later seized the legislative imagination (redundantly as to public scientists, because the same prohibition had swept within its maw 'the creation of . . . embryos for research purposes'). After its launch with private funds, embryonic stem cell research continued to sail on short reaches in provincial waters. It is of course possible that its journey, like any scientific inquiry, will not bring home results. But disparaging the nascent field of embryonic stem cell research for lack of results is analogous to criticizing a football team for failure to score prior to kickoff. On the heels of the foregoing history of constrained investigation, Cato offers the opinion that functional equivalence obtains. Of functional equivalence, we might say with Mill, 'There is the greatest difference between presuming an opinion to be true, because with every opportunity for contesting it, it has not been refuted, and assuming its truth for the purpose of not permitting its refutation.'[8]

There obtains a reasonable belief in a significant probability that embryos will yield knowledge of fundamental biology, or therapies, that differ from what other sources will yield. This suffices to motivate my present study, and to bring to bear the Duty of Beneficence.

7.3 PROCURING PLURIPOTENT CELLS

Another line of opposition to embryo use concedes the special value of pluripotent stem cells. It indulges wishful thinking in another vein. Pluripotent stem cells, we are told, can be gotten and converted to therapies without

---

[8] *On Liberty*, p. 24.

using embryos. In the following, I try to illustrate how, as such claims arise, we should go about analyzing them. In each case, we must inquire whether a proffered alternative said to be morally superior to embryo use would itself constitute or be consequent on embryo use.[9] The activated oocyte possesses properties that may be nonpareil, including its cytoplasm's ability to reprogram development. Hence the difficulty of gaining, without use of embryos, the sorts of results that embryo experiments may yield.

(1) It has been imagined that an investigator could create a mutant clone that develops to the blastocyst stage and thereupon yields pluripotent stem cells, but which clone is not an embryo. This is a contradiction in terms when 'blastocyst' is a phase sortal restricting the phase sortal 'human embryo.'

The scenario envisioned is that the investigator would alter source DNA before using it to form a clone. (This procedure has been called 'altered nuclear transfer,' although only the DNA would be altered, not the process.) The genetic alterations would be chosen in hopes of bringing about sufficient disorganization in the clone to disqualify the clone as an organism, but not so much disorganization as to scuttle derivability of pluripotent cells. It is urged that we pursue research on mutant clones, characterized as nonembryos, and refrain from embryo use.

It seems implausible that any clone at the one-cell stage would fail to be an organism. A one-cell clone's operations will integrate in the sophisticated way that makes plausible the classification of an amoeba or zygote as an organism. Concerning later stages, we saw in §3.6(b) that the modest extent of intercellular interaction in the preblastocyst embryo is such that the preblastocyst has been described as a clump of cells. Extent of organization, even if quantifiable, seems unlikely to distinguish an embryo produced by fertilization from a mutant clone that develops to the blastocyst stage. The mutant clone may by the blastocyst stage exhibit the tight junctions, desmosome-like structures, and gap junctions indicative of intercellular interaction in the zygote's successors. The reasons that we earlier encountered for characterizing an embryo produced by fertilization as an organism from activation onwards – including the simpler hypothesis that an organism exists continuously from activation – compel the same conclusion for the mutant clone by virtue of the properties with which the mutant clone begins and that bring it to the blastocyst stage. Hence the plausible conclusion that the mutant clone is an embryo, albeit a defective one.

---

[9] What I say below concerning alternatives is developed more fully in Guenin 2005d.

It might instead be imagined that a mutant clone could be disqualified as an embryo on the ground that the clone's development is not organismic. This would seem to be the point ventured when one hears an attempt to assimilate a mutant clone to either of two degenerate products of oocyte activation, the hydatidiform mole and the ovarian teratoma.[10] A hydatidiform mole sometimes forms when a sperm fertilizes an oocyte that lacks a nucleus or whose nucleus is inactive. The mole may cleave and even implant, sometimes growing to be larger than a fetus, but its growth is not organismic development. Rather the mole proceeds down a course by which it becomes a disorganized proliferation of placental tissue with little or no embryonic tissue within it. The mole's nuclear genome is all-paternal (or in some cases triploid of which two-thirds is paternal), hence abnormal from the start. An ovarian teratoma begins from an oocyte alone, possesses an all-maternal genome, and grows into a disorganized agglomeration of cells of various types. A teratoma is a proper part of a woman's body; as noted in §3.6(b), an organism is not a proper part of another organism. Neither the mole nor teratoma develops by phase changes of the sort that usually result in a human organism, hence neither is an embryo. Their development is not organismic, but a clone's is.

A clone's nuclear genome, mutant or not, is a fully diploid genome to which the source's mother and father both contributed. Upon transfer of that genome into the oocyte, organismic development began. The motivation for creating a mutant clone is to obtain pluripotent stem cells that are as close as possible to the sort of cells derivable from an embryo originated by fertilization. The investigator must forbear from any alteration of the source DNA that would defeat development of a blastocyst. This applies pressure to assure organismic development. A product of oocyte activation undergoing early organismic development is an embryo. What is more, just as the status of substantial genet or develope makes a product of fertilization an object of moral concern, a mutant clone's status as substantial genet and develope suffices for moral concern to attach to it. We cannot assume that as a clone creator attempts to steer shy of an envisioned Scylla of failure to procure stem cells, the creator will avoid the envisioned Charybdis of creating an embryo.

The creation and use of an embryo cannot be justified merely by virtue of its defects. If the cell donors have forbidden intrauterine transfer, we can

---

[10] These growths are themselves sources of pluripotent stem cells, cells that have been studied for decades, but those cells are deranged, in many cases cancerous. I thank Peter Andrews, Ralph Dittman, and William Lensch for insights into the biology of these growths.

justify the creation and use of a donated mutant clone by the argument from nonenablement. Once one accepts that argument, one has justified the use of all epidosembryos. As a mathematician would say, when we have justified the general case, we need not confine ourselves to a special case. A decision to confine research to mutant clones has no warrant. Such a decision presumably would hamper research. Even if a mutant clone creator attempts in a derived cell line to reverse genetic alterations made in the source DNA, clones are intrinsically abnormal. A compelling need arises to study not only clones, but normal embryos and their derivatives. A need arises for studies that span the genetic diversity of healthy and afflicted individuals within a population.

(2) At the outset, it is not fatuous to ask why the discussion of embryo research so quickly turns to embryo destruction. In principle, is it not feasible to experiment on an embryo, perhaps to remove some matter, without impairing its future development? The answer for now is that there is no known risk-free technique by which to perform an invasive action on a microscopic life form so delicate. Trying to develop a non-damaging technique of experimenting on an embryo selected for transfer to a uterus would be unjustified absent expected benefit to the offspring. In the case of stem cell research, incentives obtain to experiment during a pluripotency interlude that occurs after the blastocyst forms, by which time the likelihood of experimental damage appears great, and to remove multiple cells, this because blastomeres grow better with companions. Performing on an embryo selected for intrauterine transfer any experiment that will not benefit the embryo would resemble performing an appendectomy on a child that does not need the surgery but whose appendix would be useful in research. I agree with Hare's verdict that 'experimentation not involving destruction but only damage should be strictly regulated and even banned, in the interests of the person who might survive to be born damaged.'[11]

Even so, the following has been proposed. If a fertility patient has already elected preimplantation genetic diagnosis (again, 'PGD') of an embryo prior to intrauterine transfer, then the clinic could piggyback on PGD a second procedure, namely, the derivation of a stem cell line. The supposition is that if the one or two blastomeres extracted for the purpose of PGD are cultured, sufficiently many cells will eventuate such that the technician may then not only perform PGD on one or more cells, but may also derive a stem cell line from the other cells.

---

[11] Hare 1993, p. 95.

Because PGD risks damage to the embryo and to the corresponding possible person, PGD requires justification. Most embryos survive PGD, but some die, and others may suffer harm. Some patients elect PGD, but most do not. Since PGD will not in any event benefit the tested embryo or its successors in development, PGD's justification must be somewhat roundabout. One line of defense might be the following. If because of a defect detected by PGD, an embryo is not transferred, that could be considered a benefit to the parents, while being no worse for the embryo, which has not yet been enabled anyway. If the embryo is transferred, then PGD has imposed a burden and risk upon the embryo with no benefit to it, but in reply to this, it may be said that the progenitors have fulfilled a non-person-affecting duty not to select for transfer any embryo burdened by a genetic defect that would make life so miserable as not to be worth living, or that would impose a severe deformity. Because intrauterine transfer lies within progenitor discretion, testing remains permissible even if the test destroys the embryo or a removed totipotent cell. The appeal here to the not yet enabled status of the totipotent cell or embryo is less straightforward than the ground that unenabled status furnishes for epidosembryo use: at the time of the test, the progenitor has not yet decided against intrauterine transfer, so that the Duty of Noninterference then applies. It may be replied, firstly, that destruction of the embryo, if it occurs, would be accidental, and secondly, that the progenitor implicitly decided against intrauterine transfer of any totipotent blastomere when the progenitor authorized PGD, so that no possible person ever corresponded to the blastomere, and nothing could be gained by asserting Zygotic Personhood. As my purpose is only to describe a likely defense of PGD, not to maintain one, I leave the matter here.

For purposes of the piggyback proposal, we are to assume that a patient has elected PGD for reproductive reasons. Incurring the risk of PGD is a *fait accompli*. Even so, the piggyback procedure will be morally indefensible if it interposes delay. Because the rate at which cell division occurs in the cleaving ova of mammals is among the slowest in the animal kingdom, the piggyback procedure could require delaying the performance of PGD until enough cells have grown so as to leave a quantity sufficient for stem cell derivation. That delay would serve only the stem cell project, not the embryo. For the embryo's sake, the earlier the transfer into the womb, the better. Nor will parents benefit by delay. The risk associated with delay, whatever it is, cannot be justified. One can only imagine how – and whether – a physician would attempt to defend such delay to a prospective mother. Through technical improvements, it may be possible to shorten the delay, or, if single blastomeres may sometimes be induced to issue in cell lines, to avoid any delay. But if in any respect, an attempt to derive stem cells imposes, at no benefit to the embryo or even to the parents, a risk beyond that posed by PGD alone, the piggyback procedure will be objectionable.

One occasionally offered defense of the piggyback procedure is that blastomere removal in PGD has been shown safe to the extent of a high survival rate, and that thus far at least, no indication arises of adverse later consequences. This offers an *ignoratio elenchi*, the fallacy that occurs when, in Sidgwick's words, 'the journey has been safely performed, only we have got into the wrong train.' The safety of PGD is not the issue. The question that concerns us is whether, assuming a prior choice of PGD, one may subject the embryo to additional risk solely for benefit of beings other than the offspring.

(3) According to another proposal on offer, embryos that have ceased to grow should be considered dead even if some of their cells remain alive. It is imagined that from cleavage-arrested embryos, an investigator would extract such cells as remain alive, then attempt to derive pluripotent stem cells. Confirming irreversible cleavage arrest may be difficult if, for instance, an embryo appears to cease growing, goes through a resting phase, then resumes dividing. It has been suggested that cleavage arrest occurs when cellular integration ceases. As we have seen, integration in the early embryo is not well-defined. Beyond this, since cleavage arrest can occur within twenty-four hours of activation, there is the possibility that an apparently arrested embryo contains one or more live totipotent blastomeres. If the investigator cannot eliminate both the possibility that the embryo as a whole should be considered alive, and the possibility that the embryo contains live totipotent blastomeres, a consensus moral justification for using the embryo may have recourse, assuming a donor instruction barring intrauterine transfer, to the argument from nonenablement. Once one has accepted that argument, and thereby justified the use of all epidosembryos, no reason appears to restrict research to embryos so defective that growth has ceased.

(4) The last purported alternative that I shall mention is the pursuit of dedifferentiation by production of induced pluripotent stem cells, as contrasted with embryo use. Thus couched, this proposal presents a false dichotomy. Dedifferentiation consists in the transformation of specialized cells into multipotent or pluripotent cells. Dedifferentiation is the holy grail of stem cell research insofar as dedifferentiated cells may be induced to differentiate into patient-specific specialized cells with greater efficiency than, and without the complications of, nonreprocloning. The discovery that

dedifferentiation could be induced in human somatic cells was achieved not by eschewing embryo use, but by means of it. Transcription factors observed in embryonic stem cells were found to trigger reprogramming of nuclei to a pluripotent state. When investigators transferred genes encoding selected transcription factors into somatic cells, some of the cells gave rise to lines of induced pluripotent stem cells.[12] But the investigators accomplished this feat using retroviruses to transport the genes. The risks of using viral vectors are apparent from recent attempts at gene therapy. The viral genome inserts randomly and multiply in the target genome. Among the risks is insertional mutagenesis, in which an oncogene is transcribed by virtue of a viral promoter, and the cell is predisposed to cancer. Hence investigators seek nonviral ways of inducing reprogramming. Progress may be achievable by further observations of reprogramming – as it occurs in clones and in products of the fusion of embryonic stem cells and other cells – and by observing how transcription factors contribute to maintaining pluripotency in embryonic stem cells.

Embryonic stem cells remain both the standard of comparison for, as well as primary subjects for learning more about, pluripotency. It is not known whether cells that are pluripotent in consequence of dedifferentiation will behave in the same way as cells whose plasticity has never been less than pluripotent. It could obtain that investigators may more reliably direct the differentiation of embryonic stem cells than of dedifferentiated cells. It would not be surprising if cells that are similar but not exactly similar differ in their therapeutic utility. When it is not known which, if any, cell types will yield the more safe and effective therapies for a given malady, it makes sense to investigate all simultaneously. Taking the long view, embryonic stem cell research may someday be seen as the science that issued in reprogramming as a clinical technique.

Concerning any proposal of the sort just analyzed, the same technical question arises, namely, whether the technique will produce pluripotent stem cells, and if so, how the cells differ from the embryonic. While that question remains to be answered in each case, we can presently say the following. To the extent that any purported alternative to embryo use depends on the use of embryos, leans on a defense whose generality justifies the use of epidosembryos, or fails to produce therapeutically efficacious pluripotent cells or whatever else may be its humanitarian object, a choice to explore only its products and to renounce epidosembryo use would not be

---

[12] Takahashi *et al.* 2007; Yu *et al.* 2007; Park *et al.* 2008. Concerning this, I have benefited from discussions with Paul Lerou, William Lensch, and Thomas Zwaka.

a moral improvement over epidosembryo use. Such a choice would impose a moral detriment insofar as it would confine research to malengineered conceptuses, defective cells, or less efficient methods.

7.4 PARTHENOTES

Parthenogenesis consists in organismic development from an oocyte activated without insertion of foreign DNA. Parthenogenesis may be artificially induced by chemical or electrical means (which may effectively be the same process, using the same pathway). To accomplish parthenogenesis artificially, an investigator must bring about the formation of a diploid genome of 23 chromosome pairs – just as does fertilization. In fertilization, a secondary oocyte ejects one-half of its inventory of 46 chromosomes, extruding that half into the *second polar body*. That leaves 23 chromosomes to join with the sperm's 23 chromosomes. One technique for inducing parthenogenesis consists in introducing enzymes that will prevent extrusion of the second polar body upon oocyte activation. Thereby the oocyte will retain 46 chromosomes. Then if all other conditions for growth are fulfilled, the oocyte will begin dividing.

A parthenote differs notably from a product of fertilization. One conspicuous and fatal difference is that a parthenote will not develop a functional placenta. Expression of imprinted alleles, epigenetic regulation, and expression in general is thoroughly abnormal in a parthenote for want of a genetic contribution from a father. In some cases, this will result in nonexpression of a gene that should be expressed, and in other cases, in double the extent of normal gene expression.[13] So it has been considered obvious that a human parthenote will not progress beyond the blastocyst stage and cannot develop into a baby. Insofar as it is nomologically impossible for a parthenote to develop a functional placenta, if that be the case, no possible person corresponds to a parthenote. But one cannot project from this reasoning a categorical permission to use any and all parthenotes in the future. As a product of oocyte activation undergoing organismic development, a parthenote falls within my definition of 'embryo' for moral purposes. In scientific parlance, a parthenote at day 5 is a blastocyst. Pluripotent cells derived from parthenotes are referred to as 'parthenogenetic embryonic stem cells.' When legislators opposed to embryo use propose or enact statutes forbidding embryo use, they often list parthenogenesis as one of the methods of embryo creation. Moral concern may attach to parthenotes in

[13] This has been explained to me by William Lensch.

view of the nomological possibility that future genetic interventions could overcome the abnormalities in gene expression that result in placental and other problems. I proceed in the belief that it behooves us to recognize, fully and inclusively, the universe of moral concern of any view that we engage. This we may do without prejudice to the moral verdict, since we are not committed to the proposition that we must treat every embryo alike. No one need refrain from adducing facts that distinguish a particular parthenote from other embryos.

In the future, investigators creating parthenotes might employ techniques of genetic engineering that have the effect of overcoming parthenote developmental limitations. A strategy deployed in the mouse consists in mimicking a paternal genome as to particular alleles, this by initiating parthenogenesis with a primary oocyte's genome.[14] The primary oocyte is the beginning developmental stage of the oocyte; it precedes that which is ovulated, the secondary oocyte. A primary oocyte's genome has not developed long enough for full imprinting to occur. Anything that might interfere with the paternal effects to be mimicked may be deleted through genetic engineering. Whereupon the investigator transfers the altered chromosomes of the primary oocyte to a secondary oocyte, initiating activation. The parthenote thus formed has effectively been supplied with unimprinted alleles that in sexual reproduction would come from the father. This procedure differs from cloning insofar as it transfers only a haploid genome to an unenucleated recipient; it differs from parthenogenesis as traditionally understood insofar as it introduces foreign DNA, but it is still faithful to the literal sense of parthenogenesis insofar as it does not introduce any male DNA. By employing this technique as to as few as two alleles, there may occur a salutary ripple effect resulting in normal expression of many alleles. In humans, obtaining a primary oocyte from a newborn girl is not a morally permissible option, but this technique illustrates the sorts of maneuvers that scientists might use to overcome developmental failures in parthenotes. If scientists overcome those failures, thinkers of Aristotelian bent might say that inability to develop a functional placenta is an accidental attribute of a parthenote qua developing human organism. In all events, experiments with parthenote epidosembryos will be justified by the argument from nonenablement.

Parthenotes may be studied for various purposes. Parthenotes in theory could be used to achieve autologous transplantation, but only into patients from whom an oocyte can be recovered and activated, i.e., young fertile

---

[14] Kono 2004; Loebel and Tam 2004.

women. Even though not autologously, transplants without rejection may be achievable for a larger universe of patients who match closely enough to the major histocompatibility complex of a donor of a parthenogenetically activated oocyte.[15] But the question arises whether pluripotent stem cells derived from parthenotes will be as robust as those derived from products of fertilization. What defects will parthenote derivatives exhibit? Research on parthenotes is a special case that is defensible as such, but for which we need not settle when we can justify the general case.

Thus again it does not appear, any more than for the strategies discussed earlier in this chapter, that we lack a reason to tackle the morality of embryo use. Even if one or more alternatives to embryo use were to avail in stem cell biology, that would not obviate embryo use in general. Taking the long view, it seems intuitive that the salient respects in which embryos differ from other life forms will persistently draw attention to epidosembryos as permissible subjects of research.

---

[15] Kim 2007.

CHAPTER 8

Shaping norms

Once we have dealt with the primary question whether there exist embryos that may permissibly be used solely as means, we may move on to concerns that arise in connection with embryo use. We have first the matter of public policy and its confluence with such moral consensus as lies within our reach. I shall propose a policy congruent with the moral permissibility of epidosembryo use. I shall then pose some related practices that raise moral concerns, and shall attempt to construct norms that could govern such practices. I imagine a course familiar in the history of science. Innovation presents a technological advance that would enable doing good. The innovation also alarms people because it seems unnatural or susceptible of misuse. In due course there develop some consensus governing norms, and as those norms are observed, the innovation gains acceptance. In the fullness of time, the innovation results in great good, beside which any untoward consequences seem modest.

8.1 GIFTS AND CONSENTS

I begin by clarifying the practices of giving and providing informed consent. Institutions engaged in medical research operate according to the norm that in respect of a research protocol that presents some prospect of direct benefit to the subjects, or that will not seriously harm the subjects, the institution may justify using a patient as a subject if the patient provides informed consent. Conditioned to applying this norm, institutions tend to view the use of embryos as research in which the mother is the subject. They look to her, and to the coprogenitor, for consent.[1] They are apt to begin with standard documents for obtaining informed consent, documents that speak of 'selecting' and 'recruiting' subjects for clinical trials.

---

[1] E.g., National Research Council 2005, pp. 83, 101; Daley *et al.* 2007.

The fact of informed consent avails when the consenting person and the research subject are the same individual. It also avails in the circumstance in which a guardian (e.g., a parent) acts in the best interests of a subject (e.g., a minor child). In the case of embryo use, neither of these circumstances obtains. The embryo is a subject distinct from its parents. The embryo cannot consent. The contemplated research will not benefit or avoid serious harm to the embryo, but instead will sacrifice it. Embryo use does not fit the mold of 'human subjects research' as institutions have heretofore conceived it. For embryo use, the consent of the mother and coprogenitor is necessary – she is a subject insofar as oocyte retrieval is performed – but not sufficient.

Epidosembryo use is permissible not in virtue of passive parental consent, but in virtue of active conduct. The first pertinent action is a progenitor decision, communicated in a written instruction, forbidding intrauterine transfer. That decision constitutes the linchpin of a recipient institution's moral justification, within public reason as remarked at the close of §5.1, for using an embryo in experiment. Absent that decision, the only persons in the world privileged to decide the embryo's fate will not have barred intrauterine transfer. In such case a possible person will correspond to the embryo, and the justification of epidosembryo use will not apply. When consenting progenitors receive a document disclosing that contemplated experiments will consume the embryo subjects, an institution's representatives might infer that the progenitors have decided against intrauterine transfer. But an institution ought not rely on an inference when there arises the opportunity for an instruction that is explicit. The second requisite action is a gift of the embryo. When Genevieve undergoes an operation in which surgeons remove a kidney and transplant it to her ailing sister Julie, we do not merely say that Genevieve provided informed consent for the operation. Genevieve did consent after receiving pertinent information – the law would not otherwise permit the operation – but that is an altogether understated description of her generosity. We say that Genevieve *gave* her kidney to Julie.

A research institution conducting embryo research should therefore resolve to accept only epidosembryos for use in such research. It may secure this result by arranging for the following. The institution may enter into an agreement with any physician who, on behalf of a patient, proposes to deliver embryos or cells from which to form embryos. The agreement will provide that the institution will furnish to the physician a document, composed by the investigators, that describes a given research protocol in a style suitable for informing prospective donors. This document will explain how donated embryos will be consumed in experiment. Or it will explain how contributed cells will be used to form embryos, by cloning (this is not the place to do battle against ordinary usage), parthenogenesis, or fertilization, to be consumed in experiment. The document will disclose that the donor is unlikely to receive any direct benefit from the research. The agreement will provide that donations will be accepted by the institution if accompanied by a certificate from the donor's board-certified fertility physician that states, without disclosing donor identity, that both progenitors of extant embryos, or both contributors of cells donated for use in creating embryos, as the case may be, have executed a written instrument instructing that the same be donated to the institution on the condition that the institution shall use the extant or resultant embryos solely in medical research or therapy and may never transfer the embryos or any totipotent cell taken therefrom into a woman or into an artificial uterus. In the agreement, the institution will covenant for benefit of the donors to abide by these instructions. The agreement will clarify the roles of the institution and the physician. The institution will conduct research, the physician will care for the patient.

The question arises whether a fertility physician may participate in research using embryos donated by the physician's patients or received in consideration of such donations. A cautious resolution of this would preclude such involvement, thereby guaranteeing that the physician serves only the patient and that desire for research materials will not insinuate itself into advice about whether to retain or dispose of embryos. But mechanisms could be devised to minimize the effect of a conflict of interest so as to permit a physician to be an investigator. A patient could be assured that the possibility of a donation to research will not be allowed to influence the clinic's evaluation of the quality of embryos, that selection of any embryo for donation will be undertaken only after selections for intrauterine transfer have been made, and that unless the patient has declared unqualifiedly that she does not wish to bear any more children, embryo donations will be accepted from her only if she has stored some minimum number of embryos, or if the embryos selected for donation are abnormal.

The wishes of a coprogenitor may tend to be overlooked, but they demand attention. A protocol that provides for nonreprocloning must require that the person from whom source DNA originates will have been fully informed of the nature of the research and will have issued instructions that bar intrauterine transfer of, and donate to medicine, any embryo produced. This requirement would preclude use of some banked cells that vendors supply. An institution cannot reliably assume that contributors of cells for general use contemplate creation of embryos, least of all clones of themselves.

8.2 PUBLIC SUPPORT

If ever there were a public policy constituting, in Edmund Burke's phrase, 'morality enlarged,' a policy on embryo use would seem to be one. When policymakers propose measures that would fund embryo research, they often advert to a moral rationale, then unfold a list of 'strict ethical standards.' The longer the list, it seems, the better. Entries on such lists often reiterate requirements that are already law, prescribe procedures that practitioners already practice, or proscribe practices that practitioners already shun.

For citizens troubled by embryo use, the issue remains not how, but whether. The bone of contention is embryo use *per se*. A policy that rests embryo-based research on informed consent[2] will have neglected what my account depicts as constitutive of the most likely consensus ground for such research. It will have overlooked the crucial and logically prior progenitor decision. A progenitor possesses singular authority. The progenitor is the only person in the world, save for the coprogenitor, privileged to decide what will happen to embryos formed from the progenitor's cells. It is in virtue of a progenitor decision against transfer of an embryo into a uterus that it becomes permissible for a donee to use the embryo in experiment. The key premise for a government in endorsing or funding experiments that involve embryo use, as for investigators in conducting experiments, is that investigators act in consequence of permissible donor decisions barring intrauterine transfer. In reliance on the justification of epidosembryo use, I therefore propose the following rule.

> *Public Policy on Embryo Use*. Scientists may conduct, and the government shall support, biomedical research using human embryos that, before or after formation, have been donated to medicine under donor instructions forbidding intrauterine transfer.

This rule defines eligible research by reference to morally permissible research. Thereby the publicly-supported and the morally permissible coincide. Thereby the rule wears its justification on its sleeve. The more conspicuous the moral logic, the better the prospects for consensus.[3] By adoption of this rule concerning embryo use *per se*, a polity may lay a justificatory cornerstone upon which other norms may be placed.

It is possible, though not assured, that when embryo research first bears therapeutic fruit, the therapies will be unusually expensive. I subscribe to the view that a collective duty of minimal provision requires that

---

[2] As in S. 5, 110th Cong., 1st Sess. (2007).   [3] This is further discussed in Guenin 2005c.

institutions of a just society assure to all citizens throughout their lives the material requisites, including food, shelter, clothing, and health care, for sustaining the rudimentary functioning that it is reasonable to expect for each citizen's physical constitution and accidental encounters with illness and disability. I would defend this duty, though I cannot go into the details here, as a distributive principle chosen in a Rawlsian original position by rational deliberators aware of disease and disability, and as the command of a weak form of the Duty of Beneficence obliging our consent to the beneficent use of taxes collected come what may. Distribution of the benefits of epidosembryo use may be understood as a demand imposed by this duty in respect of the health care that we are obliged to assure.

8.3 OOCYTE CONTRIBUTIONS

In order that scientists may create embryos in research, they must receive oocytes. Although investigators continue to improve the process of nonreprocloning, that process is presently inefficient: for every oocyte successfully activated, many other oocytes will have failed to activate or will have issued in clones that do not survive. A need for oocytes may obtain not only in research but also in clinical medicine if it becomes feasible to perform autologous transplantation of cells derived from clones.

We earlier observed that the process of recovering oocytes imposes a significant burden on a patient – daily injections of follicle-stimulating hormone, discomforting side effects, and oocyte retrieval under anesthesia. The risks include ovarian hyperstimulation syndrome.[4] Ovarian stimulation could also adversely affect fertility, and the long-term consequences of the regimen may not be fully known. Since only a small minority of patients experience serious adverse effects during the process, young women seeking to help others may be willing to accept the burden and incur the risks. For the polity, the question is how, if at all, physicians and scientists should accept or arrange for oocyte transfers. We have here what Feinberg calls a 'two-party case' (or what Gerald Dworkin calls an occasion of 'impure paternalism').[5] That is, we have the question whether, in order to protect x, the state or a public system of rules should impose a restraint not only on the conduct of x, but on the conduct of y in dealing with x.

---

[4] 'The syndrome has a broad spectrum of clinical manifestations, from mild illness needing only careful observation to severe disease requiring hospitalization and intensive care. . . . Life-threatening complications . . . include renal failure, adult respiratory distress syndrome (ARDS), hemorrhage from ovarian rupture, and thromboembolism' (American Society for Reproductive Medicine 2003, pp. 1309–1310).
[5] Feinberg 1986, to which I am indebted for many insights concerning paternalism.

Here *x* is a woman willing to contribute oocytes and *y* may be anyone involved in procuring oocytes from her.

Two thinkers are discussing oocyte contribution. The first, Patrius, argues as follows. Offering money for oocytes runs an unacceptably high risk of inducing poor women to contribute imprudently. The prospect of receiving money is enough to induce women to neglect risk. It constitutes a good reason for the state to prohibit conduct that a prohibition will prevent harm to an agent, even if the conduct is the agent's fully voluntary and informed choice. This is the precept of *legal paternalism* (or *hard paternalism*). The state should also act to prevent an unconscionable transaction between parties of greatly disparate bargaining power. On these grounds, the state should prohibit payment of valuable consideration to women in connection with the transfer of oocytes. Consistently with Mill's harm principle,[6] the state may act to prevent not only individual but collective harm, including, in this case, harm to society from treating oocytes as commodities. A market in oocytes would produce deleterious symbolic consequences. As and when therapies such as autologous transplantation become feasible, such therapies may become the privilege of the wealthy who are able to outbid others for oocytes. It is also morally legitimate for the state to prohibit immoral conduct, this is by the precept of legal moralism. As a moral matter, no one should pay a woman to transfer an oocyte. We should follow Kant in condemning any transfer of body parts, paid or unpaid. Kant's reasoning is that the body is a part of the person. No one should treat a part of a person as a thing.[7] For Kant, selling or donating a tooth or limb falls into the same category as lying: each violates one's duty to respect humanity in one's own person. If, in Kant's metaphor, a liar 'throws away' his dignity, the transferor of a body part does so literally.[8] As it is right to prohibit payment of valuable consideration for organs,[9] it is right to do the same for oocytes.

A second discussant, Liberta, espouses a contrary view. An autonomous agent chooses her own ends. She legislates the moral law to herself. Neither the state nor any system of rules ought to curtail her liberty in respect of her body. That includes the liberty to enter into transactions concerning dispensable or renewable body parts. Women already receive money in exchange for allowing their bodies to be used in clinical trials, and more to

[6] As quoted earlier, this provides that 'the only purpose for which power can be rightfully exercised over any member of a civilized community, against his will, is to prevent harm to others.'

[7] *Lectures on Ethics* 27:346, 386–387, 602, 630.

[8] *Lectures on Ethics* 27:346, 602; *The Metaphysics of Morals* 6:423, 429.

[9] As in the National Organ Transplant Act, 42 U.S.C. §274e (2000).

the point, for contributing oocytes to fertility patients. A woman's liberty to transfer oocytes for research and to receive money therefor ought not be infringed either directly or by any restriction on those who might pay her. Nothing about the terms of an oocyte transfer shocks the conscience – unless, that is, oocyte recipients refuse to compensate transferors. For support, Liberta draws on a passage of Kant's lectures not mentioned by Patrius. Here it is said that an agent is 'at liberty to do anything in regard to his body that seems to him expedient and useful,' and further that 'to preserve our person, we have disposition over our body.'[10] On this ground, it is permissible for a woman to undergo oocyte retrieval for the purpose of therapeutic transplantation of derived cells into herself. It does not require a great leap to reach the further conclusion that it is permissible for a woman to undergo oocyte retrieval for the purpose of preserving someone else's life. Kant elsewhere allows that one will not violate a duty to oneself by giving away a nonintegral part such as hair that the body will replenish.[11] Although this is followed by a remark that 'there would still be something base' about selling hair, Kant does not give a compelling argument against selling a nonintegral part. Within his view, what alone has dignity, that which is above price, is humanity in one's person insofar as it is capable of morality. Things, on the other hand, have a market price.[12] To reason that all parts of one's body are above price because one's person is above price would commit the fallacy of division. We may honor the dignity of humanity in one's person by regarding the whole person or whole body as above price even as we regard bodily parts, especially dispensable parts, as things. In any case, Kant opposes any notion that the state or other collectivities should enforce ethical duties. He asserts concerning paternalistic interference with autonomy that 'no man can coerce me to be happy in his way . . .; instead, each may seek his happiness in the way that seems good to him.' Kant pulls no punches as he describes 'a paternalistic government' as 'the greatest despotism thinkable.'[13] In the words of Isaiah Berlin, who harkened to Kant in arguing against Fichte and others, paternalism constitutes 'an insult to my conception of myself.'[14]

Patrius rejoins that prohibiting payment for oocytes would be right even according to *soft paternalism*. This weaker precept declares that the state may prohibit conduct for the purpose of preventing harm to an agent if the conduct would be nonvoluntary, or if delay is required to establish

---

[10] *Lectures on Ethics* 27:370.   [11] *The Metaphysics of Morals* 6:423; *Lectures on Ethics* 27:630.
[12] *Groundwork* 4:435.
[13] 'On the Common Saying: That May Be Correct in Theory, But It Is of No Use in Practice,' 8:290–291.
[14] Berlin 1969, pp. 147–151, 157.

voluntariness. The prospect of money, Patrius contends, will overcome the will of a poor woman. It will render her choice not fully voluntary, or at least not voluntary enough. Liberta replies that in respect of oocyte transfers to research, no serious question about voluntariness arises. Scientists and physicians, he says, operate under self-imposed norms such that they neither coerce oocyte transfers nor accept transfers from women whose decisionmaking capability seems in any way impaired.

My own view of the matter is as follows. Soft paternalism warrants application to a circumstance such as that described by Mill of a pedestrian about to cross an unsafe bridge. If 'there were no time to warn of his danger,' a passerby may 'seize him and turn him back,' this because 'liberty consists in doing what one desires, and he does not desire to fall into the river.'[15] For soft paternalism to justify state prohibition of oocyte transfers across the board, or to justify an imposed ceiling on payment, there must loom a chronic failure of voluntariness. It is not plausible that the circumstances of oocyte transfer are inherently coercive such that the prospect of money will in every case overcome the will. Hard paternalism, on the other hand, only establishes that it *may be* legitimate to restrict liberty for benefit of an agent. Hard paternalism does not guide us *whether* to restrict liberty in a particular case. We already recognize individual liberty to decide on other medical procedures concerning one's own body. Notwithstanding paternalistic concerns and concerns about commodification of oocytes, I see no warrant for categorical prohibition of oocyte transfers. Such a prohibition would unduly restrict personal liberty.

Two moral duties seem to me decisive. A physician has a duty not to harm a patient; a prospective oocyte contributor has a duty to herself, so we may say following Kant, to care for her physical and emotional welfare. The first duty provides a nonpaternalistic rationale for professional norms governing physicians as they assist women in donating oocytes; the second duty provides a reason for a woman to respect those norms. Since the risks and burdens of oocyte retrieval, though not trivial, are reasonable, neither duty compels a physician or woman to refrain from the procedure. But each duty demands attention to whether one entering into the procedure fully appreciates the risks and burdens, and to whether the choice is fully voluntary.

A prospective oocyte transferor will fall into one of two categories: a woman who requests of a fertility physician only retrieval of oocytes (an

---

[15] 'On Liberty,' p. 117. As Feinberg notes (1986, pp. 12ff.), soft paternalism would better be named 'antipaternalism.'

oocyte retrieval patient), and a woman undergoing treatment to achieve pregnancy who contemplates the contribution of one or more retrieved oocytes to someone else (an *IVF patient*). Applicable professional norms could provide that the following will occur. Prior to any transfer of an oocyte to research, every prospective oocyte contributor will receive the investigator's aforementioned written description of the research protocol. The physician or a colleague will interview her to confirm that she has reflected on the choice, understands the risks and burdens, and is not acting under duress or in any other condition that impairs decisionmaking. The interviewer will attempt to ascertain whether a desire for money leads her to misperceive her medical condition or to underestimate risk. Screening will also occur for communicable diseases. In the case of a prospective oocyte retrieval patient, the physician will strive to ascertain whether, in view of the woman's medical history and condition, she may undergo ovarian stimulation and oocyte retrieval without unusual risk. If the woman has not yet borne children, the physician will advise of the risk that the ovarian stimulation regimen could adversely affect fertility.

It is likely that a current or prospective IVF patient willing to donate an aliquot share of her oocytes may be moved by the desire to reduce the net cost of IVF, thereby to make the procedure affordable. In IVF, clinicians usually seek to maximize the chances of pregnancy by fertilizing all oocytes recovered. Hence the interview of an IVF patient contemplating oocyte contribution will also inquire into whether she understands that relinquishing some oocytes will reduce her chances of pregnancy and increase her probable number of cycles. Because investigators performing nuclear transfer may be able to activate oocytes that have failed to fertilize, an IVF patient may also be informed of any opportunity to donate only those of her oocytes that fail to fertilize.

None of the foregoing implies that receiving compensation is wrong. It does imply concern that a physician observe any sign that a patient is not taking full account of her physical and emotional welfare, and it implies concern that her choice be fully voluntary. Other norms may be established – for example, that a physician will not assist a woman in undergoing more than some maximum number of ovarian stimulation cycles.

The question arises whether a fertility physician should participate in research using oocytes contributed by the physician's patients or received in consideration of such contributions. In the case of an oocyte retrieval patient, an incentive could obtain for a physician scientist to obtain oocytes, but the physician must remain alert to halt ovarian stimulation if things go badly for the patient. A conflict of incentives such as this is inherent, yet often reconciled, in clinical trials that enroll patients of physician scientists.[16] The scientist seeks data obtainable by observing the patients. There arguably obtains a defeasible duty to collect enough data to make the study valuable so as to make the participation of all participants worthwhile. The physician's primary obligation is to care for the patient. Sometimes for a patient's welfare, the physician must recommend that the patient withdraw from a study. In the case of oocyte retrieval, the patient is not being studied. No duty to collect data pertains. So long as the physician takes precautions to assure that the patient's welfare remains paramount, and discloses to the patient that the physician will participate in the research, it would seem that the physician could properly participate.

In the case of an IVF patient, any decision to forego fertilization of retrieved oocytes is problematic in view of the patient's goal of achieving pregnancy. If, to reduce the financial burden of IVF, a patient voluntarily chooses to transfer some oocytes to another fertility patient, the physician has no stake in the outcome of that allocation. But if the physician is a disclosed investigator in research to which donated oocytes would be given, and the patient is trying to assess the effect on her odds of pregnancy of giving up oocytes for research, will the patient have confidence in the physician's advice? It has been proposed, and caution would recommend, that 'decisions related to the creation of embryos for fertility treatment' be 'free from the influence of researchers.'[17] A case of an oocyte that has failed to fertilize presents an occasion in which decisionmaking should not be difficult. A patient may confidently believe that such an oocyte is of no value to her.

Let us delve further into the matter of compensation. I mention several principles that would not sustain a prohibition or restriction on compensation. Mill's harm principle would not, on grounds of preventing harm to the agent, allow the state to restrict liberty to pay a fully consenting agent. This follows upon applying the precept *volenti non fit injuria*. The harm principle does not warrant state prohibition of that to which an oocyte contributor consents. Since no possible person corresponds to a gamete, the Duty of Noninterference also does not apply. I shall only say concerning legal moralism that such precept is controversial – it would justify state action against taboos – and that even when applying it, transfer of oocytes for consideration does not so obviously violate a physician's duty not to harm, or a woman's duty to herself, as to warrant state prohibition.

[16] As analyzed in Merritt 2005.
[17] National Institutes of Health, 'Guidelines for Research Using Human Pluripotent Stem Cells,' 65 Fed. Reg. 51976, 51980 (2000).

The present question of remuneration is neither new nor peculiar to research. When it first became apparent that an IVF patient who does not produce healthy oocytes might achieve pregnancy using oocytes donated by someone else, fertility physicians deliberated about remuneration to oocyte contributors. They adopted a professional norm that remuneration is permissible but should be bounded. This norm states that remuneration incident to a transfer in which a fertility physician assists should approximate the amount of direct costs plus the estimated value of the time, inconvenience, discomfort, and emotional burden of ovarian stimulation and oocyte retrieval.[18] The authors distinguished 'compensation' in the foregoing amount from 'payment for the oocytes themselves.' This distinction was drawn so that the authors might join in repudiating the notion of oocytes as commodities, thus comporting with the view that body parts should not be sold. It must be said that the notion that money paid to an oocyte contributor in her capacity as such is not attributable to the oocytes is strained. In clinical trials, investigators do seek from patients only the opportunity to observe them, and take nothing from their bodies. In the case at hand, no observations are sought. Money would not be offered were there no prospect of procuring oocytes. What can tenably be said is that any remuneration is not associable with any embryo to which a possible person corresponds, or for which the assertion of Zygotic Personhood could avail, since by advance decision of the oocyte and somatic cell contributors, intrauterine transfer of any resultant embryo has been barred.

There obtain good reasons for compensating oocyte contributors. The burdensome services rendered amply merit compensation. I suggest that we see this as an instance in which it would be mistaken to condemn a transaction because it in some way makes applicable the epithet 'commodity.' Medical and life insurance both assign monetary values to the body. So do wage rates. The legal interdiction of payment for organs has recently been called into doubt. (Given an acute shortage of transplantable organs, it has been argued that the law should allow payment to people for granting that their organs may be used after their deaths. If insurers and government providers were to defray the costs of organ procurement, that would improve access to organ transplants for poor people who cannot afford black market prices. A black market presently operates as desperate affluent patients purchase organs from the poor in developing countries.) Insofar as those who donate oocytes to medicine receive valuable consideration in exchange, the humanitarian purpose served warrants the

---

[18] American Society for Reproductive Medicine 2000, p. 217.

practice.[19] Women should be offered, and may accept, payment up to the point at which a detriment would occur either in violation of a physician's duty not to harm a patient, or in violation of a woman's duty to care for her physical and emotional welfare.

Yet some legislatures and scientific societies have embraced a norm that forbids provision of valuable consideration to oocyte contributors other than relief from direct medical expenses.[20] Insofar as this norm may be thought to avoid treating oocytes as commodities, it should be said that it too treats oocytes as things. A stronger charge against the norm is that it is exploitative. The practice would allow recipients to take advantage of a woman's generosity, to reap a disproportionate gain.[21] The norm could gain no defense from the fact that the gain is a collective one; the donor would still absorb a burden with no benefit.

In clinical trials, participants often absorb burdens while realizing no medical benefit, but they do receive money. Oocyte retrieval resembles a clinical drug trial in that most of the burden and risk comes about through administration of drugs. If participants in drug trials and women who contribute oocytes to fertility patients receive payment, so should contributors of oocytes to research and therapy. Absent compensation to an oocyte contributor, the objection may lie that the patient's consent is not voluntary enough. All of which suggests a professional norm establishing a nonzero lower bound on compensation for any solicited oocyte contribution. Once it is understood that compensation for an oocyte contribution is proper, it is not an unworthy motive in offering compensation that without it, there may not become available enough oocytes to meet the need in medical research and therapy. An upper bound on compensation should also be set, this in fulfillment of the physician's duty not to harm a patient. This upper bound, if reckoned with care, may be viewed by a woman as appropriate to impose upon herself in recognition of her duty to care for her physical and emotional welfare. The upper bound should equal such amount whose imposition may reasonably be believed to minimize the frequency with which compensation induces contributions that result in a significant health or emotional problem for the patient. The lower bound should approximate the amount paid for comparable time and burden. What those amounts are is an empirical question. The answer will depend on economic circumstances that vary with time and place. One may strive for the golden mean between the extremes of compensation so great that

---

[19] Other replies to concerns about commodification are given in Resnik 2001.
[20] E.g., National Research Council 2005, pp. 84–87.
[21] On exploitation, I have benefited from Feinberg 1988, ch. 31.

many poor women are induced to damage their health, and compensation so small that generous women are exploited.

Under this norm, there will operate a market regulated by norms of the medical and scientific professions. In case it be thought that markets could easily skirt such norms, we may observe that ovarian stimulation and oocyte retrieval is a sufficiently complex procedure, both as to expertise and equipment, that only fertility physicians perform it. Scientific societies could adopt as a norm that scientists will accept only donations inter- mediated by board-certified fertility physicians. Whereupon for the vast preponderance of oocyte transfers to research and therapy, professional norms will constrain compensation.

There will remain the market in which people purchase oocytes thinking that they will fertilize them and bring forth children with desirable genomes. The targets of advertising are women in their student years, since younger women generally produce the highest quality oocytes. They too may be drawn by the money. Prices in this market, if not bounded, could exceed the upper bound set for compensation in connection with contributions to research. There obtain the same reasons, the physician's duty not to harm and the duty to oneself of a prospective contributor, for bounding remu- neration in this market. An already adopted norm of fertility physicians states that when asked to perform oocyte retrieval from a woman solely for the purpose of transfer to someone else, a fertility physician should 'attempt to ascertain' the amount of money offered. The physician 'should refuse to participate if prospective oocyte recipients or recruiting agencies have offered excessive payment that could compromise the donor's free choice.'[22] On occasion a patient could conceal the amount of payment that she expects to receive for oocytes. But since a fertility physician's assistance is needed for oocyte retrieval, a norm establishing an upper bound could constrain the size of the market, even if not preventing all instances of excessive payments. In any case, the contribution of oocytes for creation of epidosembryos in research will stand apart from these transactions.

Hard paternalism would legitimize state action to impose a bound on compensation. Both soft and hard paternalism would legitimize state action to assure voluntariness. If what I have just sketched concerning the circum- stances of oocyte retrieval and the efficacy of professional norms obtains, state action would not be needed for regulating contributions to research. Because the suitable upper and lower bounds on compensation will vary by time and place, setting them can more efficiently be done by professional

[22] American Society for Reproductive Medicine 2000, p. 219.

norms than by legislation. Given those bounds, the practice of contributing oocytes to research will minimize the problem of the rich outbidding the poor. Academic research is not generally purchasable for private use; it is an intellectual public good. At such time as autologous transplantation becomes feasible, concern may arise that wealthy people will monopolize care by purchasing oocytes for use in the procedure. In that event, professional norms could still constrain. If, for contributions to therapeutic use, a legislature were to impose a ceiling on compensation, it could cite as the rationale therefor not hard or soft paternalism, but distributive justice.

To convey an accurate sense of supply versus demand, I mention the following. Scientists may succeed in inducing embryonic stem cells to issue in oocytes. They may also succeed in performing nuclear transfer into blastomeres, into stem cells, or into epidosembryos whose chromosomes have been removed. Primary oocytes might also be retrieved from an aborted fetus (here of course supposing an abortion chosen without inducement by any thought of aiding research), then nurtured in the laboratory to a point at which the oocytes could be activated. In some non-reprocloning experiments, investigators can use oocytes from nonhuman mammals. Notwithstanding these sources, scientific reasons will doubtless continue to motivate experiments using secondary oocytes from women who represent the genetic diversity of a population. What I have sketched is an ethical framework within which to receive their contributions.

8.4 ECTOGENESIS

Two reasons have underwritten the consensus rule that an investigator may not nurture an embryo outside the human body beyond the earlier of the appearance of the primitive streak and day 14 of development. The first is that this boundary is shy of the very earliest events (e.g., formation of the neural plate) in the development of what will become the central nervous system. But there is no significant risk, so it is now generally believed, that an embryo at this early stage feels anything. The earliest embryonic reflexes do not occur until about seven weeks and they are not felt. Pleasure and pain require neural connections to the brain, which are unlikely before the fourteenth week. The cortex forms later. The second consideration that has motivated a day 14 boundary is *NA*, the argument that in Chapter 3 we found to be unsound. The Warnock Committee adverted to both reasons, then adopted *NA*.

A new rationale could be given for choosing day 14 as a boundary. By definition, an epidosembryo is barred from transfer into a natural or artificial uterus. I have defined an artificial uterus as any device capable of nurturing embryonic development past what is achievable by cell culture techniques in the dish. As day 14 is an upper bound on development in the dish, day 14 is an upper bound on epidosembryo development. As I earlier put the matter, because an epidosembryo is barred from intrauterine transfer, it follows that (1) the embryo's developmental potential is bounded such that it cannot develop to any significant further extent, hence (2) the embryo cannot acquire any morally significant property that it does not already have, hence (3a) if the embryo is not already a person, nothing can happen to make it one and therefore no possible person corresponds to it, and (3b) as to that embryo, nothing can be gained by asserting Zygotic Personhood.[23]

It will be observed that the bound on developmental potential to which I have just referred is a function of a contingent technical limitation, the properties of a tissue culture dish. Upon substituting a different device as the locus of oocyte activation, a different least upper bound might obtain. To investigate this possibility in its most robust form, let us consider an artificial uterus. Unlikely as such a device may seem, that was true of incubators and heart-lung machines a century ago. Invention of an artificial uterus would understandably evoke fears of the ramified consequences of departing from nature's method of gestation. People could also look upon an artificial uterus as a more sophisticated incubator for use in trying to save very premature infants. In theory at least, there could even exist an artificial uterus whose associated probability density function shows it to be more efficient than the womb. Whether and how to use any such device to bring forth children is a question for a future time. Here, in considering experimentation, I shall merely suppose that such a device exists, and that it is capable of gestating a conceptus from creation to maturity. Someone now proposes that we revisit the decision to specify day 14 as a normative boundary. They speak of important knowledge that scientists might gain from observing and experimenting upon embryos developed past day 14. As an example, they mention that studying differentiation of the myocardium will require embryos developed beyond day 20. The argument from nonenablement will not defend the foregoing proposal. An embryo placed in the just described artificial uterus would not be an epidosembryo. It would be nomologically possible for an embryo to develop within that device to term, and thus to become what many accounts would recognize as a person. A possible person would correspond to such embryo, and the putative Duty of Noninterference would come to bear. A choice to insist on Zygotic Personhood could gain birth for the conceptus and spare it discomfort in gestation.

---

[23] §2.3(d) and (e).

Sacrifice of the conceptus in this artificial uterus would be tantamount to an abortion.

We may consider instead a weaker proposal. It is proposed to carve an exception to the requirement that there occur no intrauterine transfer of an epidosembryo. The exception would allow transfer of an embryo into an artificial uterus if and only if (2), (3a), and (3b) above would hold. We are first to imagine one or more devices capable of nurturing a conceptus to postimplantation stages, but not to birth. In such a device, developmental potential would be decisively bounded, although the least upper bound manifested by the probability density function would be a later stage than the least upper bound for an embryo in the dish. If a device could emulate the endometrium, it might nurture an embryo through gastrulation. Progressively more complex devices might sustain gestation over various intervals of time. In considering this proposal while seeking to construct a consensus view, we must take account of what some moral views may classify as prenatal personhood-conferring properties. We, many of us, would hold human sentience sufficient for personhood for purposes of the duty not to harm. We would condemn any action that inflicts discomfort on a human conceptus. Over the course of postgastrulation development, there seems no obvious biological event, prior to sentience, with which to associate personhood. But some people may think that the end of the first trimester marks the beginning of personhood, if only because they have become habituated to that threshold as decisive for the legality of abortion. Others, in an Aristotelian vein, might take the emergence of a discernible bodily form, late in the fourth week, as indicative of a person. Within any view that recognizes some prenatal property as sufficient for personhood, the weaker proposal becomes problematic for the following reason. It seems plausible that the nurturing capabilities of artificial uteruses will graduate in discrete jumps. If a device is capable of bringing about gestation to a targeted fetal stage, say, month 5, it seems likely that the device's mechanisms for supplying nutrients and oxygenated blood to the conceptus, these substituting for the womb, placenta, maternal blood vessels, and maternal metabolism, will have attained such sophistication that the device is capable of sustaining gestation to a range of stages. That range could include the advent of sentience or the attainment of some other morally significant property that an early embryo does not possess. Within one or more moral views, it may plausibly be reasoned that, absent evidence excluding the possibility, it is nomologically possible that inside a device with such a range, a conceptus would acquire – it has the developmental potential to acquire – a personhood-conferring property. Whereupon, as in the case of the stronger proposal, it may follow within such a moral view that there corresponds to an embryo placed in such a device a possible person, or that the assertion of Zygotic Personhood would achieve a gain for that conceptus. Sacrifice of the conceptus in such a device might be assimilated to an abortion.

I am constructing an account that does not countenance any nontherapeutic action by which a conceptus would feel discomfort, and that stands independently of whatever view one takes of abortion. I do not defend experimental creation of an embryo within, or transfer into, any device within which it is nomologically possible that a conceptus would progress to sentience, and I observe that (2) is difficult to maintain for a gestating embryo after its cells have oriented in gastrulation and it possesses, in its situation, the developmental potential to acquire a recognizable anatomical shape. A modern incantation of hylomorphism could support an intuition that we ought not use in experiment an embryo that has acquired a bodily form. This would motivate drawing a line at the stage when a bodily form first appears, when the embryonic disc has developed into a cylindrical body and limb buds appear. This occurs by the end of week 4 when the embryo is about 4 mm. long. By then also occur the last events of neurulation. At about day 27, the neural plate closes to form the neural tube, the precursor of the brain and spinal cord. One drawing a line there could amend the definition of an epidosembryo (§2.2) by replacing 'an artificial uterus' with 'any device in which an embryo possesses the developmental potential to attain sentience or in which development is sustained past day 25 or such earlier stage as the progenitors have specified.' An epidosembryo could then be nurtured in a device, when such exists, that emulates the endometrium. (*In utero*, an embryo during week 4 remains embedded in the endometrium.) On the other hand, one might say that shape is an arbitrarily chosen property. As Bernard Williams saw when endorsing a boundary at day 14, this is an occasion on which there may not be a non-arbitrary or uniquely reasonable line to draw, yet it is reasonable that we draw a line. It would be prudent to err on the side of caution concerning devices capable of effecting gestation.

Alternatives and future innovations could obviate the motivation for experimental gestation. These may include the ability to obtain specialized cells for study by inducing differentiation of embryonic stem cells, the use in research of abortuses donated after abortions performed for reasons unrelated to research, advances in tissue engineering, and development of devices allowing nonintrusive observations in the womb. A full picture of appropriate norms will require further discussion at a later time when the technological context has become more clear.

An opponent of embryo use might reply that I have already condoned abortion even by defending sacrifice in the dish. An abortion, the opponent says, is any killing of a conceptus. To this I demur that nonspontaneous abortion consists in the fatal ejection of a conceptus, other than by miscarriage or birth, from a uterus, or, according to a now generalized understanding, from any artificial device in which the conceptus possesses the developmental potential to attain birth. More cautiously, in the foregoing sentence one might replace the second token of 'birth' with 'sentience.' We have considered devices in which an embryo does not have the potential to attain birth or sentience. No abortion occurs if an embryo thus situated is sacrificed. Apart from this semantic clarification, the pertinent question is how we should act. A proponent of experiments involving an artificial endometrium might argue that, with developmental potential permissibly bounded short of any stage at which experiences could be had, use of a donated embryo not nurtured to the point of attaining a bodily form is permissible to serve humanitarian ends.

Another objection would assert that a society that begins to support research using embryos in the dish will eventually travel down a slippery slope to experiments that gestate embryos to sentience in artificial uteruses. I do not think it overly sanguine to say to the contrary that a collective resolve to ban such gestational experiments may be mustered. It seems likely that a consensus would develop for a rule such as this: an embryo may not be nurtured within an artificial device capable of nurture to sentience unless the device is also capable of nurture to birth and the embryo will be nurtured to birth therein without any nontherapeutic intervention. Even if one takes a pessimistic view of humans facing temptation, even if one predicts that we shall prove incapable of resisting the unconstrained use of an artificial uterus when one exists, that prediction will not state a persuasive reason against experimental use of epidosembryos that will never enter such a device.

8.5 HYBRIDS AND CHIMERAS

When an oocyte of one species is activated by sperm or source DNA of another species, the product is a *hybrid*. Hybrid animals (e.g., a liger, the offspring of a male lion and female tiger) pique our curiosity. An alternative to activating human oocytes in nonreprocloning is to create a clone by inserting human DNA into the oocyte of a rabbit, cow, or other nonhuman mammal. The thought of human hybrids walking among us strikes many people as abominable. Hybrids, they say, would 'breach the species boundary.'

To this I first reply that, as we saw in Chapter 4, interspecies boundaries may be illusory. There may be no sudden discontinuities between species. Locke held that 'the boundaries of the species, whereby men sort them, are made by men.' After there occurred the first split into human and chimpanzee lineages, humans and chimpanzees apparently hybridized for over a million years.[24] As and when speciation again begins within our genus, members of new branches may again interbreed. Even so, let us suppose for present purposes the view that it is wrong for humans to bring forth hybrid progeny.

No challenge to that view arises from the following stance concerning hybrid epidosembryos. I classify as human, for present purposes, any embryo formed from a human gamete or from human source DNA inserted with or into the nucleus. My account justifies use of a human embryo only if the embryo is an epidosembryo. A benefactor of medical research and therapy may contribute source DNA to be used in creating an epidosembryo from a nonhuman oocyte. In so doing, the donor will bar intrauterine transfer of the resultant hybrid epidosembryo. The argument from nonenablement will justify use of the hybrid epidosembryo in experiment. The hybrid epidosembryo will not attain sentience, will not achieve birth, will not reproduce. No offspring will walk about. Should it be objected that it is unnatural to insert human DNA into a nonhuman oocyte, that objection may be met by arguing in the same vein as the refutation of the teleological objection, disputing single-purpose teleology and considering the humanitarian purpose. In due course, the question will arise whether physicians may safely transfer into humans the derivatives of hybrid epidosembryos. Light will be shed on this by future discussion of xenotransplantation as we learn more about how to deal with risks of immune rejection and transmission of retroviruses and other infectious agents.

A staple of experimentation is the *chimera*, an organism containing as cellular parts the descendants of more than one develope.[25] A chimera forms when embryos fuse, or when cells of one organism enter and become parts of another. Unlike hybridization, chimerization does not commingle DNA. Rather it leaves the organism with more than one intact genome.

One motivation for creating chimeras may be to test the safety and efficacy of transplanted cells and their issue. Tests may reveal how transplanted

---

[24] Patterson 2006.
[25] As defined in Chapter 3, a develope is a successor in development of an activated oocyte. Lest it be thought that parasites within an organism render it a chimera, we may observe that parasite life processes are not regulated by a master part of the host. Hence parasites are not parts of their host. See Hoffman and Rosenkrantz 1997, pp. 139–141.

cells migrate, respond to cues in the cellular environment, and integrate. Investigators wish to observe chimeras, particularly of apes and monkeys, from formation through adulthood. We collectively have already crossed the bridge to chimeras. Research using human–mouse chimeras has steadily contributed to medical progress on many fronts, among them bone marrow transplantation. A cardiac patient into whom a pig valve has been inserted is a chimera. Someone may still object that the creation of human–nonhuman chimeras disrespects humanity. This stance, if it is to amount to more than prejudice, would require an argument. It may be said in anticipation of one argument that condemnation of the practice of humans interbreeding with nonhumans ought not lead to conflating that practice with the experiments in point here. A scientist creating a chimera would inject cells into an *already formed* organism, this in an attempt to alleviate human afflictions.

But imagine that an investigator transplants into an early embryo of a developmentally similar species – e.g., a chimpanzee blastocyst *in vitro* – a quantity of human embryonic stem cells, a quantity that is large enough that the neuronal issue of the transplanted cells come to dominate the brain of the developed chimera. As a result, the chimera manifests some cognitive abilities that strike the investigator as humanlike. The prospect of this prompts scientists to ask themselves the following question. If investigators create such cognitively enhanced chimeras, how must they treat the chimeras? Scientists anticipate the answer that a chimera that reaches some threshold of cognition must be treated as if it were a human. It may be asserted that such a chimera should be deemed a person, or correspondent of a possible person, for purposes of some duty not to harm and duty not to experiment without the subject's consent.

In view of what we have earlier reviewed about species partiality, the reader will sense the irony in the foregoing concern. It is presumed in this scientific thinking that experiments on nonhumans that inflict pain and suffering are permissible. The usual, but contentious, rationale is that preventing harm to humans may be placed above preventing harm to nonhumans. The thought that troubles commentators is that painful experiments of the sort contemplated for the chimeras could not permissibly be performed on humans, and therefore not on beings that should be treated as if they were humans. The shortcoming of this thinking lies in its emphasis on the categorization of the chimeras as near human – this in contrast with emphasizing the actual experimental outcome for the chimeras. It may be doubted whether enhancement of cognition, notwithstanding any benefit, will much matter to how the experiments are viewed from the point of view of the chimeras. Only a minimal level of cognition seems needed for suffering, and simian primates have it. Great apes are sentient, self-conscious, and have roughly the intelligence of human children. Monkeys are also sentient and intelligent. For them, the key question about an experiment would seem to be 'How much will it hurt?' The answer may not be much affected by whether their cognition has been enhanced – even if the answer to 'Will it disrupt my listening to music?' may be affected. But in human commentary about how to treat chimeric subjects, what gives pause is that some properties of the chimeras might be classifiable as human. This reasoning rests on Property-Based Partiality ('*PBP*') as defined in §4.7. Although species membership is not explicitly mentioned, the reasoning manifests partiality toward bearers of the properties that members of one species ascribe to themselves. Those species members take for granted that properties that they think distinctive of their species warrant preferred treatment. Among the objectionable consequences of *PBP* in this case is that it furnishes a ground for inequalities in moral status, predicated on extent of cognitive ability, among humans. The application of *PBP* would not form part of an account of what it is rational for someone who cares for chimeras to want for them for their sakes. That an appeal to *PBP* occurs in discussing animal use may partially explain how humans reconcile compassion for animals and self-interest.

Three sorts of chimerization are in point. In the first, investigators transplant human cells into an extant nonhuman embryo and experiment upon it *in vitro*. In the second, they transplant human cells into an extant nonhuman embryo *in vitro*, perform an intrauterine transfer, then observe the developing or developed chimera in experiment. In the third case, investigators transplant human cells into a nonhuman fetus or adult, then observe the chimera in experiment. Although in the first case, the human cell contributor might bar intrauterine transfer of any resultant, it has been supposed by discussants disposed to species partiality that justifying a chimerization of any of these three sorts will require a showing that the investigators are not morally obliged to treat the chimera as if it were human. To avail such a showing, investigators have envisioned that they would constrain experiments so as to minimize the extent to which transplanted human cells enhance cognition. They would perform transplants into monkeys rather than into our closer relatives the great apes, into fetal and adult stages rather than into embryonic, into the cerebellum rather than into the cerebrum. They would transplant fewer cells rather than more, and, since domination is more likely after xenografts of wholes, they would transplant dissociated cells rather than whole brain regions.[26]

In a small animal such as the mouse, by virtue of brain size it would seem unlikely that any chimerization by human cells would produce significantly humanlike cognition. For primates, evidence could help clarify what happens in transplantations of the foregoing three sorts, or within the proposed constraints. But if someone is seeking to decide whether a given human–simian chimera must be treated as if it were a human, and they compare quantities of human cells and host cells, or compare cognitive feats against a list of putatively human cognitive feats, they will encounter a sorites paradox. How many grains of sand may one remove from a heap and still have a heap? How much cognition qualifies as human? The situation resembles Parfit's puzzle of the Physical Spectrum in which it is feasible to replace any proportion from 0 to 100% of the cells in my brain and body.[27] What is the proportion beyond which the resulting being would no longer be me? As we saw in Chapter 4, we cannot read off from species membership *the* properties of moral significance. If for purposes of some protective duty, resemblance to one or more humans is taken to be the criterion for membership in the set of persons, or in the set of correspondents of possible persons, the set will be fuzzy. Meanwhile an incentive impinges to choose a test subject that closely resembles the human. We face the challenge of specifying a permissible universe of chimeric subjects. This challenge is not peculiar to research concerning embryonic derivatives. The challenge already arises when investigators experimentally transfer into a nonhuman primate brain a quantity of neuronal stem cells recovered from a developed human.

8.6 PLEONEXIA AND PATENTS

We may foresee that, as progress occurs in modeling diseases, studying reprogramming, and producing stem cell lines, investigators will seek patents on newly devised products and processes. For a final challenge to our moral machinery, I turn to the question of patents on embryos.

The patent system constitutes a mechanism for coaxing the production of intellectual public goods. The two-part strategy, to whose articulation

---

[26] Karpowicz *et al.* 2004, Greene *et al.* 2005. It is argued in DeGrazia 2007 that great apes are 'borderline persons' that should not be subjected to such harmful experiments. To guard against the possibility that embryonic stem cells transferred into an early stage recipient reach the germ line, investigators could also prevent chimeras from breeding.

[27] Parfit 1984, pp. 234–236.

both Bentham and Mill contributed, is as follows. First, intellectual public goods are underprovided in perfect competition. 'He who has no hope that he shall reap,' wrote Bentham, 'will not take the trouble to sow.'[28] The availability of patents presents an incentive for creating such goods. A patent will transform an invention into a marketable public good, i.e., a good that is excludable and nonrivalrous. To a prospective inventor, this presents an opportunity to monopolize the rewards from an invention during the n-year term of a patent. The inventor may internalize the positive externalities of providing a public good. Second, a patent induces public disclosure of the invention. In the bargain struck between the applicant and the patent system, the government grants a monopoly in exchange for disclosure of the invention for all to see. The published patent teaches the invention in sufficient detail so as to allow anyone skilled in the art to practice the invention. 'Patent' derives from the Latin *patere*, 'to stand open' (thus 'patently'). What the teaching reveals may foster other innovations. When the patent expires n years later, the invention enters the public domain.

Designed to bring about the foregoing envisioned results, the criteria for grant of a patent are that the product or process is 'new,' 'useful,' 'nonobvious,' and not 'a product of nature.'[29] Insofar as cloning by nuclear transfer does not naturally occur, a clone is not a product of nature. But a clone *simpliciter*, and the process of making one, may be obvious at a given state of technology, whereupon only specially-designed clones and refinements of the cloning process would qualify as nonobvious. Beyond this, the mere suggestion that patents would issue on embryos, or on ways of creating embryos, elicits the response that no human should own another human. The creation of human individuals is not analogous to breeding in animal husbandry, to manipulation by owners of mating subjects. Ownership of a human is slavery. In Kant's view, we do not even own ourselves. A body is not a thing, not property.[30]

No patent holder does *own* the tokens of a patented type. A patent grants only a limited monopoly: it confers the right to exclude others for n years from making, using, or selling the patented product or process. A more carefully put objection to granting a patent on a human clone or process for creating a clone is that human conception, birth, and life would

---

[28] *A Manual of Political Economy*, p. 71.
[29] Thus in the US (35 U.S.C. §§101–103 [2000]). The last phrase is attributed to Thomas Jefferson. The equivalent criteria of the European Patent Convention, Articles 52 and 53, are that patentable inventions are 'new,' 'susceptible of industrial application,' 'involve an inventive step,' and are not 'plant or animal varieties.'
[30] *Lectures on Ethics* 27:386–387.

thereby become assailable as patent infringement. That would be a perverse result. Upon the birth to Alice and Bob of a clone Clara developed from an oocyte formed by the unlicensed practice of a patented invention, a cause of action for damages would lie against Alice and Bob complaining of the conception and birth of Clara. Clara, or her employer, could be liable for using a patented product, viz., herself. Infringement will occur whenever anyone creates a patented clone, or uses a patented method of cloning, without obtaining a license from the patent holder and paying whatever royalty the holder demands. From a Kantian point of view, the dignity of rational nature is above price. Licensing procreation arguably would disrespect rational nature. It would put a price on human conceptuses not barred from the womb, conceptuses that in their situations possess the developmental potential to become rational beings.

That a patent would render parents and children as such liable as infringers furnishes a compelling reason against granting the patent. Even so, we must expect the biotechnology industrialist to urge that the prospect of patents could coax valuable innovations in nonreprocloning. Let us suppose a case in which a government, seeking to foster innovations that lead to therapies, allows patents on artificially created embryos or on processes of creating them. For such a situation, I suggest the following rule by way of amendment of applicable patent law.

> *Immunity.* No claim of patent infringement shall lie against a parent or child as such.

This rule, confining the remedy available to a patent holder, will not hamper a patent holder's ability to exclude corporations from practicing its invention, nor its ability to hold corporations liable for infringement. When infringements occur of pharmaceutical and biotechnology products, patent holders do not sue consumers anyway. They sue those from whom they can recover substantial damages, namely, other companies.

A good reason for adopting Immunity has already entered from another quarter. Now recognized as patentable are complementary DNA ('cDNA') sequences. These sequences already exist, albeit interruptedly, in human chromosomes, and their uninterrupted transcripts appear in messenger RNA. I have argued against patents on cDNA sequences, notwithstanding that by historical accident firms have come to expect them, insofar as these sequences are mechanistic assemblies, not ingenious inventions.[31] One cannot invent what already exists. A consequence of ceding so much

---

[31] Guenin 1996 and Guenin 2003b, on which I draw elsewhere in this section.

of the human genome to these patents is the chance that, if Alice and Bob procure germ line intervention at the time of arranging to have a child by means of IVF, one or more DNA sequences inserted into their offspring will happen to be patented. Thereupon parents, provider, and child will be infringers unless they procure a license. We have not yet witnessed the first assertion of such a claim, this only because germ line intervention has not yet been practiced. Adoption of Immunity would prevent the pending contretemps.

Immunity would leave open a claim of infringement against a fertility physician. A polity could adopt a stronger rule immunizing providers as well. Medical procedures are not patentable in Europe,[32] and since 1862, when a patent was sought on the use of ether, a dim view has been taken of their patentability elsewhere. It seems wrong to discourage physicians from using the best means at their disposal for the relief of suffering. A polity could adopt a stronger version of Immunity by declaring simply that human reproduction cannot be a patent infringement. The reach of a patent owner ought not extend into the process of creating a human. If anything qualifies as a domain from which one would want to keep out snoopers, reproduction should. Intruding into reproduction would manifest that disrespect for what belongs to others that Plato and Aristotle called *pleonexia*. On this view, the reach of an embryo patent should extend only to nonreprocloning and to nonprocreative parthenogenesis.

From the perspective of distributive justice, the lodestar for whether to grant patents of any given sort is whether allowing them will produce a net welfare gain. Even if we lack consensus on what shall be the social welfare function defining aggregate welfare, we may observe that in embryo-based research, innovations spring forth without a patent incentive. Strongly supported by public opinion, governments have declared human organisms and human cloning unpatentable.[33] Such declarations do not appear to have diminished the enthusiasm of academic scientists for conducting embryo-based research. Unavailability of a patent, it has been said, will not curb scientific curiosity any more than Canute could command the tides.

---

[32] European Patent Convention Article 52(4).

[33] 'The human body,' 'processes for cloning human beings,' 'use of human embryos for industrial or commercial purposes,' and 'processes for modifying the germ line genetic identity of human beings' have been declared unpatentable by European Patent Convention Rules 23d and 23e(1), following European Patent Convention, Article 53, and Directive 98/44/EC of the European Parliament and of The Council of 6 July 1998 on the Legal Protection of Biotechnological Inventions, Articles 5.1 and 6. A 'human organism' has been declared unpatentable in the US by Pub. L. 108–199, §634, 118 Stat. 101 (2004), and annual reiterations thereof. A like policy is set forth in *Official Gazette of the U. S. Patent and Trademark Office* 1077: 24 (April 21, 1987).

Ample motivation seems supplied by the desire to advance fundamental knowledge and to develop therapies against crippling diseases, and in this case, applications do not lie distant from research. If we do not need patent incentives to coax exploration of this corner of nature's storehouse, a net welfare loss could occur by ceding monopolies to the first entrants. In general, a monopoly allows its possessor to constrict output and to set price above marginal cost.

I turn to embryonic derivatives. It may be argued that embryonic stem cells are not products of nature insofar as we do not find populations of such cells in humans. Embryonic stem cells are not human body parts; they are the cell culture derivatives of human body parts, namely, day 5 blastomeres that *in vivo* would differentiate. Thus may begin a case for a patent on human embryonic stem cells or on processes for deriving such cells.[34] Against such a patent, the following moral objection has been lodged: 'use of human embryos for industrial or commercial purposes' is 'contrary to *l'ordre publique* or morality,' hence any invention concerning such use is unpatentable.[35] I observe that epidosembryo use fosters humanitarian ends and only incidentally will it subserve an industrial or commercial purpose inasmuch as health care is provided in commerce, and that, according to my account, epidosembryo use is virtuous and a fulfillment of a collective duty.

Once investigators have characterized and produced embryonic stem cells, the production of one disease-specific cell line after another would seem to be mechanistic and obvious steps, hence not deserving of product patents. Other types of embryonic derivatives include cells differentiated from embryonic stem cells. These may be progenitor or other cells at various stages along the path toward specialization. Such of these cells as occur naturally would not be patentable, but a patent applicant may claim to have produced cells of a given type in an isolated and purified form not found in the body. Many process innovations are needed in order to produce therapies. Product patents, we must be aware, will block the use of improved methods of making the patented products. I have argued that a high standard of ingenuity should be demanded for issuance of product patents on human life forms and that process patents rather than product patents may yield the greater welfare gains.[36]

---

[34] E.g., U. S. Patent No. 6,200,806 on cells and method described in Thomson *et al.* 1998.
[35] The objection invokes a standard set forth in Directive 98/44/EC, Article 6, and European Patent Convention, Article 53 and Rule 23d.
[36] Guenin 1996, pp. 294–300; Guenin 2003b, pp. 331–332.

To coax supply of underprovided intellectual public goods, a recognized alternative is subsidy. The fruits of subsidized research immediately enter the public domain. Firms may use such fruits to develop beneficial products. This prospect shows to the advantage of the publicly-supported research advocated in §8.2. In default of public support, a risk arises of ceding a field to private control. Having given away part of nature's storehouse to DNA sequence patent holders, the patent system could allow the preponderance of transplantable cell types to be swept within the maw of patents. This might occur either in consequence of indulging patents on another part of the storehouse, or for lack of publicly-funded research, or both. An unsubsidized commercial patent holder may require exorbitant royalties, decline to grant licenses, use a patent as mere leverage, or become bankrupt. Public support for research will not afford free access to resulting inventions insofar as grantees of public funds are allowed to procure patents. But by suitable enactments, a government that funds research may require that its grantees place results in the public domain. It may require that grantees license patented inventions at no more than a specified maximum royalty, and it may grant nonprofit institutions a research exemption.

The contours of intellectual property remain open for discussion. The refusal of patents on embryos and processes for making them, selective immunity from patent infringement, and the other patent norms that I have just sketched constitute norms of the sort that may take effect within institutions. Here I follow Rawls in conceiving institutions as public systems of rules. The same holds for norms described earlier – a public policy specifying a morally permissible scope of embryo use, norms for facilitation and acceptance of oocyte contributions, a constraint on the type of device in which ectogenesis may occur, and constraints on forming hybrids and chimeras. Further discussion may contribute to refining these norms and to developing others.

We may sometimes hear predictions that embryo use will misdirect resources and ramify in wrongful practices. The prospect of embryo use has fueled the imaginations of some commentators purporting to project its course. They variously predict exploitation of women, 'embryo farms,' and the unleashing of social forces that will demolish respect for human dignity. They counsel that if we start using embryos as means, our descendants will inevitably fail to constrain themselves. They therefore urge that we not start.

The question of what we ought to do may be understood as the question of how we ought to shape our future. We began with metaphysical and moral considerations that usually do not concern us when thinking about humans that have begun or completed gestation. These led us to think of potential relative to a situation, of what constitutes one of our kind, of how we stand in relation to other animals, and of a justified practice and norms to govern it. The defense of epidosembryo use as a beneficent practice does not imply any priority over other beneficent practices. By virtue of our collective duties of justice and beneficence, many exigencies place moral demands upon us. To decline epidosembryo use would assure that we shall not succumb to imaginable temptations, but it would achieve this only at the price of wasting resources, resources by which good might permissibly be accomplished. According to the account of permissibly bounded developmental potential given here, epidosembryo donations present us with means by which we might assist in the relief of suffering at no cost in thwarting development of beings to which possible persons correspond, and at no cost in lives of beings for which we could achieve anything by ascribing personhood for purposes of the duty not to harm. In these circumstances, it would be uncaring of us not to attempt the work of which we are capable within the constraints that we have the ability to impose.

Bibliography

Adams, Robert M. 1999. *Finite and Infinite Goods*. Oxford: Oxford University Press.

Alexander, H. G., ed. 1956. *The Leibniz–Clarke Correspondence*. Manchester: Manchester University Press.

American Society for Reproductive Medicine Ethics Committee. 2000. 'Financial Incentives in Recruitment of Oocyte Donors.' *Fertility and Sterility* 74: 216–220.

American Society for Reproductive Medicine Practice Committee. 2003. 'Ovarian Hyperstimulation Syndrome.' *Fertility and Sterility* 80: 1309–1314.

Anscombe, G. E. M. 1985. 'Were You a Zygote?' *Philosophy* 59 Supplement 19: 111–116.

Aquinas, Thomas. *Scriptum Super Libros Sententiarum*, in Roberto Busa, ed., *Thomae Aquinatis Opera Omnia*, 2nd ed. 1996. Milan: Editoria Elettronica Editel.

Summa Theologiae, vols. 6, 11, 50, trans. Ceslaus Velecky, Timothy Suttor, Colman E. O'Neill. 2006. Cambridge: Cambridge University Press.

Aristotle. *De Interpretatione, De Anima, Historia Animalium, Parts of Animals, Progression of Animals, Metaphysics, Nicomachean Ethics*, and *Politics*, in Jonathan Barnes, ed., *The Complete Works of Aristotle, The Revised Oxford Translation*. 1984. Princeton: Princeton University Press.

Armstrong, D. M. 1989. *Universals, An Opinionated Introduction*. London: Westview.

1997. *A World of States of Affairs*. Cambridge: Cambridge University Press.

Arneson, Richard. 1999. 'What, If Anything, Renders All Humans Morally Equal?,' in Jamieson 1999, pp. 103–128.

Ayer, A. J. 1954. 'Individuals,' in *Philosophical Essays*, pp. 1–25. London: Macmillan.

Behrensmeyer, Anna K. 2006. 'Climate Change and Human Evolution.' *Science* 311: 476–478.

Bentham, Jeremy. *A Manual of Political Economy*, in John Bowring, ed., *The Works of Jeremy Bentham*, vol. 3. 1962. New York: Russell and Russell.

Berlin, Isaiah. 1969. *Four Essays on Liberty*. Oxford: Oxford University Press.

Boyd, Richard. 1988. 'How To Be a Moral Realist,' in Geoffrey Sayre-McCord, ed., *Essays on Moral Realism*, pp. 181–228. Ithaca: Cornell University Press.

1999. 'Homeostasis, Species, and Higher Taxa,' in Wilson, R. 1999, pp. 141–189.

Brinsden, Peter R., ed. 1999. *A Textbook of In Vitro Fertilization and Assisted Reproduction, The Bourn Hall Guide to Clinical and Laboratory Practice*, 2nd ed. New York: Parthenon.

Brinster, Ralph L. and Avarbock, M. R. 1994. 'Germ Line Transmission of Donor Haplotype Following Spermatogonial Transplantation.' *Proceedings of the National Academy of Sciences* 91: 11303–11307.

Brogaard, Berit. 2004. 'Species as Individuals.' *Biology and Philosophy* 19: 223–242.

Buchanan, A. *et al.* 2000. *From Chance to Choice.* Cambridge: Cambridge University Press.

Casati, Roberto and Varzi, Achille C. 1999. *Parts and Places, The Structure of Spatial Representation.* Cambridge: MIT Press.

Cavalieri, Paola and Singer, Peter. 1993. *The Great Ape Project.* New York: St. Martin's.

Chisholm, Roderick. 1976. *Person and Object.* London: Allen & Unwin.

Choo, K. H. A. 2001. 'Engineering Human Chromosomes for Gene Therapy Studies.' *Trends in Molecular Medicine* 7: 235–237.

Copi, Irving M. 1954. 'Essence and Accident.' *Journal of Philosophy* 51: 706–719. Reprinted in Schwartz 1977, pp. 176–191.

Dale, B. *et al.* 1991. 'Intercellular Communication in the Early Embryo.' *Molecular Reproduction and Development* 29: 22–28 (1991).

Daley, George Q. 2003. 'Cloning and Stem Cells – Handicapping the Political and Scientific Debates.' *New England Journal of Medicine* 349: 211–212.

Daley, George Q. *et al.* 2007. 'The ISSCR Guidelines for Human Embryonic Stem Cell Research.' *Science* 315: 603–604.

Darwall, Stephen L. 2002. *Welfare and Rational Care.* Princeton: Princeton University Press.

Davidson, Donald. 2001. 'Rational Animals,' in *Subjective, Intersubjective, Objective*, pp. 95–106. Oxford: Clarendon Press.

Dawkins, Richard. 1998. 'What's Wrong with Cloning?,' in Nussbaum and Sunstein 1998, pp. 54–66.

De Coppi, Paolo *et al.* 2007. 'Isolation of Amniotic Stem Cell Lines with Potential for Therapy.' *Nature Biotechnology* 25: 100–106.

DeGrazia, David. 2007. 'Human-Animal Chimeras: Human Dignity, Moral Status, and Species Prejudice.' *Metaphilosophy* 38: 309–329.

de Queiroz, Kevin. 1999. 'The General Lineage Concept of Species and the Defining Properties of the Species Category,' in Wilson, R. 1999, pp. 49–89.

Donceel, Joseph, S. J. 1970. 'Immediate Animation and Delayed Hominization.' *Theological Studies* 31: 76–105.

Dunstan, G. R. 1988. 'The Human Embryo in the Western Moral Tradition,' in Dunstan and Seller 1988, pp. 39–57.

Dunstan, G. R. and Seller, Mary J., eds. 1988. *The Status of the Human Embryo.* London: King Edward's Hospital Fund.

Dupré, John. 1981. 'Natural Kinds and Biological Taxa.' *Philosophical Review* 90: 66–90.

　1993. *The Disorder of Things.* Cambridge: Harvard University Press.

Dworkin, Ronald. 1993. *Life's Dominion*. New York: Alfred A. Knopf.

Eberle, Rolf A. 1970. *Nominalistic Systems*. Dordrecht: Reidel.

Engelhardt, H. Tristram, Jr. 1974. 'The Ontology of Abortion.' *Ethics* 84: 217–234.

Ereshefsky, Marc. 1991. 'Species, Higher Taxa, and the Units of Evolution.' *Philosophy of Science* 58: 84–101. Reprinted in Ereshefsky 1992a, pp. 381–398.

 1992a. ed. *The Units of Evolution, Essays on the Nature of Species*. Cambridge: MIT Press.

 1992b. 'Eliminative Pluralism.' *Philosophy of Science* 59: 671–690. Reprinted in Hull and Ruse 1998, pp. 348–368.

 1999. 'Species and the Linnean Hierarchy,' in Wilson, R. 1999, pp. 285–305.

Feinberg, Joel. 1984. *Harm to Others*. Oxford: Oxford University Press.

 1986. *Harm to Self*. Oxford: Oxford University Press.

 1988. *Harmless Wrongdoing*. Oxford: Oxford University Press.

Fine, Kit. 1994. 'Essence and Modality.' *Philosophical Perspectives* 8: 1–16.

Ford, Norman M. 1988. *When Did I Begin?* Cambridge: Cambridge University Press.

Gensler, Harry J. 1986. 'A Kantian Argument Against Abortion.' *Philosophical Studies* 49: 83–98.

Ghiselin, Michael T. 1974. 'A Radical Solution to the Species Problem.' *Systematic Zoology* 23: 536–544. Reprinted in Ereshefsky 1992a, pp. 279–291.

 1997. *Metaphysics and the Origin of Species*. Albany, NY: State University of New York Press.

Glock, Hans-Johann. 2000. 'Animals, Thoughts, and Concepts.' *Synthese* 123: 35–64.

Goodman, Nelson and Quine, W. V. 1947. 'Steps Toward a Constructive Nominalism.' *Journal of Symbolic Logic* 12: 105–122. Reprinted in Goodman 1972, pp. 173–200.

Goodman, Nelson. 1972. *Problems and Projects*. Indianapolis: Bobbs-Merrill.

 1977. *The Structure of Appearance*. 3rd ed. (1st ed. 1951). Dordrecht: Reidel.

Gould, Stephen Jay. 1977. *Ontogeny and Phylogeny*. Cambridge: Harvard University Press.

 1998. 'Dolly's Fashion and Louis's Passion,' in Nussbaum and Sunstein 1998, pp. 41–53.

Gracia, Jorge J. E. 1988. *Individuality, An Essay on the Foundations of Metaphysics*. Albany, NY: State University of New York Press.

Graft, Donald. 1997. 'Against Strong Speciesism.' *Journal of Applied Philosophy* 14: 107–118.

Greene, Mark *et al.* 2005. 'Moral Issues of Human–Non-Human Primate Neural Grafting.' *Science* 309: 385–386.

Griffiths, Paul E. 1999. 'Squaring the Circle: Natural Kinds with Historical Essences,' in Wilson, R. 1999, pp. 209–228.

Guenin, Louis M. 1996. 'Norms for Patents Concerning Human and Other Life Forms.' *Theoretical Medicine* 17: 279–314.

 2001a. 'Morals and Primordials.' *Science* 292: 1659–1660.

2001b. Testimony at Hearing, Subcommittee on Health of the Committee on Energy and Commerce, U.S. House of Representatives, on The Human Cloning Prohibition Act of 2001 and The Cloning Prohibition Act of 2001, Ser. No. 107–41, 58–67.

2001c. 'The Set Theoretic Ambit of Arrow's Theorem.' *Synthese* 126: 443–472.

2003a. 'The Set of Embryo Subjects.' *Nature Biotechnology* 21: 482–483.

2003b. 'Dialogue Concerning Natural Appropriation.' *Synthese* 136: 321–336.

2004. 'A Failed Noncomplicity Scheme.' *Stem Cells and Development* 13: 456–459.

2005a. 'Stem Cells, Cloning, and Regulation.' *Mayo Clinic Proceedings* 80: 241–250.

2005b. 'Intellectual Honesty.' *Synthese* 145: 177–232.

2005c. 'A Proposed Stem Cell Research Policy.' *Stem Cells* 23: 1023–1027.

2005d. 'Wishful Thinking Will Not Obviate Embryo Use.' *Stem Cell Reviews* 1: 309–315.

2006. 'The Nonindividuation Argument Against Zygotic Personhood.' *Philosophy* 81: 463–503.

2008. 'Species Are Structures' [forthcoming].

Haldane, John and Lee, Patrick. 2003. 'Aquinas on Human Ensoulment, Abortion and the Value of Life.' *Philosophy* 78: 255–278.

Handyside, Alan H. *et al.* 1992. 'Birth of a Normal Girl After In Vitro Fertilization and Preimplantation Diagnostic Testing for Cystic Fibrosis.' *New England Journal of Medicine* 327: 905–909.

Hardy, Kate *et al.* 1990. 'Human Preimplantation Development *In Vitro* Is Not Adversely Affected by Biopsy at the 8-Cell Stage.' *Human Reproduction* 5: 708–714.

Hare, Richard M. 1981. *Moral Thinking*. Oxford: Clarendon Press.

1993. *Essays on Bioethics*. Oxford: Clarendon Press.

1997. *Sorting Out Ethics*. Oxford: Clarendon Press.

Harman, Elizabeth. 2007. 'How Is the Ethics of Stem Cell Research Different from the Ethics of Abortion?' *Metaphilosophy* 38: 207–225.

Heller, Mark. 1990. *The Ontology of Physical Objects: Four-Dimensional Hunks of Matter*. Cambridge: Cambridge University Press.

Hoffman, Joshua and Rosenkrantz, Gary S. 1997. *Substance, Its Nature and Existence*. London: Routledge.

Hull, David L. 1965. 'The Effect of Essentialism on Taxonomy: Two Thousand Years of Stasis (I).' *British Journal for the Philosophy of Science* 15: 314–326. Reprinted in Ereshefsky 1992a, pp. 199–225.

1978. 'A Matter of Individuality.' *Philosophy of Science* 45: 335–360. Reprinted in Ereshefsky 1992a, pp. 293–316.

1986. 'On Human Nature.' *Proceedings of the Biennial Meeting of the Philosophy of Science Association 1986*, vol. 2, pp. 3–13. Reprinted in Hull and Ruse 1998, pp. 383–397.

1999. 'On the Plurality of Species: Questioning the Party Line,' in Wilson, R. 1999, pp. 23–48.

Hull, David L. and Ruse, Michael, eds. 1998. *The Philosophy of Biology*. Oxford: Oxford University Press.

Huxley, Thomas H. 1894. 'The Origin of Species,' in *Collected Essays*, vol. 2, *Darwinia*, pp. 22–79. New York: D. Appleton.

Jamieson, Dale, ed. 1999. *Singer and His Critics*. Oxford: Blackwell.

John Paul II. 1981. 'Cosmology and Fundamental Physics,' in Paul Haffner, ed., *Discourses of the Popes from Pius XI to John Paul II to the Pontifical Academy of Sciences 1936–1986*. 1986. Vatican City: Pontifica Academia Scientiarum.

 1995. *Evangelium Vitae*. Vatican City: The Holy See.

Jones, D. A. 2005. 'The Human Embryo in the Christian Tradition: A Reconsideration.' *Journal of Medical Ethics* 31: 710–714.

Jonsen, Albert R. and Toulmin, Stephen. 1988. *The Abuse of Casuistry*. Berkeley: University of California Press.

Kant, I. *Critique of Pure Reason*, in Paul Guyer and Allen W. Wood, trans. and ed., *The Cambridge Edition of the Works of Immanuel Kant*. 1998. Cambridge: Cambridge University Press.

 Groundwork of the Metaphysics of Morals, The Metaphysics of Morals, and 'On the Common Saying: That May Be Correct in Theory, But It Is of No Use in Practice,' in Mary J. Gregor, trans. and ed., *The Cambridge Edition of the Works of Immanuel Kant, Practical Philosophy*. 1996. Cambridge: Cambridge University Press.

 Lectures on Ethics, in Peter Heath and J. B. Schneewind, trans. and ed., *The Cambridge Edition of the Works of Immanuel Kant*. 1997. Cambridge: Cambridge University Press.

Karpowicz, Philip *et al.* 2004. 'It Is Ethical to Transplant Human Stem Cells into Nonhuman Embryos.' *Nature Medicine* 10: 331–335.

Kavka, Gregory. 1982. 'The Paradox of Future Individuals.' *Philosophy and Public Affairs* 11: 93–112.

Kim, Kitai. 2007. 'Histocompatible Embryonic Stem Cells by Parthenogenesis.' *Science* 315: 482–486.

Kitcher, Philip. 1984a. 'Species.' *Philosophy of Science* 51: 308–333. Reprinted in Ereshefsky 1992a, pp. 317–341.

 1984b. 'Against the Monism of the Moment: A Reply to Elliott Sober.' *Philosophy of Science* 51: 616–630.

Kono, Tomohiro. 2004. 'Birth of Parthenogenetic Mice That Can Develop to Adulthood.' *Nature* 428: 860–864.

Korsgaard, Christine. 2005. 'Fellow Creatures: Kantian Ethics and Our Duties to Animals,' in Grethe B. Peterson, ed., *The Tanner Lectures on Human Values*, vol. 25, pp. 77–110. Salt Lake City: University of Utah Press.

Kripke, Saul A. 1971. 'Identity and Necessity,' in Milton K. Munitz, *Identity and Individuation*, pp. 135–164. New York: New York University Press. Reprinted in Schwartz 1977, pp. 66–101.

 1980. *Naming and Necessity*. Cambridge: Harvard University Press.

Kuhn, Thomas. 1970. *The Structure of Scientific Revolutions*, 2nd ed. Chicago: University of Chicago Press.

Kuhse, Helga and Singer, Peter. 1990. 'Individuals, Humans, and Persons: The Issue of Moral Status,' in Singer *et al.* 1990, pp. 65–75.

Larmore, Charles. 2003. 'Public Reason,' in Samuel Freeman, ed., *The Cambridge Companion to Rawls*, pp. 368–393. Cambridge: Cambridge University Press.

Leibniz, G. W. F. *Fragmente zur Logik*, trans. and ed. Franz Schmidt. 1960. Berlin: Akademie-Verlag.

Leonard, Henry S. and Goodman, Nelson. 1940. 'The Calculus of Individuals and Its Uses.' *Journal of Symbolic Logic* 5: 45–55.

Leśniewski, Stanislaw. 1983. 'On the Foundations of Mathematics,' trans. Vito F. Sinisi. *Topoi* 2: 3–52.

Locke, John. *An Essay Concerning Human Understanding*, 5th ed., ed. John W. Yolton. 1965. New York: Dutton.

Loebel, David A. F. and Tam, Patrick P. L. 2004. 'Mice without a Father.' *Nature* 428: 809–811.

Lowe, E. J. 1983. 'On the Identity of Artifacts.' *Journal of Philosophy* 80: 220–232.

1989. *Kinds of Being*. Oxford: Blackwell.

1996. *Subjects of Experience*. Cambridge: Cambridge University Press.

1998. *The Possibility of Metaphysics*. Oxford: Clarendon Press.

2003a. 'Individuation,' in Michael J. Loux and Dean W. Zimmerman, eds., *The Oxford Handbook of Metaphysics*, pp. 75–95. Oxford: Oxford University Press.

2003b. 'Identity, Individuality, and Unity.' *Philosophy* 78: 321–336.

2003c. 'Substantial Change and Spatiotemporal Coincidence.' *Ratio* 16: 140–160.

2006. *The Four-Category Ontology*. Oxford: Clarendon Press.

2008. 'Two Notions of Being: Entity and Essence,' in Robin Le Poidevin, ed., *Being: Developments in Contemporary Metaphysics*. Cambridge: Cambridge University Press.

Machin, Geoffrey A. 1996. 'Some Causes of Genotypic and Phenotypic Discordance in Monozygotic Twin Pairs.' *American Journal of Medical Genetics* 61: 216–228.

Macleod, Colin M. 2001. Review of Casiano Hacker-Cordon and Ian Shapiro, eds., *Democracy's Edges. Ethics* 112: 151–155.

Maddy, Penelope. 1990. *Realism in Mathematics*. Oxford: Clarendon Press.

Martin, C. B. 1980. 'Substance Substantiated.' *Australasian Journal of Philosophy* 58: 3–10.

Martin, C. B. and Heil, John. 1999. 'The Ontological Turn.' *Midwest Studies in Philosophy* 23: 34–60.

Mayr, Ernst. 1982. *The Growth of Biological Thought*. Cambridge: Harvard University Press.

McIntyre, Alison. 1994. 'Guilty Bystanders? On the Legitimacy of Duty to Rescue Statutes.' *Philosophy and Public Affairs* 23: 157–191.

McLaren, Anne. 1986. 'Prelude to Embryogenesis,' in The Ciba Foundation 1986, pp. 5–23.

2000. 'Cloning: Pathways to a Pluripotent Future.' *Science* 288: 1775–1780.

McMahan, Jeff. 2002. *The Ethics of Killing*. Oxford: Oxford University Press.

Mellor, D. H. 1977. 'Natural Kinds.' *British Journal for the Philosophy of Science* 28: 299–312.

Merritt, Maria. 2005. 'Moral Conflict in Clinical Trials.' *Ethics* 115: 306–330.

Mill, J. S. *On Liberty and Other Essays*, ed. John Gray. 1991. Oxford: Oxford University Press.

Millikan, Ruth G. 1999. 'Historical Kinds and the "Special Sciences".' *Philosophical Studies* 95: 45–65.

Mills, Eugene. 1993. 'Dividing without Reducing: Bodily Fission and Personal Identity.' *Mind* 102: 37–51.

Mishler, Brent D. 1999. 'Getting Rid of Species?,' in Wilson, R. 1999, pp. 307–315.

Nagel, Thomas. 1975. 'Brain Bisection and the Unity of Consciousness,' in John Perry, ed., *Personal Identity*, pp. 227–245. Berkeley: University of California Press.

National Research Council and Institute of Medicine. 2005. *Guidelines for Human Embryonic Stem Cell Research*. Washington: National Academies Press.

Nozick, Robert. 1997. 'Do Animals Have Rights?,' in *Socratic Puzzles*, pp. 305–310. Cambridge: Harvard University Press.

Nussbaum, Martha C. and Sunstein, Cass R., eds. 1998. *Clones and Clones, Facts and Fantasies About Human Cloning*. New York: W. W. Norton & Co.

Oderberg, David. 1997. 'Modal Properties, Moral Status, and Identity.' *Philosophy and Public Affairs* 26: 259–298.

Parfit, Derek. 1976. 'Rights, Interests, and Possible People,' in Samuel Gorovitz, ed., *Moral Problems in Medicine*, pp. 369–375. Englewood Cliffs, NJ: Prentice-Hall.

Park, In-Hyun *et al.* 2008. 'Reprogramming of Human Somatic Cells to Pluripotency with Defined Factors.' *Nature* 451: 141–146.

1984. *Reasons and Persons*. Oxford: Clarendon Press.

Park, Woosuk. 1988. 'The Problem of Individuation for Scotus: A Principle of Indivisibility or a Principle of Distinction?' *Franciscan Studies* 48: 105–123.

Patterson, Nick *et al.* 2006. 'Genetic Evidence for Complex Speciation of Humans and Chimpanzees.' *Nature* 441: 1103–1108.

Pius IX. 1869. *Apostolicae Sedis Moderationi, in Acta Apostolicae Sedis*, vol. 5, pp. 305–331. Vatican City: The Holy See.

Plantinga, Alvin. 1974. *The Nature of Necessity*. Oxford: Clarendon Press.

Putnam, Hilary. 1975. 'Is Semantics Possible?' and 'The Meaning of Meaning,' in *Mind, Language, and Reality. Philosophical Papers*, vol. 2, pp. 139–152, 215–271. Cambridge: Cambridge University Press.

Quine, W. V. 1959. *Methods of Logic*, rev. ed. New York: Holt, Rinehart, and Winston.

1960. *Word and Object*. Cambridge: MIT Press.

1961. 'On What There Is,' 'Identity, Ostension, and Hypostasis,' and 'Reference and Modality,' in *From a Logical Point of View*, 2nd ed., pp. 1–19, 65–79, 139–159. New York: Harper and Row.

1969. 'Speaking of Objects' and 'Natural Kinds,' in *Ontological Relativity and Other Essays*, pp. 1–25, 114–138. New York: Columbia University Press.

1970. *Philosophy of Logic*, Englewood Cliffs, NJ: Prentice Hall.

1972. Review of M. O. Munitz, ed., *Identity and Individuation. Journal of Philosophy* 69: 488–497.

1976. 'Three Grades of Modal Involvement,' in *The Ways of Paradox and Other Essays*, rev. ed., pp. 156–174. Cambridge: Harvard University Press.

1981. 'On the Individuation of Attributes,' in *Theories and Things*, pp. 100–112. Cambridge: Harvard University Press.

1987. *Quiddities*. Cambridge: Harvard University Press.

1995. *From Stimulus to Science*. Cambridge: Harvard University Press.

Rawls, John. 1971a. *A Theory of Justice*. Cambridge: Harvard University Press.

1971b. 'Justice as Reciprocity,' in Rawls 1999, pp. 190–224.

1996. *Political Liberalism*, paperback ed. [pagination of the main text of which coincides with that of the original edition of 1993]. New York: Columbia University Press.

1997. 'The Idea of Public Reason Revisited,' in Rawls 1999, pp. 573–615.

1999. *Collected Papers*, ed. Samuel Freeman. Cambridge: Harvard University Press.

2000. *Lectures on the History of Moral Philosophy*, ed. Barbara Herman. Cambridge: Harvard University Press.

2001. *Justice as Fairness, A Restatement*, ed. Erin Kelly. Cambridge: Harvard University Press.

Reid, Thomas. *Essays on the Intellectual Powers of Man*, ed. Baruch Brody. 1969. Cambridge: MIT Press.

Resnik, David B. 2001. 'Regulating the Market for Human Eggs.' *Bioethics* 15: 1–25.

Roemer, John E. 1996. *Theories of Distributive Justice*. Cambridge: Harvard University Press.

Rosenkrantz, Gary S. 2001. 'What is Life,' in Tian Yu Cao, ed., *Proceedings of the Twentieth World Congress of Philosophy*, vol. 10, pp. 125–134. Bowling Green, OH: Philosophy Documentation Center.

Ruse, Michael. 1987. 'Biological Species: Natural Kinds, Individuals, or What?,' *British Journal for the Philosophy of Science* 38: 225–242. Reprinted in Ereshefsky 1992a, pp. 343–361.

Sacred Congregation for the Doctrine of the Faith. 1974. *Declaration on Procured Abortion*. Vatican City: The Holy See. Reprinted in Austin Flannery, ed., *Vatican Council II: More Postconciliar Documents*, vol. 2, pp. 441–453. 1982. Collegeville, MN: The Liturgical Press.

1987. *Donum Vitae*. Vatican City: The Holy See. Reprinted in Kevin W. Wilkes, ed., *Infertility: A Crossroad of Faith, Medicine, and Technology*, pp. 209–238. 1997. Dordrecht: Kluwer.

Sainsbury, Mark. 1995. *Paradoxes*, 2nd ed. Cambridge: Cambridge University Press.

Salmon, Nathan U. 2005. *Reference and Essence*, 2nd ed. Amherst, NY: Prometheus Books.

Scheffler, Israel. 2001. 'My Quarrels with Nelson Goodman.' *Philosophy and Phenomenological Research* 62: 665–677.

Schwartz, Stephen, ed. 1977. *Naming, Necessity, and Natural Kinds*. Ithaca: Cornell University Press.

Shamblott, Michael J. *et al.* 1998. 'Derivation of Pluripotent Stem Cells from Cultured Human Primordial Germ Cells.' *Proceedings of the National Academy of Sciences* 95: 13726–13731.

Sider, Theodore. 2001. *Four-Dimensionalism: An Ontology of Persistence and Time.* Oxford: Clarendon Press.

Silver, Lee. 1997. *Remaking Eden.* New York: Avon Books.

Simerly, Calvin *et al.* 2003. 'Molecular Correlates of Primate Nuclear Transfer Failures.' *Science* 300: 297.

Simons, Peter. 1987. *Parts: A Study in Ontology.* Oxford: Clarendon Press.

Singer, Peter *et al.*, eds. 1990. *Embryo Experimentation.* Cambridge: Cambridge University Press.

Singer, Peter. 2002. *Unsanctifying Human Life,* ed. Helga Kuhse. Oxford: Blackwell.

Smith, Barry and Brogaard, Berit. 2003. 'Sixteen Days.' *Journal of Medicine and Philosophy* 28: 45–78.

Smith, M., Bruhn, J., and Anderson, J. 1992. 'The Fungus *Armillaria bulbosa* Is Among the Largest and Oldest Living Organisms.' *Nature* 356: 428–431.

Soane, Brendan. 1988. 'Roman Catholic Casuistry and the Moral Standing of the Human Embryo,' in Dunstan and Seller 1988, pp. 74–85.

Sober, Elliott. 1980. 'Evolution, Population Thinking, and Essentialism.' *Philosophy of Science* 47: 350–383. Reprinted in Ereshefsky 1992a, pp. 247–278.

　1984a. 'Sets, Species, and Evolution: Comments on Philip Kitcher's "Species".' *Philosophy of Science* 51: 334–341.

　1984b. *The Nature of Selection.* Chicago: University of Chicago Press.

Solter, David and Knowles, Barbara B. 1975. 'Immunosurgery of Mouse Blastocyst.' *Proceedings of the National Academy of Sciences* 72: 5099–5102.

Stock, Gregory. 2002. *Redesigning Humans: Our Inevitable Genetic Future.* Boston: Houghton Mifflin.

Strasnick, Steven. 1981. 'Neo-utilitarian Ethics and the Ordinal Representation Theorem,' in Joseph C. Pitt, ed., *Philosophy in Economics,* pp. 63–92. Dordrecht: Reidel.

Strawson, P. F. 1959. *Individuals.* London: Methuen.

Takahashi, Kazutoshi *et al.* 2007. 'Induction of Pluripotent Stem Cells from Adult Human Fibroblasts by Defined Factors.' *Cell* 131: 1–12.

Tauer, Carol A. 1984. 'The Tradition of Probabilism and the Moral Status of the Early Embryo.' *Theological Studies* 45: 3–33.

Tendler, Moshe. 2000. Testimony, in National Bioethics Advisory Commission, *Ethical Issues in Human Stem Cell Research,* vol. 3, *Religious Perspectives.* Rockville, MD: National Bioethics Advisory Commission.

Testa, Giuseppe and Harris, John. 2004. 'Ethical Aspects of ES Cell-Derived Gametes.' *Science* 305: 1719.

The Ciba Foundation. 1986. *Human Embryo Research, Yes or No?* London: Tavistock.

Thomson, James A. *et al.* 1998. 'Embryonic Stem Cell Lines Derived from Human Blastocysts.' *Science* 282: 1145–1147.

Tooley, Michael. 1972. 'Abortion and Infanticide.' *Philosophy and Public Affairs* 2: 37–65.

Tye, Michael. 2003. *Consciousness and Persons*. Cambridge: MIT Press.

Van Cleve, James. 1995. 'Essence/Accident,' in Jaegwon Kim and Ernest Sosa, eds., *A Companion to Metaphysics*, pp. 136–138. Oxford: Blackwell.

van der Kooy, Derek and Weiss, Samuel. 2000. 'Why Stem Cells?' *Science* 287: 1439–1441.

van Inwagen, Peter. 1990. *Material Beings*. Ithaca: Cornell University Press.

Ward, Keith. 1990. 'An Irresolvable Dispute?,' in Anthony Dyson and John Harris, eds., *Experiments on Embryos*, pp. 106–119. London: Routledge.

Warnock, Mary. 1983. '*In Vitro* Fertilization: The Ethical Issues (II).' *Philosophical Quarterly* 33: 238–249.

  1985. *A Question of Life*. Oxford: Basil Blackwell.

Watt, Fiona M. and Hogan, Brigid L. M. 2000. 'Out of Eden: Stem Cells and Their Niches.' *Science* 287: 1427–1430.

Wiggins, David. 1967. *Identity and Spatio-Temporal Continuity*. Oxford: Basil Blackwell.

  2001. *Sameness and Substance Renewed*. Cambridge: Cambridge University Press.

Willard, Huntington F. 2000. 'Artificial Chromosomes Coming to Life.' *Science* 290: 1308–1310.

Williams, Bernard. 1986. 'Types of Moral Argument Against Embryo Research,' in The Ciba Foundation 1986, pp. 185–212.

  1995. *Ethics and the Limits of Philosophy*. Cambridge: Harvard University Press.

Wilmut, Ian. 2002. 'Are There Any Normal Cloned Mammals?' *Nature Medicine* 8: 215–216.

Wilson, Bryan. 1988. 'On a Kantian Argument Against Abortion.' *Philosophical Studies* 53: 119–130.

Wilson, Jack. 1999. *Biological Individuality, The Identity and Persistence of Living Entities*. Cambridge: Cambridge University Press.

Wilson, Robert A., ed. 1999. *Species, New Interdisciplinary Essays*. Cambridge: MIT Press.

Wittgenstein, Ludwig. 1961. *Tractatus Logico Philosophicus*, trans. D. F. Pears and B. F. McGuiness. London: Routledge & Kegan Paul.

Wood, Allen W. 1998. 'Kant on Duties Regarding Nonrational Nature.' *Proceedings of the Aristotelian Society Supplement*, vol. 72, pp. 189–208.

  1999. *Kant's Ethical Thought*. Cambridge: Cambridge University Press.

  2005. 'Ethics and Embryonic Stem Cell Research.' *Stem Cell Reviews* 1: 317–324.

Woodger, J. H. 1937. *The Axiomatic Method in Biology*. Cambridge: Cambridge University Press.

  1970. 'The Technique of Theory Construction,' in Otto Neurath, Rudolph Carnap, and Charles Morris, eds., *Foundations of the Unity of Science*, vol. 2, pp. 449–531. Chicago: University of Chicago Press.

Yu, Junying *et al.* 2007. 'Induced Pluripotent Stem Cell Lines Derived from Human Somatic Cells.' *Science* 318: 1917–1920.

Index